DYSRHYTHMIA INTERPRETATION BASED ON CARDIAC SUPPRESSION AND IRRITABILITY

CECILE HURST, R.N., B.S.N.
Coronary Care Training Coordinator
Medical Center of Delaware
Wilmington, Delaware

DYSRHYTHMIA INTERPRETATION

BASED ON CARDIAC SUPPRESSION AND IRRITABILITY

J.B. LIPPINCOTT COMPANY Philadelphia
LONDON MEXICO CITY NEW YORK
ST. LOUIS SÃO PAULO SYDNEY

Sponsoring Editor: Diana Intenzo
Manuscript Editor: Virginia M. Barishek
Indexer: Angela Holt
Design Director: Tracy Baldwin
Designer: Anne O'Donnell
Production Supervisor: Kathleen Dunn
Production Coordinator: George V. Gordon
Compositor: Waldman Graphics, Inc.
Printer/Binder: Malloy Lithographing, Inc.
Cover Printer: Malloy Lithographing, Inc.

6 5 4 3 2 1

Library of Congress Cataloging in Publication Data

Hurst, Cecile.
Dysrhythmia interpretation based on cardiac suppression and irritability.

Includes bibliographies and index.
1. Arrhythmia—Diagnosis. 2. Electrocardiography. 3. Patient monitoring. 4. Cardiovascular disease nursing. I. Title. [DNLM: 1. Arrhythmia. 2. Electrocardiography. 4. Monitoring, Physiologic—methods. WG 330 P966d]
RC685.A65H87 1986 616.1'28'07547 85-10122
ISBN 0-397-54433-2

The author and publisher have exerted every effort to ensure that drug selection and dosage set forth in this text are in accord with current recommendations and practice at the time of publication. However, in view of ongoing research, changes in government regulations, and the constant flow of information relating to drug therapy and drug reactions, the reader is urged to check the package insert for each drug for any change in indications and dosage and for added warnings and precautions. This is particularly important when the recommended agent is a new or infrequently employed drug.

To Steve for the love and caring,
and to Corey and Jeff

PREFACE

You're new in the coronary care unit. The alarm on the monitor goes off. You look at the monitor screen. What do you see? Are those funny looking beats dangerous or not? Why aren't there QRS complexes after the P waves?

I have been teaching a coronary care course for nurses and paramedical personnel at the Medical Center of Delaware in Wilmington, Delaware for the last twelve years. Over this period of time, I found that although the available textbooks on electrocardiography provide a wealth of information, on their own they do not succeed in teaching dysrhythmia interpretation, particularly to the neophyte. Most students need supplemental and individual help from an instructor to make the dysrhythmias understandable. There also seemed to be a huge gap between the criteria learned in the classroom and the application of this knowledge in the clinical setting. I finally realized that the problem was not in the material, but in its organization. Most textbooks categorize the rhythms by site of origin: SA node, atria, AV node, or ventricles. This approach seems logical but, unfortunately, when the alarm on the monitor goes off, it only beeps and flashes. There is no little voice saying, "This dysrhythmia originates in the ventricles." When faced with a rhythm strip, the abnormalities you notice first are the obvious ones, such as fast rates, late beats, pauses, missing P waves or QRS complexes, and so on. Another problem is that when the eye is drawn to the obvious, other more subtle changes can be overlooked, which may be more dangerous than the abnormalities that leap out at you. I have found that by presenting these dysrhythmias as they are seen on the monitor's scope, a lot of the confusion in the interpretation process is eliminated. By presenting an orderly approach to the interpretation, all abnormalities are uncovered, ensuring the correct therapy.

If you pay particular attention to Chapter 4, which explains the reasons dysrhythmias develop and the configuration of different beats, and use the easy five-step approach to a systematic interpretation of any dysrhythmia, I think you will find that you can examine any EKG strip confidently and interpret it precisely.

The reasoning process used to interpret dysrhythmias is very close to the process used to solve crossword or jigsaw puzzles, where you fit together separate pieces of information to come up with an answer. In fact, I have noticed that the students in my classes who are really interested in the rhythm strips are usually those who can't wait for the next Sunday *New York Times* crossword. However, even if you can't stand puzzles I think you will find that this book finally will clear up the mystery of all those little bumps and wiggles on the monitor screen.

This text is mainly about the dysrhythmias, but you need a base of information about the heart and how it works, both electrically and mechanically, before you can understand clearly what happens when the pattern on the monitor has funny looking beats, and how hemodynamics can be influenced by abnormalities in rhythm. Of course, to be complete, a text also must cover therapy for the dysrhythmias.

Although this book will not make you a junior cardiologist, I sincerely hope it will help you to provide complete and comprehensive care for your patients. I feel sure that by the time you have finished reading the book and working the rhythm strips in Chapters 5 and 6 and in the Appendix, you will be comfortable enough to look on the monitor not as an enemy but as a valuable tool that benefits both you and your patient.

Cecile E. Hurst, R.N., B.S.N.

ACKNOWLEDGMENTS

There are so many people who have helped with this project. First, I would like to thank Christine Cannon R.N., M.S.N. who began the development of this concept with me many years ago, and whose help and encouragement have been so very important. For their support and advice I would like to thank Catharine Eten Kuhner, R.N., M.S.N.; Deborah Cebenka, R.N., B.S.N.; and Lynda Juell Carpenito, R.N., M.S.N. I also sincerely appreciate the time that the following people spent in reviewing selected parts of the manuscript: Alfred E. Bacon, M.D.; A. Henry Clagett, M.D.; Richard F. Gordon, M.D.; Joseph T. West, M.D.; Paul C. Pennock, M.D.; Francis P. Parker, M.D.; Jerry Castellano, Pharm.D.; and Gary E. Sloskey, Pharm.D. I am very grateful to the nurses in the various critical care units of the Wilmington Medical Center who remembered and took the time to send interesting rhythm strips to me.

I also thank Margaret Fitzpatrick for typing the manuscript quickly and accurately despite the fact that she was working around the demands of two munchkins.

Last, but far from least, I would like to give special thanks and love to my mother, Dorothy Hurst, for her professional copyediting, support, and encouragement all through the last two years.

CONTENTS

DYSRHYTHMIA INTERPRETATION BASED ON CARDIAC SUPPRESSION AND IRRITABILITY

1

ANATOMY AND PHYSIOLOGY OF THE HEART

Every nurse, at some time or another, has studied the basic anatomy and physiology of the cardiovascular system, either in great detail or perhaps in a more basic presentation. However, anatomy and physiology are subjects that you tend to forget, since they are not the kind of knowledge that you use every day. Unfortunately, to really understand the heart and how it works, you must have a solid base of information on its anatomy and physiology before you can begin to comprehend how the electrophysiology operates, how the dysrhythmias develop, and how the dysrhythmias can affect the hemodynamic status of your patient. Because of this, we will first provide you with a basic review of the anatomy and physiology of the heart before we begin the presentation of electrophysiology and the dysrhythmias.

THE ANATOMY OF THE HEART

Basically, the heart is a four-chambered pump, approximately the size of your fist, with valves between the chambers to prevent a backflow of blood (Fig. 1-1). The four chambers are the right and left atria and the right and left ventricles. There are four valves: the mitral, tricuspid, aortic, and pulmonic. Breaking this down further, the heart is actually two synchronized pumps, a low-pressure pump on the right, which pushes blood through the pulmonary circuit, and a high-pressure pump on the left, which supplies the rest of the body. This pump, which normally weighs 250 to 400 grams, beats continuously, 60 to 100 times a minute for approximately 70 years.

The heart (Fig. 1-2) is positioned in the thoracic cavity, just behind the sternum. The base of the heart, where the great vessels and nerves

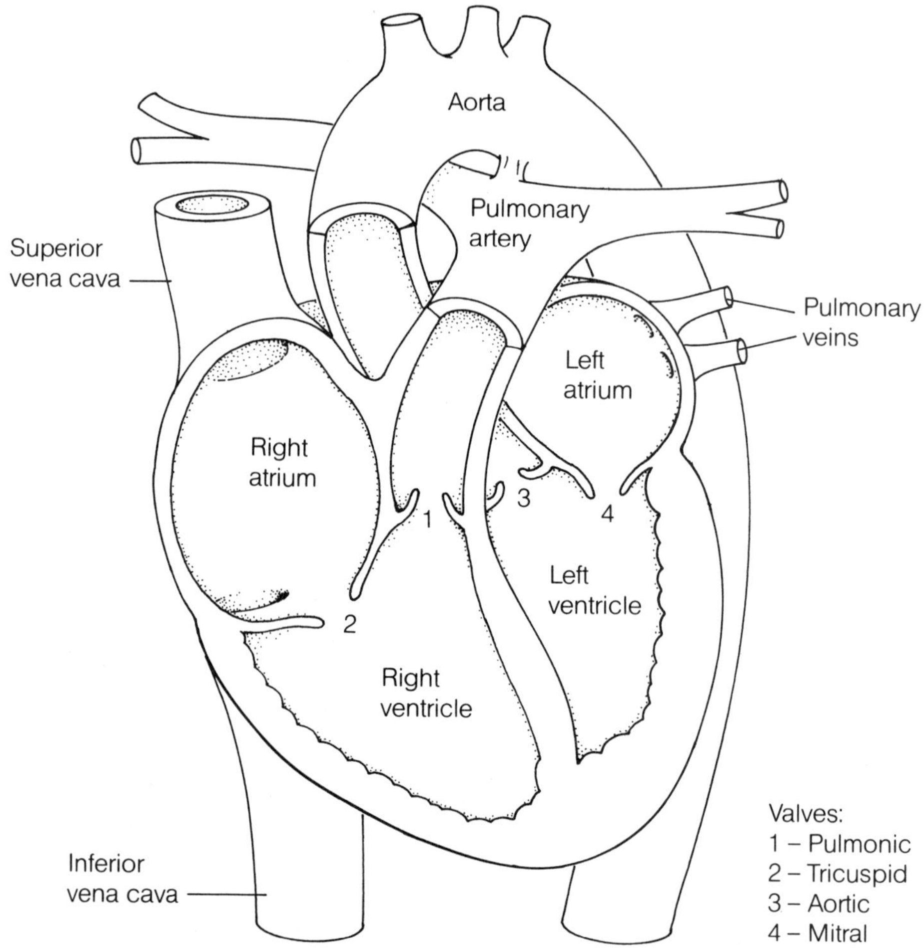

Figure 1-1 Chambers and major vessels of the heart.

enter and leave, is at the level of the second intercostal space. The apex of the heart is at the fifth intercostal space on the mid-clavicular line. On a normal chest x-ray, the cardiac silhouette extends from 1 to 2 cm beyond the right of the sternum, and 4 to 5 cm to the left of the sternum. As the heart contracts and relaxes, the apex of the ventricles taps the chest wall at the fifth intercostal space on the mid-clavicular line, producing a pulsation known as the point of maximal impulse (PMI). Most diagrams of the heart show the right and left portions sitting side-by-side, but in actuality, the right side of the heart is located to the right and anteriorly (Fig. 1-3), and the left side is sitting to the left and posteriorly.

THE LAYERS OF THE HEART (Fig. 1-4)

The Pericardium

The pericardium is a tough fibrous sac that completely surrounds the heart. There is a potential space between the heart and pericardium, which contains approximately 10 to 15 ml of fluid that acts as a lubri-

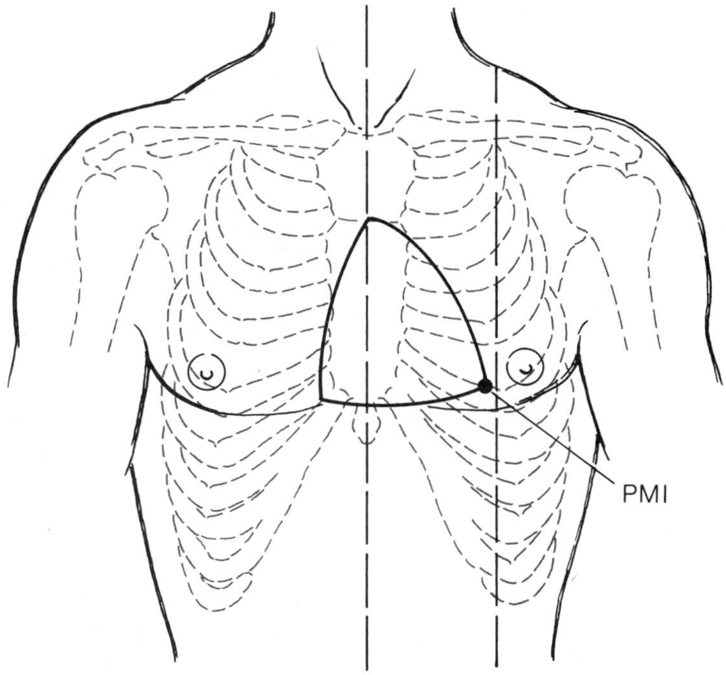

Figure 1-2 Position of the heart in the chest.

Figure 1-3 Position of the chambers.

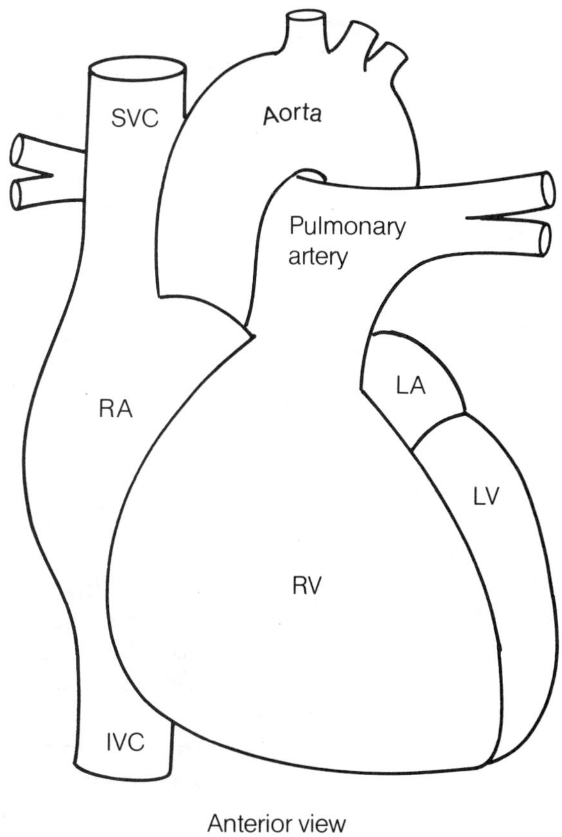

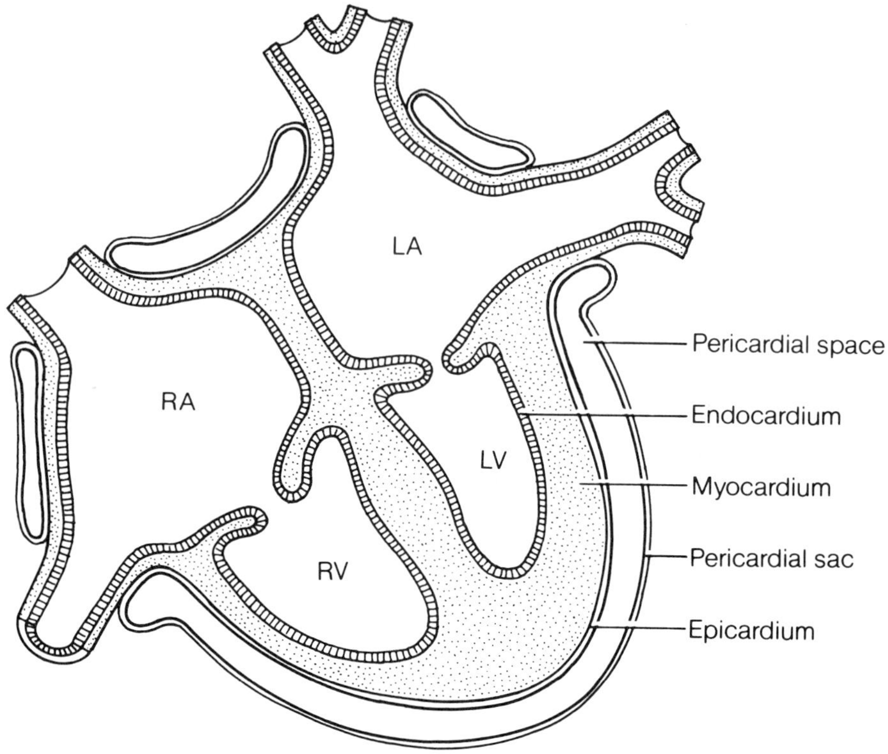

Figure 1-4 Diagram of the layers of the heart.

cant. This lubrication is necessary since the two surfaces are in constant contact and are also in motion due to contraction and relaxation of the heart. Since the pericardium is a fibrous sac, it is relatively nondistensible and cannot stretch quickly. If the heart wall ruptures or is punctured, blood rapidly fills the pericardial space and compresses the heart—a pericardial tamponade. Venous blood, returning to the heart, cannot be accommodated, and death will result unless the pressure is quickly relieved by aspiration.

If an inflammatory process occurs, such as an acute myocardial infarction or an infection, an excess of pericardial fluid may accumulate in the pericardial space—a pericardial effusion. If this happens slowly, the pericardium may stretch to accommodate the added volume of fluid, and this is not as life-threatening an emergency as is tamponade.

The Epicardium

The epicardium is the outermost layer of the heart. It is actually the visceral layer of the pericardium. If an inflammatory process occurs, the swelling and inflammatory exudate may produce increased contact between the pericardium and the epicardium and decreased lubrication. The contact between the two layers of tissue produces pain, as well as a sound known as a pericardial friction rub.

The Myocardium

The myocardium is the muscular layer of the heart between the epicardium and endocardium. The myocardium consists of a fibrous skel-

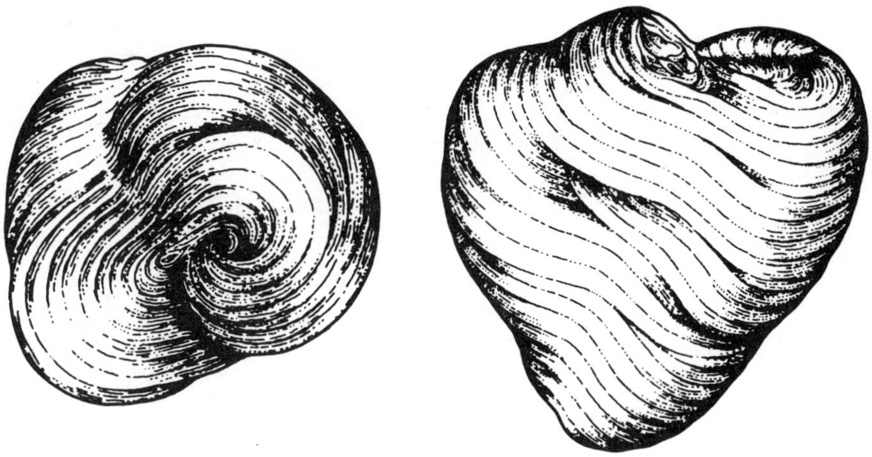

Figure 1-5 Schematic view of spiral arrangement of ventricular muscle fibers. (Katz A: Physiology of the Heart, p 4. New York, Raven Press, 1977)

eton, smooth muscle, the conduction system, and the arteries and veins. The fibrous skeleton forms the framework for both atrial and ventricular muscle and valvular structures. The heart muscle or myocardium comprises about 95% of the weight of the heart. The muscle fibers are arranged in concentric rings that run in different longitudinal planes, and are cone-shaped (Fig. 1-5). When these concentric rings of muscle contract, they pump the blood up and out of the heart in a wringing or milking motion. The myocardial smooth muscle differs from the skeletal muscle in that it extracts a much higher percent of oxygen from the blood, and it also has the special property of conductivity, which will be covered in detail in the discussion of electrophysiology.

The Endocardium

The endocardium is the smooth layer of tissue that lines the inner surfaces of the atria and ventricles. Endocardial tissue also covers the surfaces of the valves. There are a number of infectious processes that may involve the endocardium, for example, rheumatic fever and acute or subacute bacterial endocarditis. These conditions can be difficult to treat and may result in actual damage to the valves.

CHAMBERS

Blood Flow Through the Heart (Fig. 1-6)

Venous blood returns from the body through the superior and inferior vena cavae. It flows into the right atrium and through the tricuspid valve, into the right ventricle. The right ventricle pumps the blood out through the pulmonic valve and into the pulmonary artery and pulmonary capillaries where it is reoxygenated. Then, the oxygen-saturated blood returns through the pulmonary veins to the left atrium. This is the only place in the body that normally has unoxygenated blood flowing through an artery and oxygenated blood flowing through a vein. From the left atrium, it flows across the mitral valve and into the left

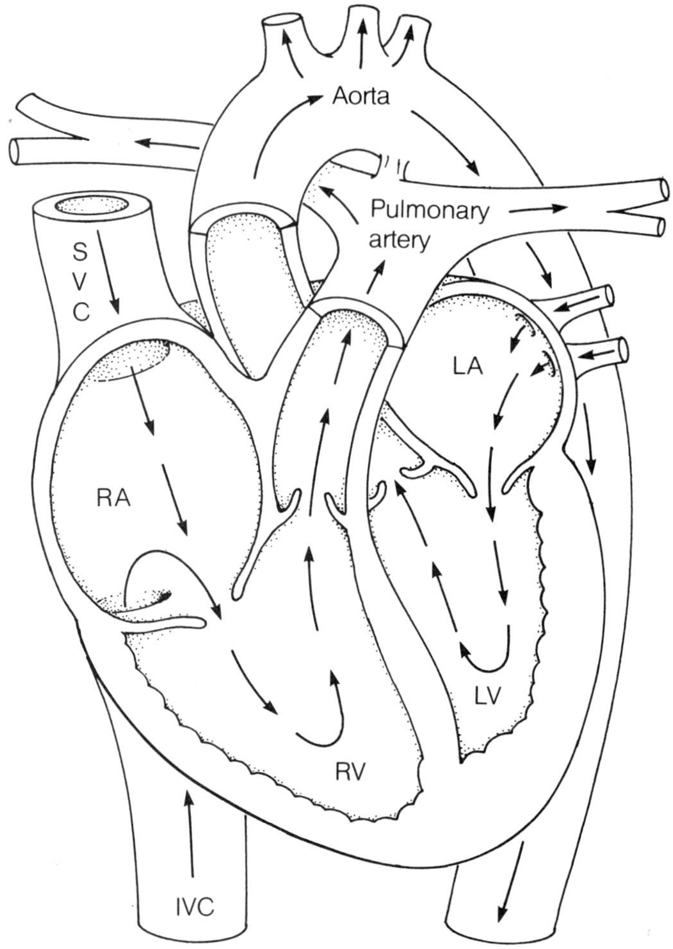

Figure 1-6 Schematic diagram of the course of blood through the heart.

ventricle. The left ventricle pumps the blood out of the aortic valve into the aorta and throughout the entire body.

The Right Atrium

The right atrium forms the right lateral cardiac border and is located above and slightly behind the right ventricle. The right atrium contains important structures such as the sinoatrial (SA) node and atrioventricular (AV) node, the orifices for the superior and inferior vena cava, and the coronary sinus. The right atrium is the site of return of venous blood from all areas of the body. Blood returns from the head and upper extremities through the superior vena cava. The inferior vena cava drains the trunk and lower extremities. The venous blood from the heart itself returns to the right atrium from the great cardiac vein through the coronary sinus. The right atrium is a low-pressure chamber, with a normal mean pressure of 5 mm Hg.

The Right Ventricle

The right ventricle is a relatively thin-walled chamber that receives blood from the right atrium. The right ventricle is the most anterior chamber. It has three papillary muscles that anchor the three leaflets of the tricuspid valve. The wall of the right ventricle is only 3 to 6 mm thick since it is normally pumping against low resistance in the pulmonary vasculature. Normal pressures generated by the right ventricle are 25/5 mm Hg.

The Left Atrium

The left atrium is the most posterior chamber, located near the midline. Four pulmonary veins bring the oxygenated blood returning from the lungs: two from the right lung and two from the left. Mean pressure in the left atrium normally is around 12 mm Hg.

The Left Ventricle

The thick-walled, left ventricle forms the left lateral border of the heart, but the main bulk of the left ventricle is located behind the right ventricle. There are two papillary muscles to anchor the two leaflets of the mitral valve. Essentially, your heart is your left ventricle, because the left ventricle is the primary pump that works the hardest. The left ventricle has to pump against the high resistance of the peripheral circulation, and thus has a wall that is 10 to 20 mm thick. It normally develops pressures of approximately 120/10 mm Hg.

THE VALVES

The Semilunar Valves

The two semilunar valves are the aortic valve on the left side and the pulmonic valve on the right side of the heart (Fig. 1-7). The semilunar valves are so named because each cusp has the shape of a half moon. Their function is to prevent backflow or regurgitation of blood from the aorta and pulmonary artery into the left and right ventricles, respectively, during the relaxation phase, or diastole, of each cardiac cycle. The aortic and pulmonic valves are similar in that they both are formed of three triangular-shaped cusps of equal size. They lie at the top of the outflow tracts of each ventricle. They are made of a tough fibrous tissue, and each triangular cusp has two free edges that project into the lumens of the aorta and pulmonary artery.

During systole, the pressure generated by the contracting ventricle pushes the free edges of the cusps back into the vessel, permitting the ejection of blood (Fig. 1-8). Behind each cusp is a pouch-like dilitation known as the sinus of Valsalva. One important difference between the aortic and pulmonic valves is that two of the three aortic sinuses of Valsalva contain the ostia for the right and left coronary arteries.

During diastole, the pressure in the relaxing ventricle drops, and blood in the aorta and pulmonary arteries tries to flow back into the ventricles (Fig. 1-8). This backflow of blood fills the cusps of the semilunar valves, much as the wind fills the sails of a boat, and the free edges of the valves move together, down into the center of the lumens of the vessels, thus sealing the outflow tract and preventing the backflow of blood into the ventricles. It is during this phase of the cardiac cycle (diastole) that the majority of coronary blood flow occurs. The semilunar valves are open in systole and closed during diastole.

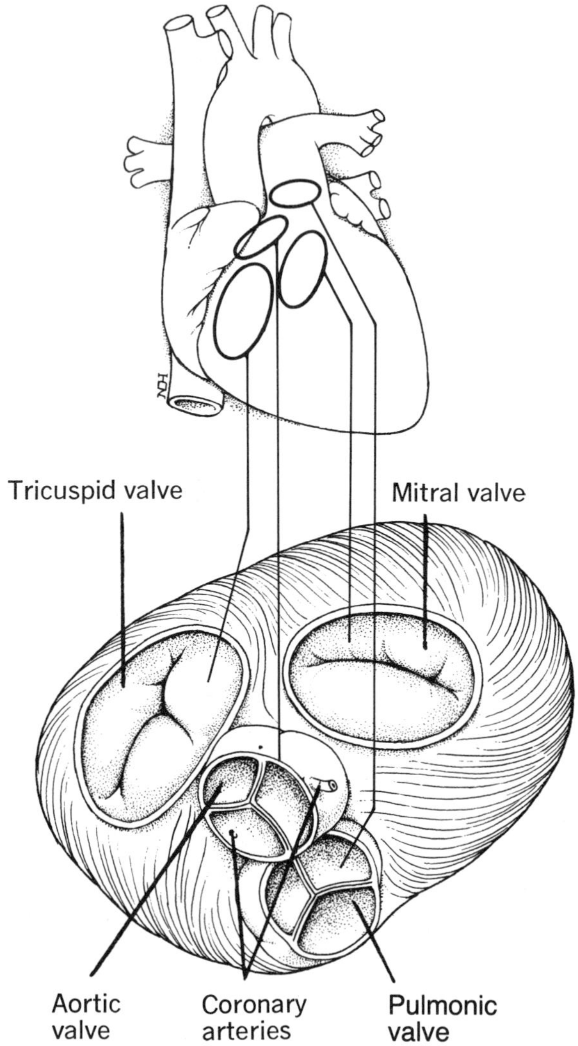

Figure 1-7 Valves of the heart. In the lower drawing, the atria have been removed and the heart tilted forward; thus, the valves are seen from above.

The Atrioventricular Valves

The atrioventricular valves are inflow valves that are located between the atria and the ventricles. The tricuspid valve is on the right and the mitral valve on the left (Fig. 1-7). The mitral valve has two leaflets; the tricuspid has three. The atrioventricular valves are closed during systole and open during diastole. They differ structurally from the semilunar valves in that they are comprised of leaflets of thin fibrous tissue. One edge of each leaflet is attached to a fibrous ring, and the free edge is anchored to a papillary muscle on the ventricular wall by strings of tissue called the chordae tendinae.

During diastole, or the relaxation phase of the ventricle, the greater pressure of the blood in the atria forces the leaflets of the atrioventricular valves to open, and the blood flows into the ventricles (Fig. 1-8). During ventricular systole, or the contraction phase, the papillary muscles contract first, thus putting tension on the chordae tendinae. The

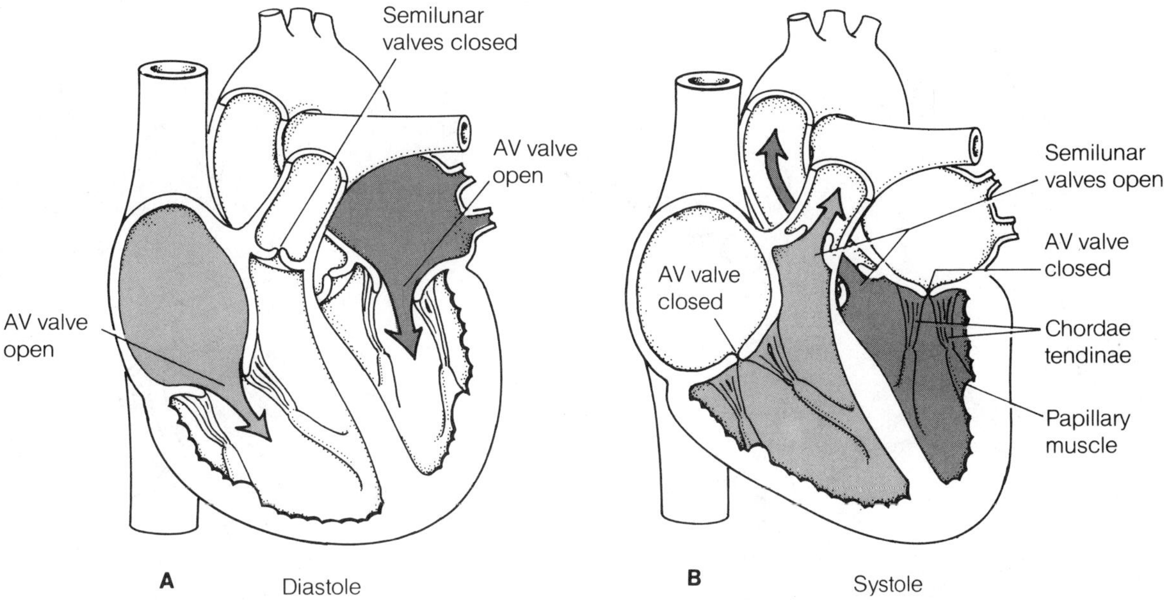

Figure 1-8 Diagram of valve action in the heart. (*A*) *Ventricular diastole.* As ventricular pressure falls, the AV valves open as a result of higher pressure of blood in the atria. The semilunar valves close because of higher pressure of blood in the aorta and pulmonary artery, thus preventing backflow into ventricles. (*B*) *Ventricular systole.* With rising ventricular pressure, the AV valves close and prevent backflow into the atria. When ventricular pressure exceeds arterial pressure, the semilunar valves open and blood is pumped into the arteries.

chordae must be attached to the papillary muscles rather than to the ventricular wall, because the ventricle becomes smaller as it contracts and would allow the chordae to loosen. As the ventricle contracts and the pressure increases, the blood tries to flow back through the atrioventricular valves into the atria. However, the blood fills the leaflets of the valves, pushing them closed. The tensing of the chordae holds the leaflets closed so that they cannot flip back into the atria during ventricular systole.

It is the abrupt closing of the atrioventricular valves at the beginning of ventricular systole that produces the first heart sound (S_1). The closing of the semilunar valves at the beginning of the ventricular diastole produces the second heart sound (S_2). Normal valves do not make a sound when opening.

Valves may become damaged because of inflammation resulting from a variety of diseases, such as rheumatic fever, or because of injury to the papillary muscles following acute myocardial infarction. If scarring of the valve is severe enough, the cusps or leaflets may calcify, preventing the valve from opening completely, producing stenosis, or from closing completely, causing insufficiency. Papillary muscle rupture or dysfunction will allow the affected leaflet to flip back up into the atria during ventricular systole, causing regurgitation or backflow of blood. Any abnormal blood flow across a valve that is stenosed or insufficient produces a characteristic sound known as a murmur.

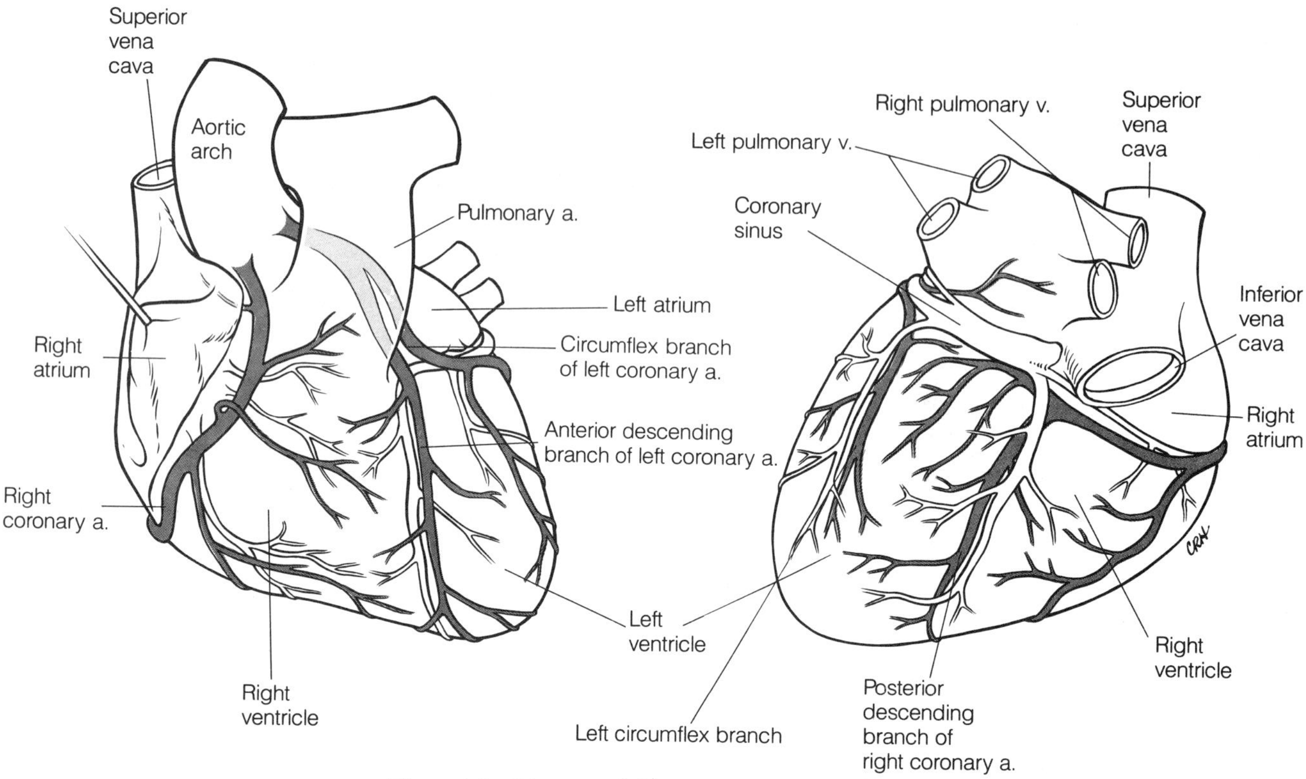

Figure 1-9 Diagram of the coronary arteries that arise from the aorta and some of the coronary veins.

THE CORONARY ARTERIES

Disease of the coronary blood vessels is the leading cause of death in the United States. A knowledge of the anatomy of the coronary arteries is necessary in order to understand how a lesion in a particular vessel can affect the important structures of the heart (Fig. 1-9). Although there are numerous anatomic variations from person to person, generally speaking, there are two main coronary arteries—the left coronary artery and right coronary artery, whose ostia are located in the sinuses of Valsalva behind two of the three cusps of the aortic valve.

The Right Coronary Artery

Normally, the right coronary artery arises from an ostia in the right sinus of Valsalva of the aortic valve. From there, it begins its course over the anterior surface of the heart in the groove between the right atrium and right ventricle. It then travels down the diaphragmatic surface of the heart. During its course, it supplies several branches to the anterior surface of the right atrium and right ventricular wall. Most people have branches off the right coronary artery that supply the major structures of the conduction system, the SA and AV nodes. As it travels around from the anterior to the diaphragmatic surface, a major branch known as the right posterior descending artery, splits off to supply the inferior and posterior walls of both the right and left ventricles in a right dominant system. This branch is less commonly supplied by the left circumflex coronary artery. In one-third of all people, double posterior descending arteries arise from both the right coronary artery and the left circumflex coronary artery. This dual blood supply to the posterior wall of the heart is called a balanced system, and is the reason that true posterior wall myocardial infarctions rarely occur.

In summary, the right coronary artery usually supplies the right atrium, the sinoatrial and atrioventricular nodes, the right ventricle, the inferior portion of the left ventricle, and the intraventricular septum. Occlusion of the right coronary artery may be less of a clinical problem than occlusion of the left coronary artery. Damage to the right ventricle is not as critical as damage to the left ventricle, which is the main pump of the heart. The right ventricle doesn't have to work as hard and it needs less oxygen than does the left ventricle. Although right ventricular failure can result from a right ventricular infarction, the usual problems that are seen stem from damage to the conduction system and the dysrhythmias that result.

The Left Coronary Artery

The left coronary artery arises from an ostia in the left sinus of Valsalva of the aortic valve. The left mainstem coronary artery is very short, and it quickly bifurcates into two branches, namely the left anterior descending and the left circumflex. A mainstem lesion is a life-threatening occurrence since occlusion at this level reduces or interrupts the blood supply to most of the left ventricle which is, of course, the main pump. When a mainstem lesion is discovered, the patient usually is taken to surgery as quickly as possible for a coronary artery bypass graft.

The left anterior descending branch is affected by atherosclerosis more often than any other coronary vessel, but the reason for this is not clear. The left anterior descending branch supplies blood to the anterior surface of the left ventricle, the intraventricular septum, and some of the anterior surface of the right ventricle. The left circumflex branch follows the left atrioventricular groove around the waist of the heart, and supplies the myocardium of the lateral and posterior surfaces of the left atrium and ventricle. Lesions of the left anterior descending and circumflex arteries will produce anterior septal and lateral infarctions, which may be complicated by acute left ventricular failure resulting from decreased pumping ability of ischemic or injured myocardium.

Because the ostia of the coronary arteries are located behind the cusps of the aortic valve, they do not fill as well during ventricular systole as do all the other arteries in the body. During systole, the aortic valve is open and the ostia are partially occluded by the valve cusps. The flow increases in coronary arteries during ventricular diastole. During systole, the myocardium is contracted and the vessels are constricted by muscle, which comprises blood flow. Thus, the coronary arterial circuit is designed as a low- (diastolic) rather than a high- (systolic) pressure system.

Coronary Artery Disease

Coronary artery disease is the leading killer in America today. It strikes people in the prime of their lives and causes untold suffering, not only physically, but also financially and emotionally. Coronary artery disease is viewed as an unavoidable part of the aging process, occurring primarily in men over the age of 40 years. However, with today's rapid pace of living, stressful occupations, and sedentary life-styles, more and more younger people, both men and women, are becoming victims of this disease. The American Heart Association lists many factors that are thought to contribute to the incidence of coronary artery disease. These are termed risk factors. Some of these are age, sex, race, diet, obesity, and stress, but the three major risk factors are considered to be cigarette smoking, high serum lipid levels and hypertension.

Coronary artery disease occurs when free fatty acids that are circulating in the blood are deposited in the intimal layer of an artery. These fatty deposits harden and become calcific plaques that will increase in size until the inner lumen of the vessel is partially or completely obstructed. This process may begin as early as the late teens, especially in men.

As the plaque begins to occlude the artery, the blood flow becomes insufficient to supply the oxygen necessary to meet the metabolic demands of the muscle tissue—coronary insufficiency. Muscle that is not getting enough oxygenated blood is said to be ischemic. Ischemia of the myocardium triggers an alarm that warns of the lack of oxygen. This warning is the classic, well-known chest pain known as angina pectoris. As the disease progresses, the vessel finally becomes occluded, and the tissue dies—a myocardial infarction (MI). This loss of functioning cardiac muscle tissue can cause sudden death, of course, but what most people do not realize is that coronary artery disease can also become a chronic, debilitating condition, like diabetes, which is just as lethal as cancer. They feel that someone who has had an infarction and survives the initial attack is "cured," an idea that is quite far from the truth.

Although exhaustive research is being conducted to discover the cause of coronary artery disease, thus far nothing has been found to reverse the course of this insidious disease. At the present time, the most hope lies in prevention. Successful prevention depends primarily upon education of the public in prudent heart living, which includes a healthy diet, weight control, exercise, not smoking, control of hypertension, and effective stress management. By controlling or eliminating risk factors from your life, the chance of developing heart disease can be reduced. However, risk-factor intervention in an adult usually requires a change in life-style and habits, a very difficult thing to accomplish. The way to achieve a successful education program is to aim the teaching at children, so that they will learn the healthy way of life and thus never develop the habits that inevitably lead to heart disease.

THE CONDUCTION SYSTEM

The heart has a specialized network of nervous tissue that initiates and distributes electrical impulses that cause contraction of the myocar-

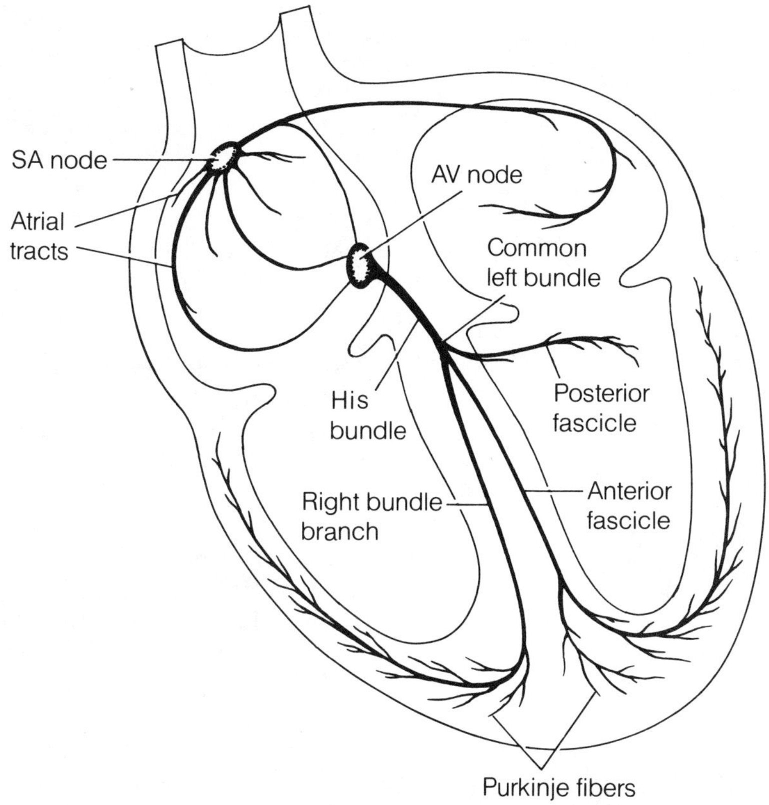

Figure 1-10 The conduction system.

dium (Fig. 1-10). Unlike skeletal muscle, which needs an impulse from the central nervous system to be electrically stimulated and contract, cardiac conduction tissue can spontaneously initiate its own electrical activity. This property of cardiac tissue is known as automaticity. Each portion of the conduction system has its own inherent rate of spontaneous or automatic depolarization. The area that has the fastest automatic rate controls the heart's electrical activity, and is called the pacemaker. Any area of the conduction system can act as the pacemaker, but usually the fastest is the SA node. The SA node acts like a spark plug; it initiates the electrical impulse, which travels through the rest of the conduction system, the intra-atrial tracts, the AV node, bundle of His, right and left bundle branches, and the Purkinje fibers in the ventricles.

The Sinoatrial Node

The SA node is a specialized area of conduction tissue where the normal cardiac cycle is initiated. It has the fastest rate of inherent automaticity and normally spontaneously depolarizes at a rate of 60 to 100 times a minute. It is 10 to 20 mm long, and is located in the right atrium, just under the endocardium close to the orifice of the superior vena cava. Blood supply to the SA node is from the SA nodal artery, which is a branch of the right coronary artery in 60% and the left coronary artery in 40% of the population. If the SA node is in control of the heart's electrical activity, the patient is said to be in normal sinus rhythm (NSR).

The Intra-atrial Tracts

The intra-atrial or intranodal tracts are described as three conduction pathways in the atria, between the SA and the AV nodes. They are Bachmann's tract, which is the shortest; Wenckebach's tract, the middle one; and Thorel's tract, which is the longest and most posterior. The tracts serve two purposes: to spread the impulse through the atrial myocardium, causing contraction, and to deliver the impulse to the AV junction.

The Atrioventricular Junction

The AV junction consists of the AV node and the bundle of His. The AV node is the only normal conduction pathway between the atria and the ventricles. It is located beneath the endocardium on the floor of the right atrium, just anterior to the coronary sinus. Blood supply to the AV node is from a branch of the right coronary artery in 90% of the population. The bundle of His penetrates the atrioventricular septum and bifurcates to become the right and left bundle branches. In the past, it was believed that all areas of the AV junction could spontaneously depolarize and act as the pacemaker. However, the development of His bundle recordings proved that the AV node proper was devoid of pacing cells.

The AV junction has several important functions. First and foremost, it is the only normal route for an impulse to be conducted from the atria to the ventricles. The AV node itself delays conduction of a normal impulse to allow time for atrial contraction to occur before the ventricles are stimulated. This area of the AV node also acts as a filter to limit the number of rapid impulses from the atria that can make it through to the ventricles. The areas just above and below the AV node and the His bundle also have the ability to act as pacemakers. The automatic rate of spontaneous depolarization inherent in AV junctional tissue is 40 to 60 beats per minute.

The Bundle Branches

The fibers of the His bundle descend along the posterior margin of the intraventricular septum, and then branch into the right and left bundle branches. The right bundle branch appears as a direct continuation of the His bundle, after the fibers of the left bundle branch have split off. The right bundle branch is a long, thin strand of fibers that fans out over the free, right ventricular wall. Because it is such a thin fiber, a small lesion can block conduction through the right bundle branch. The left bundle branch is a vertical sheet of fibers that is much larger than the right branch, and thus is more resistant to blockage since a large lesion must be present to alter conduction significantly. The left bundle branch arises from the bundle of His in an orderly fashion, as the left common bundle, which penetrates the intraventricular septum. This then divides into two fascicles, the left anterior division and the left posterior division, which form direct pathways to the anterior and posterior papillary muscles of the mitral valve. This permits the earliest transmission of the electrical impulse to the papillary muscles, so that their contraction slightly precedes that of the ventricular wall. The impulse is conducted through the ventricles in a rapid and organized fashion to allow an effective contraction.

The Purkinje Fibers

The terminal portions of the bundle branches are the Purkinje fibers. These fibers deliver the impulse directly to the ventricular muscle to produce contractions. The fibers can also act as the pacemaker at an inherent rate of 20 to 40 beats per minute. These fibers are located just under the endocardial surface and stimulate the myocardium from the inner or endocardial layer, outward to the epicardium.

The Physiology of the Conduction System

Normally, the electrical wave of activation begins in the SA node by spontaneous depolarization. It travels through the atrial tracts, AV junction, bundle branches, and Purkinje fibers, to the ventricular muscle. The mechanical contraction of the heart follows the pattern of the electrical wave. If the heart beats at a rate of 60 to 100 times a minute with normal conduction patterns, it is said to be in normal sinus rhythm (NSR).

There are many hemodynamic advantages to NSR. The delay at the AV node provides time for the atria to contract and finish filling the ventricles before they contract. The rapid transmission of the impulse through the His bundle, bundle branches, and Purkinje fibers results in the apex of the ventricle being stimulated first. Since contraction follows depolarization, the apex contracts first, moving the blood up to the base of the heart where the outflow tracts and aortic and pulmonic valves are located.

You will be exposed to many dysrhythmias in the following discussions, and you must always be acutely aware of what is happening to the heart's pumping action in response to various electrical abnormalities.

THE AUTONOMIC NERVOUS SYSTEM

As you have just seen, the heart has the property of automaticity and needs no outside stimulus to cause depolarization and contraction. However, the heart does have autonomic supply from the sympathetic and parasympathetic systems, which can regulate rate, rhythm, and strength of contraction (Fig. 1-11). Autonomic regulation helps the heart adapt to increases or decreases in metabolic demands placed on it by the body.

Both the sympathetic and parasympathetic nervous systems have sensory endings in the myocardium. Anatomically, their nerve fibers enter the cardiac plexus that entwines around the great vessels at the base of the heart. Sympathetic receptors are located throughout the heart, traveling principally along the coronary blood vessels. Parasympathetic fibers are mostly found in the atria clustered around the SA and AV nodes. If you have a problem remembering what the sympathetic or parasympathetic systems do to the heart, just remember

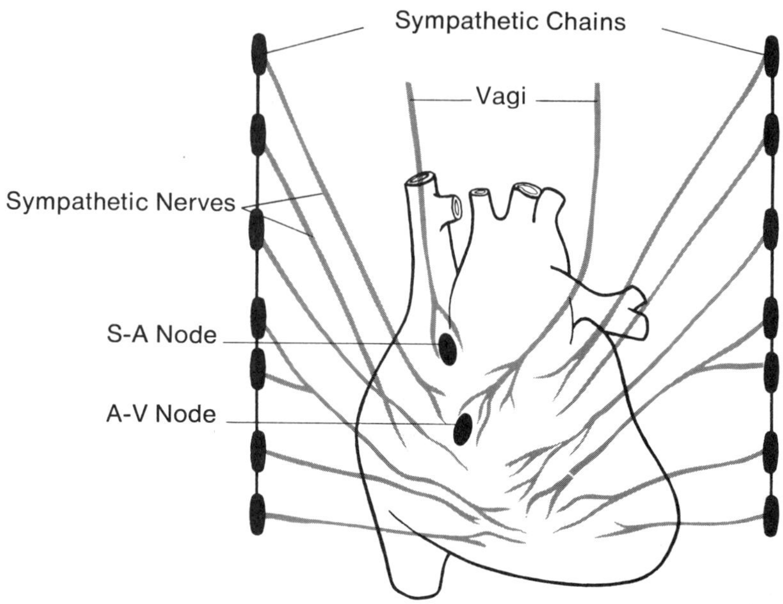

Figure 1-11 Distribution of autonomic nerve fibers to the human heart.

that the sympathetic system is in sympathy with the needs of the body and acts like an accelerator on the heart; the parasympathetic system acts like a brake.

Sympathetic Stimulation

The sympathetic nervous system controls cardiovascular and respiratory functions to ensure that there will be an adequate supply of oxygenated blood to meet the body's demands. Sympathetic control is a complicated neural and chemical interaction of four different receptors that have varying effects on different areas of the cardiovascular system. The four types of sympathetic receptors are alpha, $beta_1$, $beta_2$, and dopa. They control the amount of vasoconstriction, vasodilitation, heart rate and conduction, contractility, and bronchodilatation. The following chart is a very basic list of the four receptor types and their effects on the body.

Receptor	Site	Action
Alpha	Smooth muscle of all vascular tissue	Vasoconstriction of all arteries and veins
$Beta_1$	Myocardium	Increases heart rate, contractility, automaticity, and conductivity
$Beta_2$	Peripheral vessels Lungs	Vasodilates Bronchodilates
Dopa	Renal, mesenteric, cerebral, and coronary artery	Vasodilates

Increasing sympathetic tone to the heart causes everything to speed up. Sympathetic stimulation is caused by many different factors, such as fright, stress, exercise, fever, and drugs such as caffeine, nicotine, adrenalin, dopamine, and norepinepherine. Their effects prepare the individual's heart to meet increased demands for oxygenated blood. Sympathetic stimulation (1) increases heart rate by speeding the automatic depolarization of the SA node, and the conduction rate of the AV node ($beta_1$); (2) increases the force of ventricular contraction ($beta_1$); (3) dilates the coronary arteries because muscle that is contracting harder and faster obviously will require a larger supply of oxygenated blood (dopa); and (4) increases the excitability and automaticity of all portions of the heart ($beta_1$).

Additionally, a drop in blood pressure will cause an increase in sympathetic stimulation. There are special types of nerve endings, called baroreceptors, in the aortic arch and the carotid sinus in the neck at the base of the jaw. They are pressure receptors that sense changes in blood pressure. If the blood pressure decreases, the baroreceptors initiate sympathetic ($beta_1$) stimulation to increase heart rate and force of contraction, and also cause peripheral vasoconstriction (alpha), which will bring the blood pressure back up to a normal level.

Parasympathetic Stimulation

Parasympathetic stimulation to the heart is supplied through the vagus nerve. Vagal mediation has a slowing effect on the heart. Since the vagal fibers in the heart are located in the atria, increased vagal tone slows the automatic rate of the SA node and slows down the speed of impulse conduction through the AV node. Vagal fibers have little direct effect on the myocardium or the coronary arteries.

Factors that increase vagal tone include carotid sinus massage, Valsalva maneuver, hypertension, pain, ocular pressure, nausea and vomiting, and drugs such as digitalis, morphine, and Demerol. Increased blood pressure stretches the baroreceptors in the carotid sinus and the aortic arch, which sense the higher pressure, and slows the heart rate, thus decreasing the cardiac output and blood pressure. This baroreceptor reflex is the mechanism behind the carotid sinus massage, which frequently is used to slow a heart that is beating too rapidly.

There is normally a balance between sympathetic and parasympathetic influence on the heart which keeps the rate and speed of conduction at a reasonable level. To speed up the heart, you can either increase sympathetic tone by giving epinephrine or isoproterenol, or you can decrease vagal tone by using atropine. To slow the heart, you can increase vagal tone by giving digitalis or morphine or by using carotid sinus massage. Or, you can decrease sympathetic tone by giving a beta-blocker such as propranolol.

THE PHYSIOLOGY OF THE HEART

MECHANICAL EVENTS IN THE CARDIAC CYCLE

One cardiac cycle, or heart beat, is comprised of two parts—systole and diastole. The following discussion will refer mainly to ventricular systole and diastole. Atrial systole and diastole are in synchrony with ventricular events, occurring just prior to ventricular systole and diastole, respectively.

Diastole

Diastole is the passive or relaxation phase when the ventricles are filling with blood. Ventricular diastole accounts for about 60% of each cardiac cycle. Diastole has four separate stages: isovolumetric relaxation, rapid filling, slowed filling, and atrial contraction.

ISOVOLUMETRIC RELAXATION At the beginning of diastole, all the valves, both inflow and outflow, are closed so that no blood can enter or leave the ventricles. As the ventricular muscle relaxes, the size of the chamber increases, but since the valves remain closed and the volume of blood remains the same, the pressure in the ventricle drops. As soon as ventricular pressures drop below pressures in the atria, which have been filling during ventricular systole, the AV valves are forced open, and the next stage of diastole begins.

RAPID FILLING As the AV valves open, there is a higher pressure in the atria than in the ventricles. This relatively large difference produces a pressure gradient across the AV valves. Fluids must flow from areas of higher pressure to areas of lower pressure; the greater the pressure gradient, the faster will be the flow. Because of this, ventricular filling is rapid when the AV valves first open.

SLOW FILLING As the ventricles fill with blood, the pressure gradient between the two chambers lessens and the flow of blood slows down.

ATRIAL CONTRACTION At the end of ventricular diastole, atrial systole occurs. This is the active filling stage in which the atria contract to finish filling the ventricles. Atrial contraction provides approximately 15% to 30% of ventricular volume at the end of diastole. This volume of blood added by atrial contraction is called "atrial kick."

Systole

Ventricular systole is the active ejection phase that comprises 40% of the cardiac cycle. The ventricles contract and expel the blood that has accumulated during diastole into the aorta and pulmonary artery. Systole also has four stages: isovolumetric contraction, rapid ejection, reduced ejection, and protodiastole.

ISOVOLUMETRIC CONTRACTION At the beginning of ventricular systole, the muscle starts contracting, and the blood tries to flow back into the atria. But the AV valve leaflets close and the chordae tendinae tense to prevent regurgitation of blood. The closing of these valves produces the first heart sound, S_1, which signals the beginning of systole. With both the inflow and outflow valves closed, the ventricular muscle contracts on a fixed volume of blood and causes the intraventricular pressure to rise. When the pressures have risen to the point that they exceed diastolic pressures in the aorta and pulmonary artery, the aortic and pulmonic valves open, and the next stage begins.

RAPID EJECTION When the semilunar valves open, pressure in the ventricles quickly becomes much greater than pressure in the vessels. This high-pressure gradient across the aortic and pulmonic valves causes a rapid ejection of blood into the aorta and pulmonary artery.

REDUCED EJECTION With the reduced volume of blood remaining in the ventricles, there is a smaller pressure gradient, and although ventricular ejection continues, it is at a slower rate.

PROTODIASTOLE At the protodiastole stage of the cardiac cycle, the ventricular muscle begins to relax and ventricular pressures drop until they are less than those in the aorta and pulmonary artery. The blood tries to return to the ventricles but the backward flow catches in the cusps of the semilunar valves and closes them. Closure of the aortic and pulmonic valves produces the second heart sound, S_2, and signals the end of systole.

THE SYSTEMIC CIRCULATION

The remaining parts of the cardiovascular system are the peripheral vessels that comprise the systemic circulation (Fig. 1-12). These vessels are the aorta, the arteries and arterioles, the capillaries, the venules and veins, and the vena cavae. Their function is to transport the blood to the cells in the body, deliver the oxygen and nutrients to meet the cell's metabolic demands, remove carbon dioxide and waste products that are the end result of metabolic processes, and return the blood to the heart and lungs.

The Aorta and Arteries

The aorta and arteries are the major pipelines of the circuit. Their walls are thick, elastic, and very distensible, and are responsible for propelling the blood forward, even when the heart is in the diastolic phase of each cardiac cycle. As the left ventricle contracts, it expels a bolus of blood into the aorta whose elastic wall stretches to accommodate that amount of blood. The aortic wall then snaps back to push the blood forward. This stretching and contracting of the aortic and arterial walls moves the blood through the circuit into the arterioles. The pressure wave that moves through the arterial circuit is the pulsation that you feel under your finger when you take someone's pulse.

The Arterioles

The arterioles are the smallest branches of the arteries. Their walls are chiefly composed of smooth muscle, which has the ability to either constrict or dilate in order to control blood flow to different areas of the body. The sympathetic nervous system regulates flow by causing vasodilatation ($beta_2$ stimulation) in an area that requires increased blood supply, or by promoting vasoconstriction (alpha stimulation) that shunts blood away from areas that need less blood. The sum of all vasodilatation and vasoconstriction in the body is termed the total peripheral resistance (TPR). TPR increases with vasoconstriction and de-

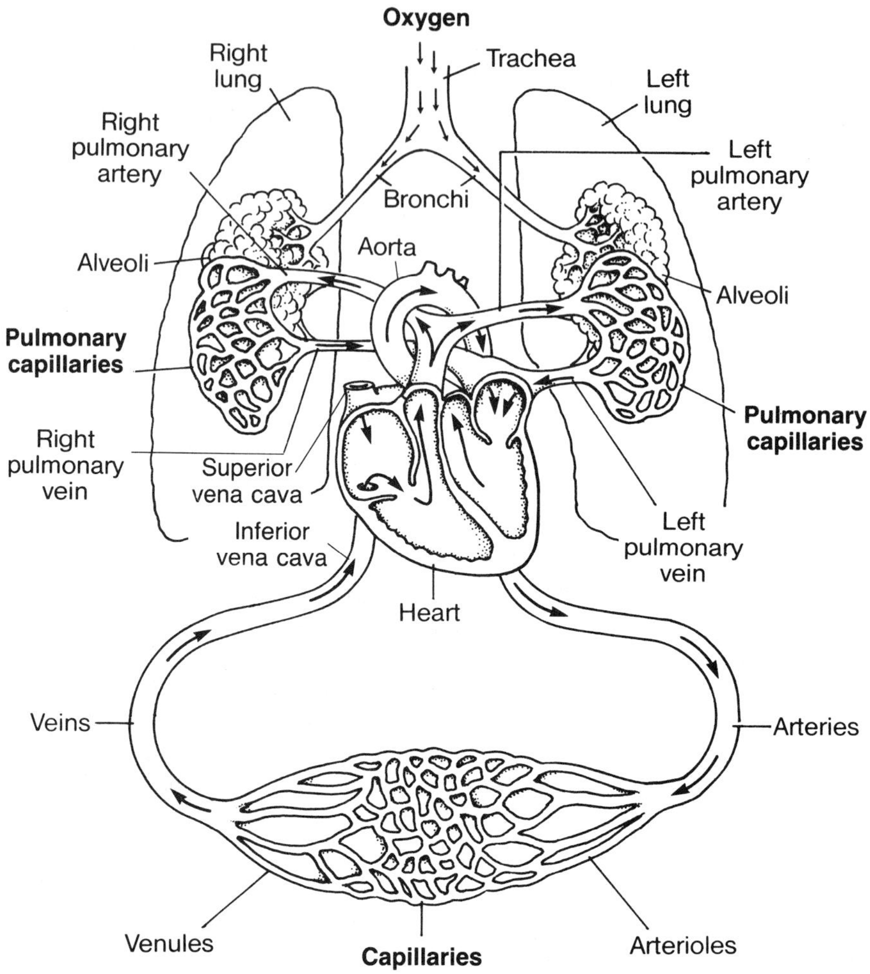

Figure 1-12 Schematic drawing of systemic circulation. (Start at bottom of diagram.) Loaded with carbon dioxide, blood from the capillaries goes through venules and veins into the right side of the heart (*arrows*). It is pumped into the two lungs. Having dropped carbon dioxide and picked up oxygen, it goes back to the left side of the heart (*arrows*). From there it is pumped through the aorta into the arteries and arterioles until it reaches the capillaries, where it gives up oxygen and picks up carbon dioxide. (National Tuberculosis and Respiratory Disease Association)

creases with vasodilitation. The TPR is actually the workload that the left ventricle is pumping against.

The Capillaries

The arterioles divide into capillaries, which are tiny vessels whose walls are one cell-layer thick. Capillaries bring the blood supply to the cellular level where the exchange of fluids, gases, nutrients, and waste products occurs. The exchange is accomplished by the processes of diffusion, osmosis, and hydrostatic pressure gradients between the intra- and extravascular spaces.

The Venous Circuit

The de-oxygenated blood moves from the capillaries into the venules, to the veins and the inferior and superior vena cavae, and then to the right atrium. Veins are thin-walled vessels containing smooth muscle and small intraluminal valves. Veins can either dilate or constrict. When dilated, they act as a reservoir for the pooling of blood in the periphery, and thus retard venous return to the heart. When constricted, they promote venous return. Blood moves from the veins to the heart in three ways:

1. As a result of gravity, particularly from the head and arms
2. From contraction of skeletal muscles that move the blood flow against gravity toward the heart. The small valves prevent back flow.
3. As a result of changing intrathoracic pressures due to respiration. On inspiration, a negative pressure develops in the chest cavity. This is what pulls the air into the body through the airways; however, it also pulls the venous blood into the thoracic cavity as well, and it returns to the right heart.

CARDIAC OUTPUT

Cardiac output is defined as the amount of blood pumped out of the heart in 1 minute, and is measured in liters per minute. A normal cardiac output at rest ranges from 4 to 6 liters/minute. The cardiac output may be altered through various neural and chemical interactions to meet the body's changing metabolic needs. When the body is at rest, its metabolic requirements for oxygen lessen, so the cardiac output will drop. During exercise, the oxygen requirements are greater, so the cardiac output increases.

The parameters that control cardiac output are stroke volume and heart rate. The heart rate is obviously the number of times the heart contracts in 1 minute, normally 60 to 100 contractions per minute. The stroke volume is the amount of blood ejected by the left ventricle with each beat, normally around 50 to 70 ml per beat. Both these determinants are directly proportional to the cardiac output. If you increase either the stroke volume or the heart rate, or both, the cardiac output will increase, too. Decreasing one or both parameters will decrease the cardiac output. The formula to determine cardiac output is:

$$\text{Cardiac output} = \text{heart rate} \times \text{stroke volume}$$

Using this formula, if the rate is 80 and the stroke volume is 50 ml, the cardiac output is 4 liters/minute.

Heart Rate

Changing the heart rate is one of the easiest ways of controlling cardiac output. If the body's need for oxygenated blood increases, the heart rate will increase.

$$\text{Heart rate (120)} \times \text{stroke volume (50 ml)} = \text{cardiac output (6 liters/min)}$$

As the rate increases, so does the cardiac output, until a certain rate is reached, usually around 160 to 180 beats/minute. At this point, the cardiac output will start to drop. The output decreases because the stroke volume begins to decrease. The stroke volume depends, in part, on the length of the diastolic filling interval (the amount of time between beats). As the rate increases, the filling interval decreases, thus diminishing the stroke volume. Patients with cardiac disease who have decreased left ventricular function may start to have a drop in output at a rate slower than the 160 to 180 range.

If the heart rate decreases, the cardiac output will decrease as well.

Heart rate (30) × stroke volume (50 ml)
= cardiac output (1.5 liters/min)

However, the diastolic filling interval also has an effect when the rate slows. As the rate drops, the filling time increases, the stroke volume increases, and the cardiac output is maintained. Eventually, the maximal stroke volume is reached and the left ventricle cannot hold any more blood. If the rate continues to drop, the cardiac output will decrease dramatically.

FACTORS AFFECTING HEART RATE

Location of the Pacemaker If the cells in the SA node are the pacemaker, the heart rate will be in the normal range of 60 to 100 beats/minute. However, if the pacemaker is located lower in the conduction system of the heart, the rate will be slower. Generally speaking, the lower in the heart the pacer is located, the slower the heart rate will be.

Autonomic Influences Any of the factors previously mentioned, such as fright, stress, exercise, nausea, and so forth, that influence the amount of sympathetic or parasympathetic tone will cause a change in the heart rate. Excess sympathetic stimulation or decreased vagal stimulation will speed up the heart. Increased vagal tone or decreased sympathetic tone will cause the heart to slow down.

Injury, Ischemia, or Infarction Coronary artery disease, with the resulting injury, ischemia, and infarction of the myocardium, can also profoundly influence the heart rate. The areas of injury and ischemia become electrically unstable and produce an increased irritability or automaticity of the myocardium. This will cause premature beats, tachycardias, flutter, or fibrillation. If the injured or infarcted areas are located in or near the conduction system, particularly the SA or AV nodes, bradycardias, AV blocks, or bundle branch block may result.

Stroke Volume

There are three determinants that affect the stroke volume: preload, contractility, and afterload. These three factors, although separate, are closely interrelated, and anything that affects one may well have an effect on one or both of the others.

PRELOAD Preload is determined by the amount of blood in the left ventricle at the end of diastole, which is termed the left ventricular end diastolic volume (LVEDV). Preload is the way the heart meets increased demands that are placed upon it. It is a reserve mechanism that allows the left ventricle to increase its output when there are greater body demands, as in stress, exercise, or fever. LVEDV controls the amount of stretch put on the individual muscle fibers in the ventricle before they contract.

Starling's Law How preload affects the stroke volume is explained by Starling's Law, which states "... that within physiologic limits, a larger diastolic cardiac volume results in a greater energy of contraction." In other words, the longer the initial fiber length before contraction (preload), the stronger will be the force of contraction. If this is unclear, an analogy may make Starling's Law easier to understand. Think of a rubber band. If you stretch the rubber band a short distance (small preload), it will snap back with a small amount of force. If you stretch the rubber band a longer distance (greater preload), it will snap back with much greater force. When a patient goes into congestive heart failure, there is too much preload, the initial fiber length becomes too long, and the muscle doesn't contract as well. In other words, the rubber band has been overstretched too many times, and it loses its elasticity. You have exceeded the physiologic limit that will provide a good strong contraction.

Many things can affect the LVEDV, and therefore the preload. Rapid heart rates that decrease the ventricular filling time will decrease the preload. Hemorrhage or dehydration decreases the total circulating blood volume, and thus decreases the preload. Overhydration or renal failure will increase preload. The rate of venous return to the heart also influences preload. Congestive heart failure or cardiogenic shock both increase preload because the failing left ventricle cannot eject all of the blood with each beat, and the circuit will eventually become overloaded. Atrial kick is another factor that influences preload. When atrial systole occurs in synchrony with ventricular systole, that 30% of LVEDV supplied by the contracting atria puts the last bit of stretch on the ventricular muscle to produce a good, strong contraction. Loss of atrial kick in a healthy heart may not be a problem because of the many available compensatory mechanisms. But, in the injured heart, whose ventricular muscle is only contracting well enough to barely maintain the patient's hemodynamic status, loss of atrial kick may be enough to cause the patient's heart to decompensate, and congestive failure or cardiogenic shock will ensue. The ventricular muscle needed the LVEDV provided by the atrial kick to produce the stretch on the initial fiber length, in order to allow a strong enough contraction to maintain the cardiac output.

Preload Measurement and Adjustment Preload is best measured in an indirect fashion through the use of a Swan-Ganz catheter located in the pulmonary artery. When the Swan-Ganz catheter is monitoring pulmonary artery pressures, it is really looking at right heart function. However, when the balloon at the catheter tip is inflated and the catheter is wedged into the pulmonary capillary bed, right heart pressures are not seen. Instead, the catheter tip is monitoring left heart pressures, reflected back through the pulmonary vasculature and the left atrium. If the LVEDV is normal, the Swan-Ganz catheter will see this reflected as a normal left ventricular end diastolic *pressure* (LVEDP) of 8 to 12 mm Hg. However, if the left ventricle begins to fail, and the LVEDV starts to increase, the LVEDP will rise and be seen as an elevated pulmonary capillary wedge pressure (PCWP).

Preload adjustment must be tailored to correct the cause of the abnormality. If the preload is too low, it is usually a result of inadequate circulating volume. To correct a low preload, volume expanders such as Dextran, plasma, or intravenous fluids might be given, or the patient could be placed in a Trendelenburg position. When preload is too high, usually because of congestive heart failure, many different methods are available and necessary to make the adjustment. Volume reduction, such as diureses or, in extreme cases, phlebotomy, may be used. Methods to retard venous return to the heart are also used. These methods include rotating tourniquets to trap venous blood in the extremities; semi or high Fowler's position, which uses gravity to slow return; vasodilators to promote peripheral pooling of blood; and intermittant positive pressure breathing to decrease the effect of negative intrathoracic pressure on venous return. Positive inotropic agents such as digitalis or dopamine will increase contractility and promote more complete emptying of the left ventricle, thus indirectly reducing preload.

CONTRACTILITY Contractility, or the inotropic state of the myocardium, is the second major determinant of stroke volume. The greater the contractility of the ventricular muscle, the faster and more forceful will be the ejection of blood, and the larger the stroke volume. Although it has already been demonstrated how preload affects contractility, the inotropic state of the ventricle is mainly controlled by the beta sympathetic receptors in the heart.

Increasing beta sympathetic tone increases contractility. Sympathomimetic drugs such as epinephrine, isoproterenol, or dopamine cause increased beta stimulation and thus contractility. Digitalis is also a positive inotropic agent, but it doesn't work through beta mediation. Digitalis' effect is at the cellular level, where it shortens the overstretched, inelastic, muscle fibers, and brings them back into the physiologic range that provides efficient contraction according to Starling's Law. Digitalis works only on damaged tissue.

On the other hand, decreasing beta sympathetic tone will decrease contractility. The pharmacologic agents known as beta blockers that are used to treat certain dysrhythmias, angina, and hypertension, also have the occasional unwanted effect of decreasing contractility, and may even cause congestive failure in a heart with little cardiac reserve. Some available beta blockers are propranolol, metaprolol, nadolol, atenolol, timolol, and pindolol.

Cardiac contractility is also decreased in myocardium that is injured, ischemic, infarcted, acidotic, or hypoxic.

AFTERLOAD The last determinant of stroke volume is afterload. Afterload is the resistance to ejection of blood, or the impedance to blood flow from the heart after the aortic valve opens and the contracting left ventricle propels the blood into the aorta. Afterload, the workload the heart is pumping against, is determined by the amount of constriction or dilitation of the arterioles, the TPR. Because the pressure generated by the left ventricle must exceed the pressure in the aorta in order to open the aortic valve and eject blood, an increase in TPR means an increase in the workload for the heart. Increasing TPR will cause a decrease in stroke volume, particularly in the diseased heart. As with contractility, TPR is controlled by the sympathetic nervous system. How the sympathetic nervous system affects resistance is explained in the discussions of the circulatory system and autonomic supply to the heart.

Afterload reduction is accomplished with vasodilating agents such as sodium nitroprusside or IV nitroglycerine, which are frequently used because of their potent action to drastically decrease TPR. Another method of afterload reduction is provided by the intra-aortic balloon pump. Both of these methods, pharmacologic and mechanical, decrease the afterload which facilitates ejection of the blood, and thus increases the stroke volume and the cardiac output. (See the following chart for a summary of the determinants of cardiac output.)

Summary of the Major Determinants of Cardiac Output.

Cardiac Output = Heart Rate × Stroke Volume

DETERMINANTS OF HEART RATE	DETERMINANTS OF STROKE VOLUME
The integrity and location of the pacemaker cell Junctional and ventricular rhythms—↓ Rate	Preload—end-diastolic fiber length ↓ Fiber length—↓ Stroke volume ↑ Fiber length—↑ Stroke volume ↑ ↑ ↑ Fiber length—↓ Stroke volume
Autonomic nervous system Sympathetic stimulation–↑ Rate Parasympathetic—vagus stimulation—↓ Rate	Contractility—inotropic state of the myocardium ↑ Contractility—↑ Stroke volume ↓ Contractility—↓ Stroke volume
Ischemia or infarction leading to irritability or conduction defects Rapid initiation of impulses due to irritability–↑ Rate Heart block–↓ Rate	Afterload—peripheral resistance to the ejection of blood from the left ventricle ↑ Afterload–↓ Stroke volume ↓ Afterload–↑ Stroke volume

Clinical Signs of Reduced Cardiac Output

The previous discussion of factors that determine and alter cardiac output explains what happens during changes in a hemodynamic status. But what clinical symptoms and signs will the patient exhibit as a result of reduction in cardiac output? Naturally, the blood pressure will drop, and massive release of catecholamines to preserve the blood pressure and cardiac output results in signs and symptoms. Also, many of the symptoms that are seen are caused by decreased perfusion of different areas of the body. The cerebral blood flow (CBF) is reduced, so there will be a change in the level of consciousness. There may be restlessness and confusion, or if the cardiac output is severely compromised, loss of consciousness. Decreased perfusion of the kidneys will diminish urinary output. Drops in cardiac output and blood pressure produce a compensatory reflex vasoconstriction in the peripheral arterioles in an attempt to maintain central arterial pressure to the vital organs. This will cause the skin to become cool and clammy, with an ashen color, and diminished peripheral pulses. And finally, the heart muscle itself is not being adequately perfused and is beating harder and faster to try to compensate for the decreased cardiac output. Thus, this increase in myocardial oxygen demand, coupled with a restricted supply of oxygenated blood, can produce angina, infarction, ECG changes, and irritability dysrhythmias.

BLOOD PRESSURE

The blood pressure in a closed system is equal to the resistance of the system times the flow. More specifically, mean blood pressure equals cardiac output times total peripheral resistance (BP = CO × TPR). We have already mentioned the determinants of both cardiac output and peripheral resistance, so let's look at the determinants of systolic and diastolic arterial pressures.

Systolic Blood Pressure

Blood ejected into the aorta from the left ventricle during systole causes an increase of pressure in the aorta, which is partly absorbed by the elasticity of the walls. The maximum pressure reached during ventricular contraction is called the peak systolic pressure. Its level depends on the rate and amount of systolic ejection and the distensibility of the aorta. The faster and larger the stroke volume ejected from the left ventricle, the higher the systolic pressure will be. Normally, the force of ejection is partially absorbed by the elasticity of the aortic wall. If the walls of the aorta are atherosclerotic, making them rigid and less distensible than normal, then the same stroke volume ejected at peak rate will generate a higher systolic pressure. Thus, in older persons with widespread atherosclerosis, the systolic pressure may be quite elevated, while the diastolic pressure is within normal limits.

Diastolic Blood Pressure

When systolic ejection is completed, and the pressure within the left ventricle falls below that within the aorta, the aortic valve closes. As the distended aortic walls begin to contract and collapse, blood continues to flow through the many arteries and arterioles into the vascular bed as the aortic pressure falls. The pressure during this interval of ventricular relaxation is the diastolic pressure. Factors that affect the diastolic pressure are the peripheral resistance and the diastolic interval. The rate of outflow or runoff from the systemic arterial system depends on the state of the peripheral resistance through which the blood flows. The arterioles are the vessels that are responsible for the major portion of the peripheral resistance. Their state of contraction or relaxation, although influenced by local metabolic factors, is largely controlled by the activity of the sympathetic nervous system as previously described. In states of vasoconstriction, there is a slower runoff of blood than in states of vasodilitation, so diastolic pressure will be higher. The level to which the diastolic pressure falls depends on the length of the diastolic interval. The slower the heart rate, the longer the diastolic interval during which the aortic pressure continues to fall, and the lower the diastolic pressure will be.

Pulse Pressure

The pulse pressure represents the difference between the systolic and diastolic pressures. Thus, factors that increase the systolic pressure or decrease the diastolic pressure will widen or increase the pulse pressure. The magnitude of the pulse pressure largely determines the forcefulness and the volume of the peripheral pulses.

Let us examine what happens to the patient who develops a tachycardia. Because of the decreased diastolic interval, diastolic filling is impaired, and there is less blood in the left ventricle to be ejected with the next contraction. Thus, stroke volume decreases as a result of reduced preload. Reduced preload, by the Starling mechanism, reduces the force of contraction. This, too, decreases the stroke volume and therefore the systolic pressure. The decreased systolic pressure initiates a regulatory reflex in the baroreceptors, which results in increased activity of the sympathetic nerves, thus producing increased vasoconstriction. The resulting increase in the peripheral resistance, which opposes the easy outflow of blood from the arterial system, leads to an increased diastolic pressure. Also, as a result of the decreased diastolic interval, the diastolic pressure does not fall to as low a level as before the tachycardia, and thus, diastolic pressure rises secondarily. Thus, several factors operate during tachycardias to decrease systolic pressure and to increase diastolic blood pressure. The typical weak, rapid, thready pulse, which is felt at the wrist during tachycardias, reflects this decreased pulse pressure and hints at the complex physiologic alterations that are occurring.

2

ELECTROPHYSIOLOGY AND ELECTROCARDIOGRAPHY

Now that we have reviewed the anatomy and physiology of the heart and the circulatory system, the discussion will turn to electrophysiology and electrocardiography. The mechanical events of the cardiac cycle were presented in detail in Chapter 1, and now emphasis will be placed on electrical activity and the methods and equipment available for observing and recording it.

ELECTROPHYSIOLOGY

Electrophysiology is the study of the electrical activity generated and transmitted by the conduction system. This activity, which causes the mechanical contraction of the atrial and ventricular myocardium, is called depolarization and repolarization.

DEPOLARIZATION AND REPOLARIZATION

Depolarization is the electrical activation of a myocardial cell that initiates mechanical contraction. The term depolarization seems to have the connotation that the cell, when activated, loses its charge and becomes electrically neutral; but that is not the case. The cell is actually changing its electrical polarity. If a miniature electrode could be positioned in such a way that it was looking at the electrical charge on one cell, it would show that the fully repolarized cell is relatively positive outside the cell and negative inside the cell. As the cell depolarizes,

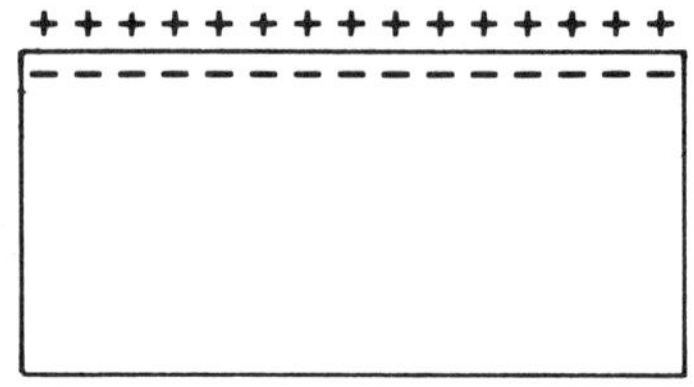

the charge changes, and the cell becomes relatively negative outside and positive inside the cell.

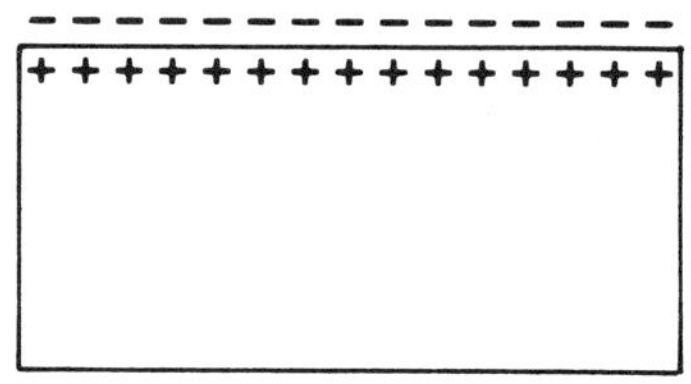

Repolarization returns the charge on the cell back to negative inside the cell and positive outside. This change in electrical polarity is caused by the movement of sodium and potassium ions across the cell membrane. The repolarized cell's membrane is somewhat impermeable to sodium. There is a large concentration of sodium ions outside the

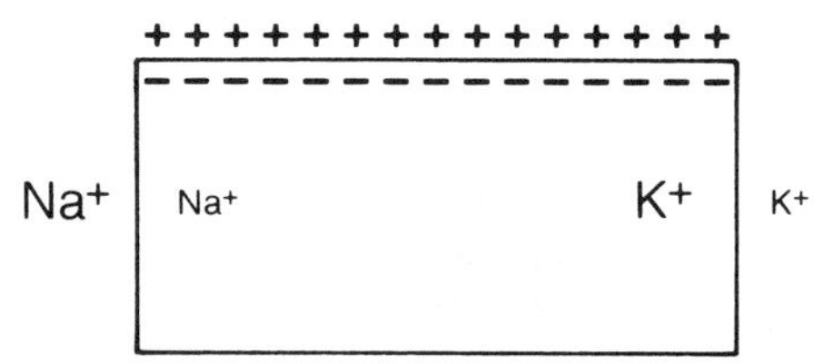

cell, and a small concentration inside the cell. The potassium ion ratio is just the opposite, with a large concentration inside and a smaller concentration outside the cell. The ability of the cell to regulate concentrations of charged particles makes the cell relatively positive outside and negative inside.

When the cell depolarizes, the sodium moves into the cell through gates or openings known as the fast channels, bringing the positive charge in with it. The cell is now positive inside and negative outside.

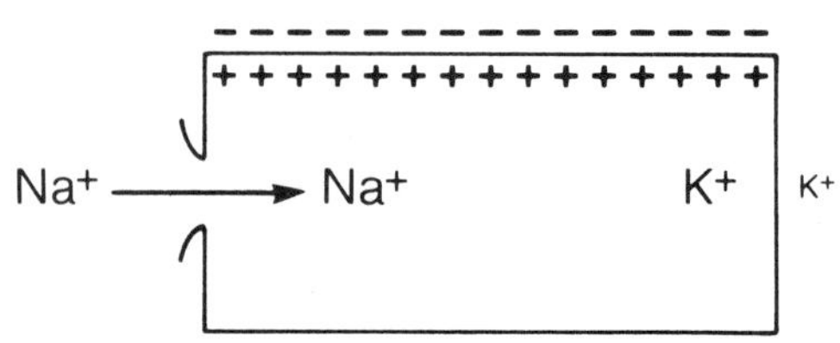

The next step in depolarization occurs when calcium moves into the cell through other gates called the slow channels. The role that calcium plays in depolarization is not fully understood, but it is known that calcium has the important job of linking the electrical activity of depolarization to the mechanical activity of contraction.

Repolarization is accomplished in two stages. First, potassium ions move out of the cell, taking the positive charge out with them. The cell

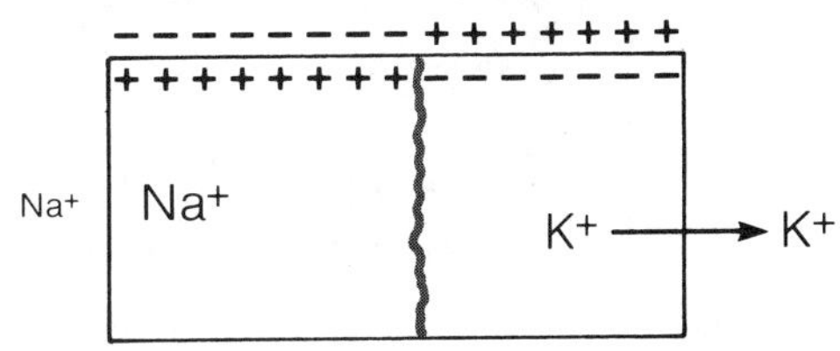

has now returned to its repolarized electrical state, with a positive charge outside and a negative charge inside. The cell is now electrically rebalanced. But, the electrolyte concentrations are not back to normal. There is too much sodium inside the cell, and too much potassium outside.

The second part of repolarization is achieved by the action of the

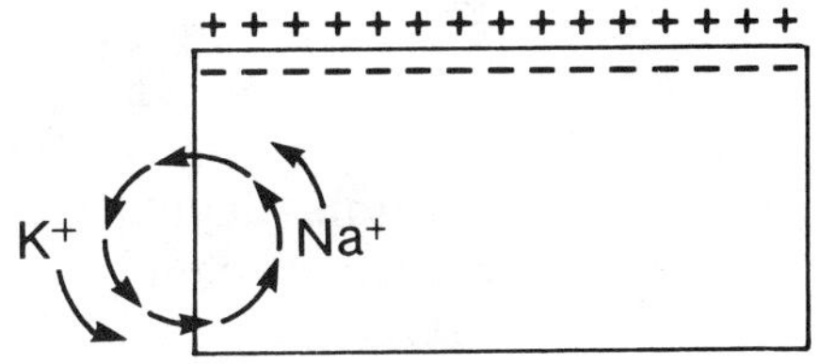

sodium pump, which pushes the excess sodium out of the cell in exchange for potassium. At this point, both the electrical charge and the electrolyte concentrations are rebalanced, and the cell is fully repolarized and ready to be activated again. This electrical activity moves from cell to cell and fiber to fiber, until the entire heart has been depolarized and repolarized.

Mechanical contraction follows the wave of depolarization through the heart. Cardiac muscle has two special properties that allow the heart to generate its own depolarization stimulus and spread this stimulus throughout the heart. These properties are automaticity and conductivity.

AUTOMATICITY

Automaticity is that characteristic property of myocardial tissue that allows almost any part of the electrical system of the heart to initiate the impulse that begins the wave of electrical stimulation. Skeletal muscle cannot activate itself, and therefore must await an electrical stimulus from the central nervous system (CNS) in order to depolarize and contract. Normal cardiac depolarization is initiated by the automatic or spontaneous firing of a cell. All cells in the conduction system, with the possible exception of those in the AV node, are able to initiate an electrical impulse. The cell that automatically depolarizes at the fastest rate will control the electrical activity of all other cells in the heart, and is said to be the pacemaker. If we take the miniature electrode and watch the pacemaker cell as it automatically depolarizes and repolarizes, we will see a waveform produced that is called the spontaneous discharge cycle (SDC).

Spontaneous Discharge Cycle

The SDC has four phases: slow diastolic depolarization, rapid depolar-

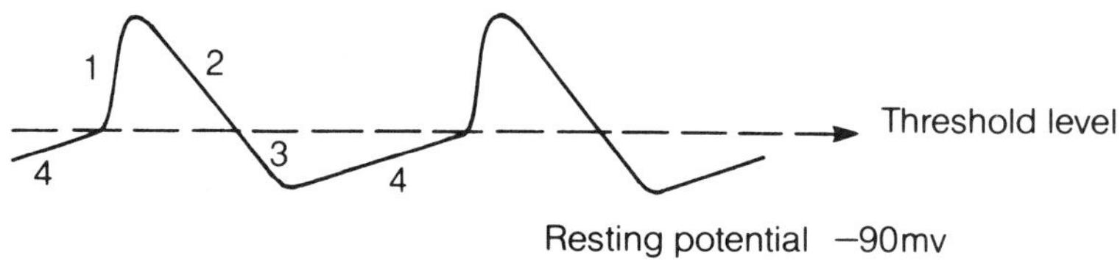

ization, and two stages of repolarization. The fully repolarized cell is said to have reached its resting potential when the charge inside the cell is relatively negative and the electrolytes have achieved their balanced ratio. The normal negative charge on the cell at its resting potential is −90 millivolts. Once the cell has reached the resting potential, slow diastolic depolarization or Phase 4 begins. Sodium begins to move across the cell membrane through the slow channels, bringing a positive charge with it. This causes the cell to become less negative inside. The charge inside the cell continues to become more and more positive until the electrical threshold level is reached. The electrical threshold is that point at which the next phase, Phase 1 or rapid depolarization, begins.

The threshold level can differ from person to person, and also will vary in the same person from time to time. Some factors influencing the threshold level are drugs, sympathetic and parasympathetic tone, and injury or ischemia of the myocardium. When the threshold is reached, Phase 1 occurs. At threshold, the cell membrane suddenly becomes very permeable to sodium, which rushes into the cell through the fast channels and gives the cell a relatively positive charge of +30 millivolts.

Repolarization occurs during Phases 2 and 3. Phase 2 is the absolute refractory period. At this time, calcium is entering the cell through the slow channels. The cell is absolutely refractory, which means that if it is stimulated, it could not respond because it is not sufficiently repolarized. Phase 3 is the relative refractory period when the cell is approaching its resting potential. Potassium is leaving the cell and taking the positive charge with it. The charge inside the cell starts to become relatively more negative. Phase 3 is called the relative refractory period because at some point in this period, the cell will have recovered enough to respond if stimulated sufficiently. After repolarization is completed, and the cell has reached its resting potential, Phase

4 begins again. The sodium pump actively rebalances the sodium–potassium ratio during this stage.

Inherent Rates

As previously mentioned, all the conductive tissue in the heart, except those cells in the AV node, are going through a SDC. It is the cell with the shortest cycle length which fires first, and thus becomes the pacemaker. Usually, the cells in the SA node have the most automaticity and are firing faster than any others in the heart, at a rate of 60 to 100 times per minute. The SA node is normally the pacemaker because it has the fastest inherent rate. The other cells in the heart have slower spontaneous discharge cycles, and usually never reach their threshold levels because the impulse initiated by the SA node discharges them before they can activate themselves. The AV junction is the next fastest pacemaker with a SDC length that produces an inherent rate of 40 to 60 beats/minute. The slowest spontaneous discharge cycle is found in the Purkinje fibers at an inherent rate of 20 to 40 beats/minute.

Ectopic Pacemakers

Because the SA node normally has the fastest SDC, and because the other cells in the heart are usually never allowed to reach their threshold level, it should follow logically that every heart should always be in normal sinus rhythm (NSR). But, as you well know, this is not the case. How, then, can other areas of the heart become the pacemaker? Basically, the SA node loses control in one of two ways.

Something can slow down the SA node, so it no longer has the shortest SDC; the next fastest pacemaker then will take over. The SA node can be slowed by raising its threshold so that it takes longer to

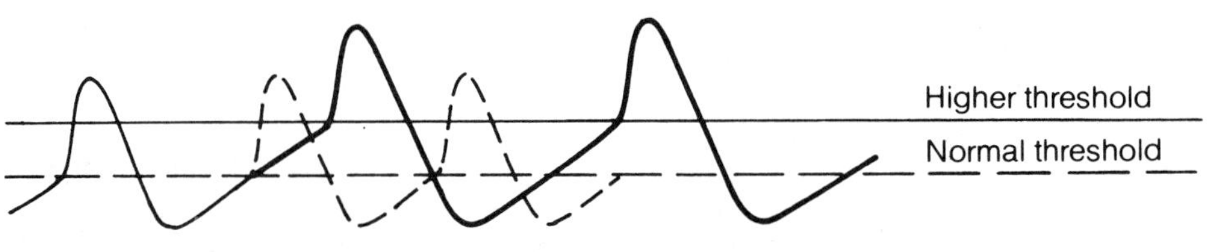

reach the higher level. The SA node can also be suppressed by slowing the rate at which sodium is leaking into the cell during slow diastolic

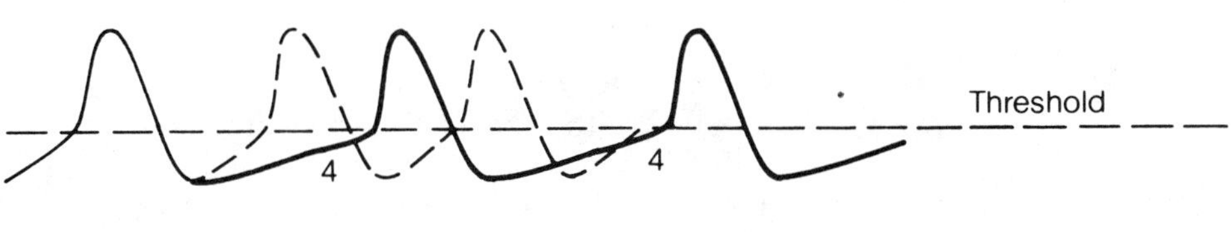

depolarization, thus decreasing the angle of the Phase 4 slope, and delaying the SA node in reaching its threshold.

Something can also speed up the SDC of an ectopic focus, so that it will fire before the SA node can, and thus usurp the pacing function.

An ectopic focus is a cell that is located anywhere in the heart other than the SA node. The SDC of an ectopic focus is accelerated in two ways, either by lowering its threshold so that the lower level is reached

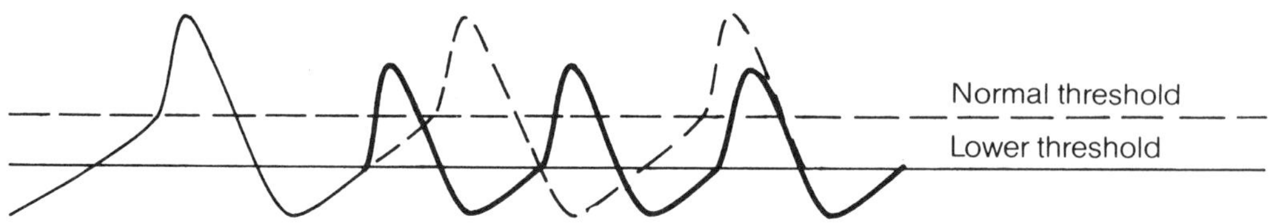

more quickly than the SA node does, or by increasing the rate at which sodium is leaking into the cell during slow diastolic depolarization,

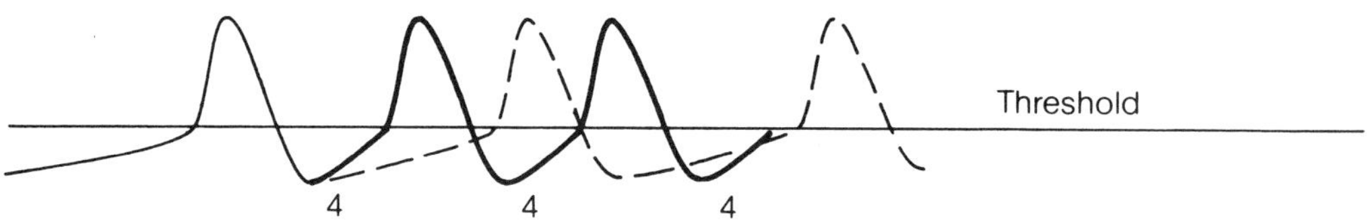

thus increasing the slope of Phase 4 and allowing the ectopic focus to reach its threshold sooner than the SA node can.

Many things can suppress or accelerate the SDC. Drugs, ischemia, injury, or varying sympathetic or parasympathetic tone are common causes of SDC alteration.

CONDUCTIVITY

Conductivity is the other characteristic property that is unique to myocardial tissue. It allows the electrical stimulus initiated by spontaneous depolarization to move from cell to cell and fiber to fiber, until the wave of propagated discharge reaches all of the cells in the heart. Skeletal muscle cells cannot be activated by this conducted wave of depolarization, and each separate fiber must have a nerve ending to transmit the electrical stimulus that arises in the CNS.

Action Potential Curve

If we were to take a miniature electrode and watch the electrical activity of one cell being discharged by a stimulus that is conducted from another cell, the shape of the waveform would differ from that of the SDC. The waveform produced by conducted or propagated discharge is known as the action potential curve, and it consists of five phases (0–4).

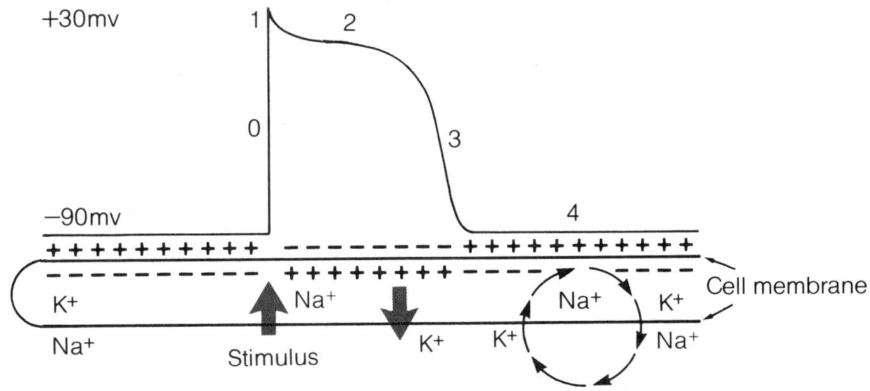

Phases 0 and 1. Phases 0 and 1 occur at the beginning of the action potential curve when the cell is fully repolarized and is at its resting potential of −90 millivolts. An electrical stimulus hits the cell and Phases 0 and 1 begin. When the wave of depolarization reaches the cell, the cell membrane suddenly becomes permeable to sodium. The sodium ions rush into the cell through the fast channels, bringing the positive charge in with them, and the cell rapidly depolarizes, producing the rapid upstroke and the spike of the action potential curve.

Phase 2. Phase 2 is the plateau of the action potential curve and corresponds to the absolute refractory period. At this point, calcium is entering the cell through the slow channels.

Phase 3. Phase 3 is the repolarization period when the potassium is moving out of the cell taking the positive charge out with it. The gradually sloping curve of Phase 3 shows the cell becoming more negative inside. As in the SDC, Phase 3 is the relative refractory period.

Phase 4. Phase 4 of the action potential curve begins when the cell has again reached its resting potential and is fully repolarized. The difference between the SDC and the action potential curve is most apparent during Phase 4, which is sloping gradually upward in the SDC but is flattened in the action potential curve. Most cells are depolarized by a propagated wave from an automatic cell during Phase 4, and never can reach their thresholds to fire themselves off.

Conduction Velocity

As the propagated wave of electrical activity known as depolarization moves from cell to cell and fiber to fiber through the heart, it varies in speed, moving slowly through some areas and faster through others. The rate at which the impulse travels is known as the conduction velocity. The slowest conduction velocity in the heart is found in the AV node. This fact becomes logical when you remember that one of the main functions of the AV node is to delay the impulse so that the atria are stimulated before the ventricles are activated. The next fastest conduction velocity is through the ventricular muscle at a rate six times faster than conduction through the AV node. Conduction through the atrial muscle is the next fastest, at 20 times the speed of conduction through the AV node. Conduction through muscle is by necessity slower because the wave is traveling from cell to cell rather than through the specialized tissue of the conduction system. The fastest conduction velocity in the heart is through the bundle branches and Purkinje fibers, at 40 times the rate through the AV node. This rapid conduction is necessary for the ventricular muscle to receive the impulse in a fast, organized fashion, so that the resulting contraction is also organized and efficient.

ELECTROCARDIOGRAPHY

Electrocardiography is the recording and measurement of the electrophysiologic events of depolarization and repolarization. It provides a means of observing the electrical activity of the heart to discover any abnormalities in the generation or conduction of impulses that may well affect the hemodynamic status of the patient. Basically, the electrical activity of the heart is observed by placement of electrodes on the skin. These electrodes pick up the ebb and flow of the weak currents produced by depolarization and repolarization. These weak currents are transmitted to an electrocardiogram (ECG) machine or monitor that amplifies them and displays them as waveforms, either on an oscilloscope or on ECG paper.

WAVES AND DEFLECTIONS

When a cardiac muscle cell is electrically activated, the wave of depolarization spreads along the cell, away from the point of stimulation.

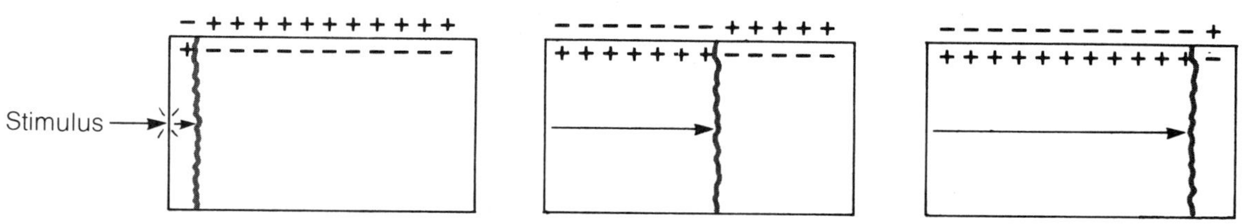

The wave front moves from cell to cell and fiber to fiber until the whole heart is depolarized. The wave of depolarization can vary in the direction it is flowing and in the amount of electrical activity being generated in different areas of the heart. The larger the portion of tissue being activated, the greater the amount of electrical activity produced.

The direction of current flow and the amount of electrical activity being produced can be diagrammed as an arrow. The arrowhead points

in the direction of the current flow. The length of the arrow's shaft denotes the amount of activity present. A short arrow means that only

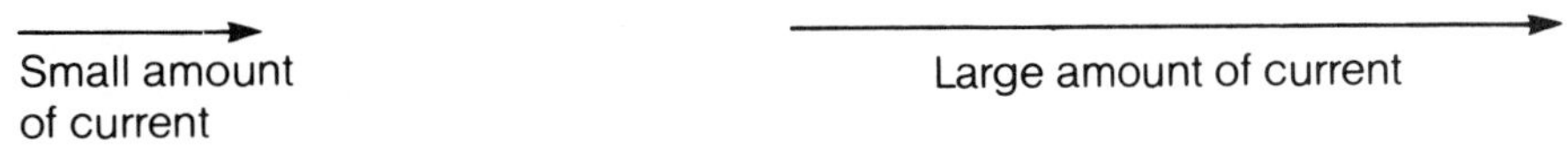

a small amount of current is being generated; a longer arrow shows a large amount.

Deflections

If a positive electrode is positioned so that the wave of depolarization

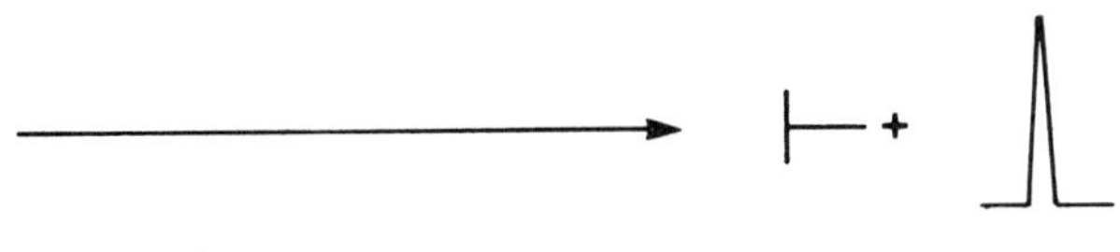

is proceeding toward it, a positive or upward deflection is produced on the ECG.

If the positive electrode is positioned so that the wave of depolarization

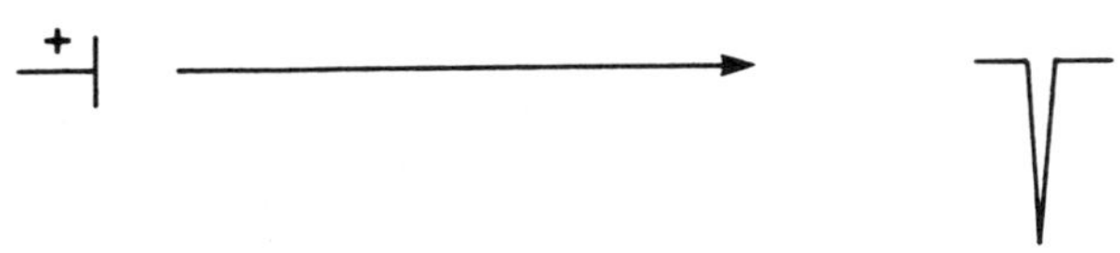

ization is receding away from it, a negative or downward deflection will be seen.

If the positive electrode is positioned so that the wave of depolarization first moves toward it, then moves away from it, a diphasic de-

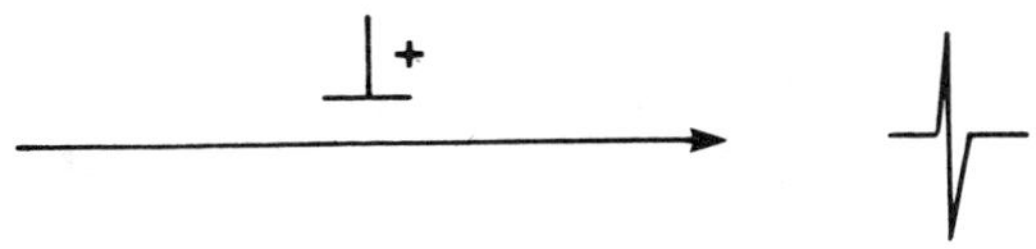

flection is produced that is initially positive as the wave proceeds toward the electrode, then negative as the wave recedes away from it.

If there is no electrical activity being generated, or if the amount of activity is too small to be perceived by the electrode, no deflection

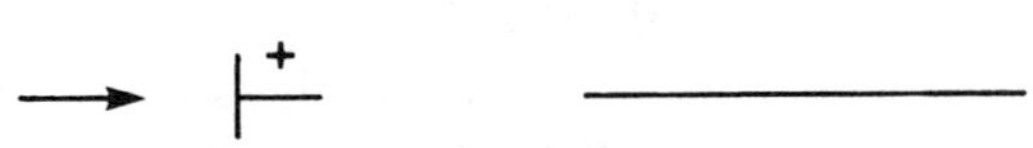

will be produced and the ECG will return to the isoelectric or base line.

If the amount of voltage being produced by the electrical activity

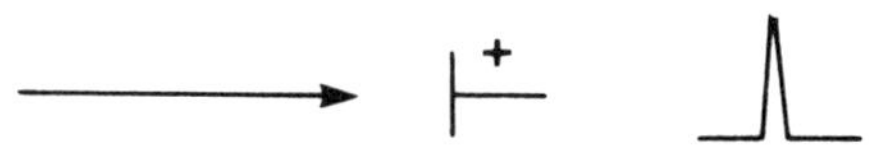

is small, the deflection will be shallow.

If a greater amount of voltage is being produced, the deflection

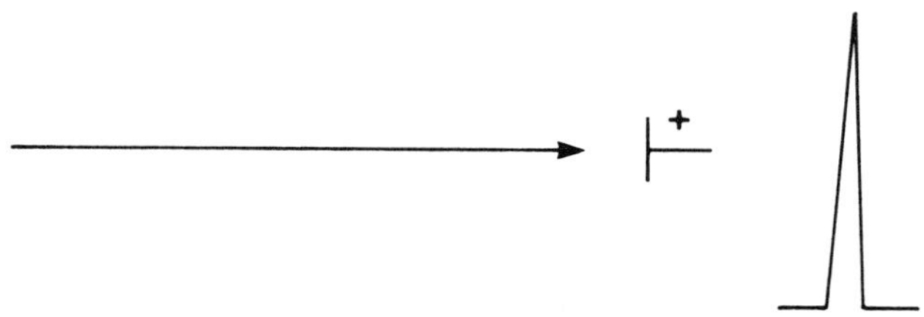

will be larger.

Cancellation

As was previously stated, the larger the piece of muscle being depolarized, the greater the amount of electrical current produced. If you have two equal strips of muscle sitting side by side, and you deliver a stimulus where the two strips are joined, the wave of depolarization will

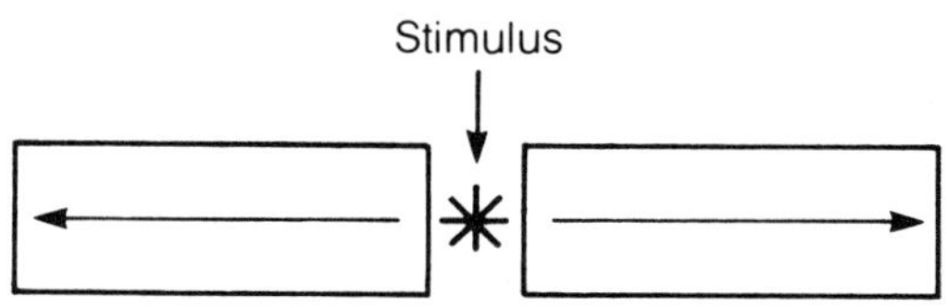

spread away from the point of stimulation through each strip, one wave to the right and one to the left. If you position two positive electrodes on either end of the two strips, each electrode will see the wave coming

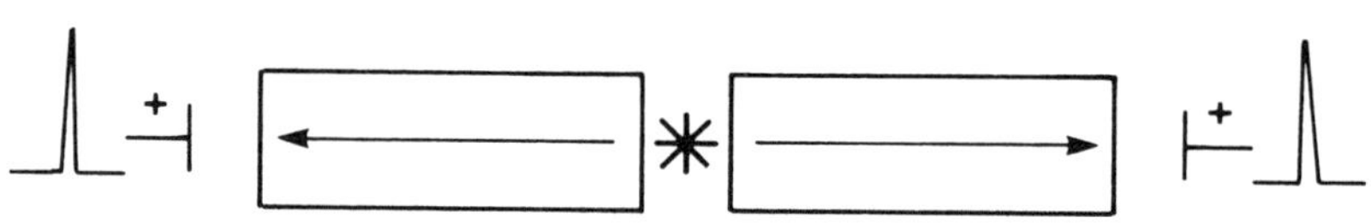

toward it through the nearest strip, and each will produce an upward deflection.

However, if you have two strips of muscle of unequal size, one much larger than the other, sitting side by side, and you deliver the same stimulus, the results on the ECG will be quite different.

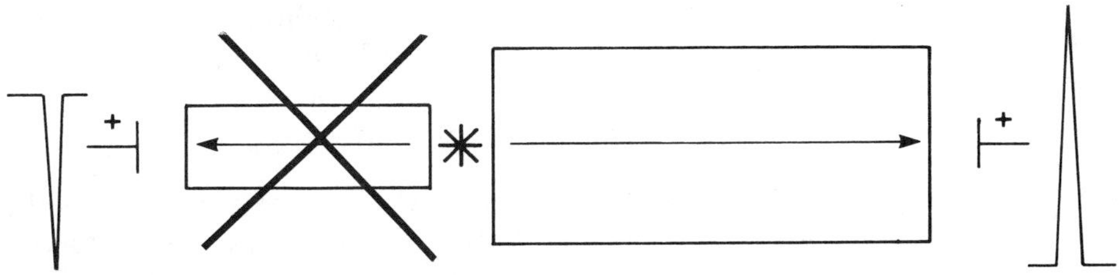

The electrode positioned by the large piece of muscle will see the greater wave coming toward it, and produce a large upward deflection. But the electrode positioned by the smaller piece of muscle will probably not perceive the lesser amount of electrical activity moving toward it at all. The much greater amount of activity in the large muscle strip overshadows the lesser activity in the small strip and cancels it out. Thus, the electrode near the small strip will only see the large amount of activity moving away from it and produce a negative deflection.

If you apply this concept of cancellation to what you have learned about the anatomy of the heart, you will see an analogy between the small and large strips of muscle, and the right and left ventricles. The electrical activity generated by the thin-walled right ventricle is normally cancelled out by the huge amount of activity in the thick-walled left ventricle. Therefore, the QRS complex that is produced by the wave of depolarization moving through the ventricles is generated primarily by the left ventricular activity. Right ventricular activity will be seen only if the right ventricle hypertrophies to the point where its size is equal to, or greater than, the muscle mass of the left ventricle. Right ventricular activity may also be seen if the right ventricle is activated after the left ventricle, so that the wave through the right ventricle is

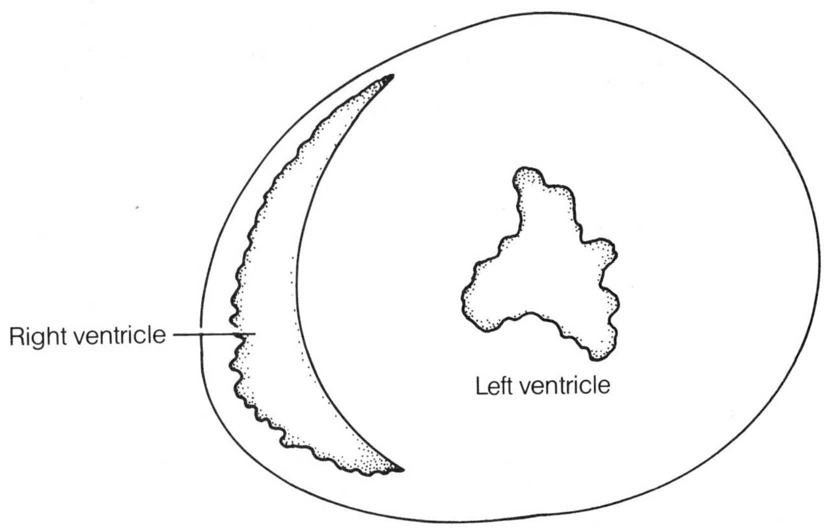

unopposed by left ventricular forces, an occurrence commonly seen in right bundle branch block.

THE GENESIS OF THE PQRST

Now, let's apply what we have just learned about the wave of depolarization and the deflections produced to the electrical activity of one cardiac cycle. As you have seen, the SDC or action potential is the waveform produced by the electrical activity of one cell. But, the waveform produced when all the cells in the heart are activated is called the PQRST.

The Wave Through the Heart

As a brief review, the wave of depolarization begins with the spontaneous depolarization of the SA node. The stimulus is conducted by a propagated wave through the intra-atrial tracts, which deliver the impulse to the atrial muscle and the AV node. The AV node delays the impulse, then conducts it rapidly through the His bundle, the bundle branches, and the Purkinje fibers. Next, the wave of depolarization activates the ventricular myocardium from the endocardial surface where the Purkinje fibers are located, outward toward the epicardial surface. The wave of repolarization follows the same path as depolarization, and the cardiac cycle is complete. Surface electrodes, watching this electrical activity originating in the heart, see the waves of depolarization and repolarization as the PQRST complex.

PQRST Production

SA node activity is not picked up by the surface ECG because it is a tiny piece of tissue that generates a very small electrical current as it automatically depolarizes. As the wave travels through the intra-atrial tracts, again too little activity is generated to be picked up on the ECG. However, you know that the SA node and intra-atrial depolarization has occurred when you see the appearance of the rounded shape of the

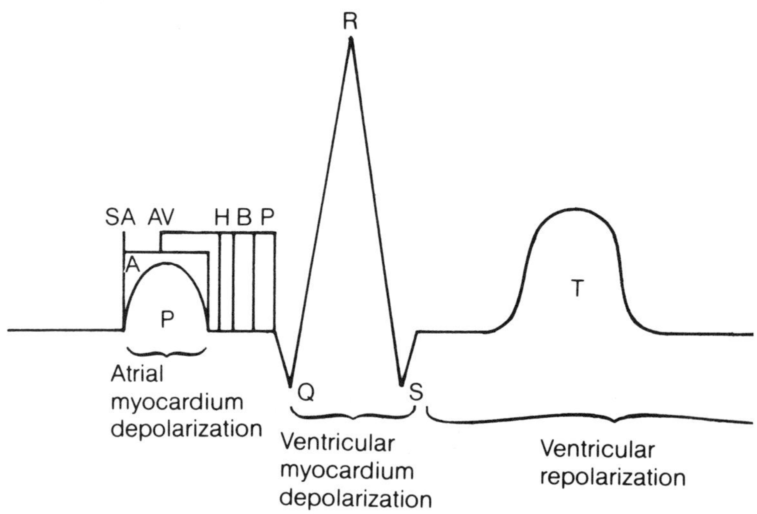

P wave, which is produced by the wave being delivered to and activating the atrial muscle. The wave of depolarization reaches the AV node about mid-way through atrial depolarization. It is delayed in the AV node, and then very rapidly transmitted through the His bundle, bundle branches, and the Purkinje fibers. Since the electrical activity generated in the ventricular conduction system is small, it is not seen as a waveform, but it does produce a time delay between the P wave and the QRS complex that is known as the PR segment. As soon as the impulse reaches the ventricular myocardium, the QRS complex begins. As the last of the ventricular muscle depolarizes, the QRS complex ends. Ventricular activation corresponds to Phases 0 and 1 of the action potential

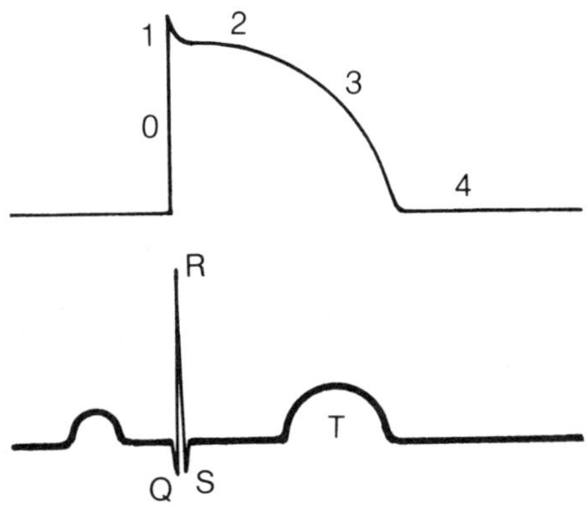

curve. Phase 2, the absolute refractory period, corresponds to the ST segment between the QRS and the T wave. Phases 3 and 4, the repolarization of the ventricular muscle, corresponds to the T wave of the surface ECG.

The wave of depolarization stimulates the ventricles in a very specific pattern. The first part of the ventricular myocardium to be activated is the intraventricular septum, which is stimulated by the left bundle branch. The impulse can move more quickly down the left bundle branch than the right because it is a shorter, thicker fiber that gives less resistance to the flow of current. The impulse then spreads down

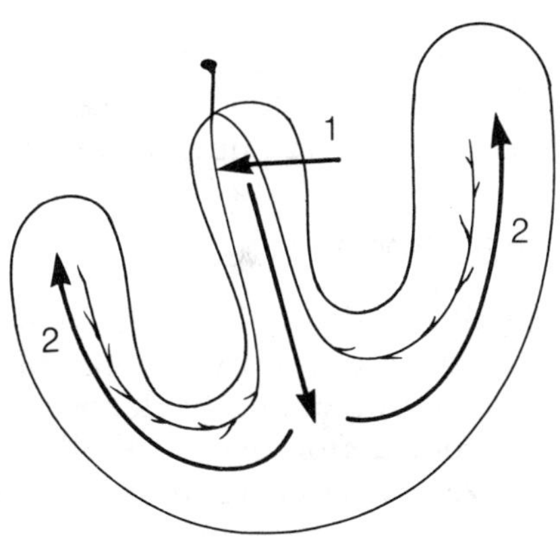

1. Septal depolarization
2. Ventricular activation

the septum and stimulates both right and left ventricles from the apex to the base, and from the endocardium to the epicardium.

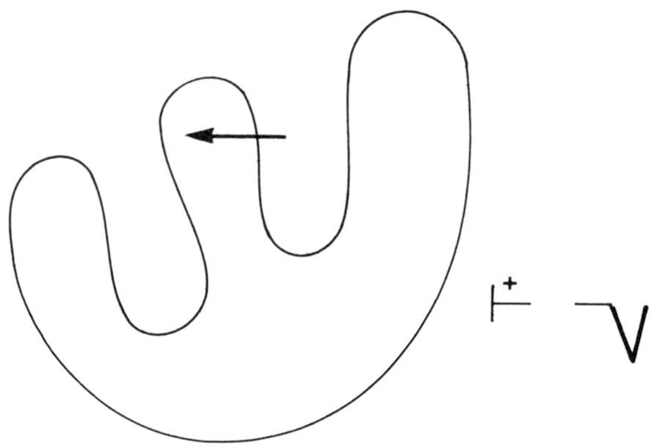

A positive electrode positioned to the left of the heart will see the initial wave of septal activation moving from left to right away from it, and will record a downward deflection that will be small in amplitude since only a small amount of tissue is being activated.

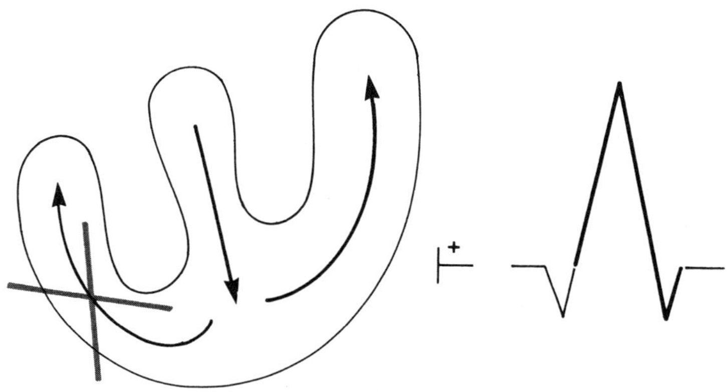

The wave of depolarization then moves simultaneously through the right and left ventricles. However, right ventricular forces are cancelled out, so only left ventricular activation is seen by the electrode, which writes a large upward deflection as the wave comes toward it.

THE ELECTROCARDIOGRAM

The ECG is basically just a graphic representation of the ebb and flow of currents produced by depolarization and repolarization of the heart. It is a recording of purely electrical activity that can tell nothing of the force of contraction that normally follows. As the heart depolarizes and repolarizes, weak currents spread throughout the body and are picked up by silver electrodes on the skin and transmitted to the ECG machine.

The ECG machine amplifies these waves over 1,000 times, and records them as deflections on a graph.

To have a graph, you must compare two different types of information; the ECG is no exception. The two things being compared by the ECG are the timing of the events in one cardiac cycle and the amount of voltage being produced. The voltage is shown on the vertical axis of the graph and the timing is measured on the horizontal axis. ECG paper

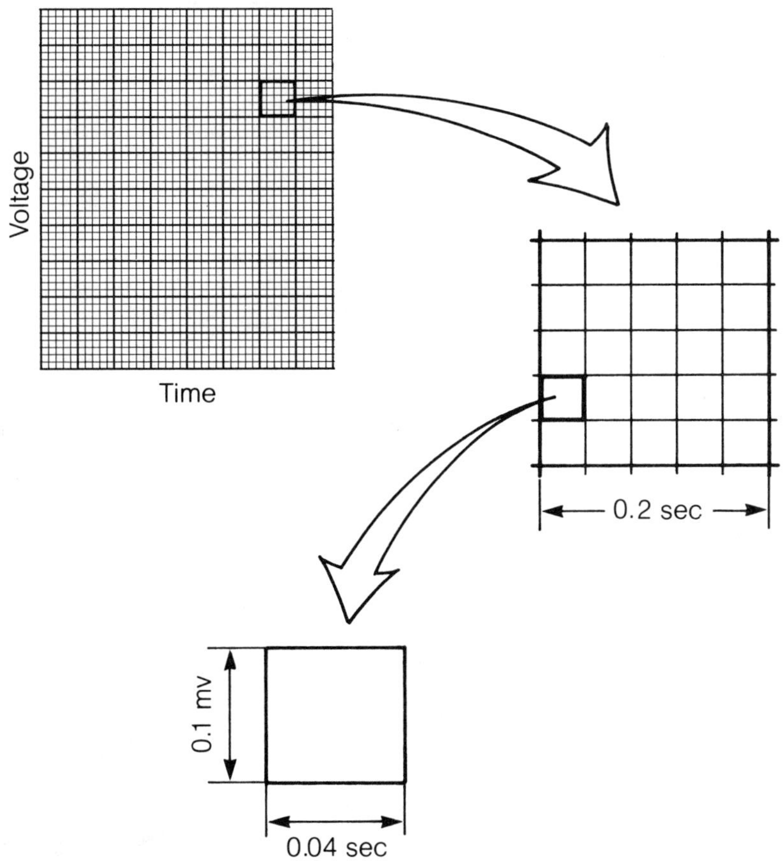

is comprised of small, 1-mm squares, with darker lines forming 5-mm squares. Basically, the paper is made with a dark background that is coated with a lighter waxy substance. The deflections are recorded by a thin stylus that is heated so that it melts the light waxy coating, thus leaving a dark line on the paper. The paper is moving under the stylus at a predetermined rate of 25 mm per second.

The 1-mm squares on the horizontal axis are measuring the time it takes to complete a cardiac cycle. Since the paper is moving at 25 mm per second, it will take the stylus 0.04 second to move across one small, 1-mm square, or 0.2 second to move across one large, 5-mm square.

The 1-mm squares on the vertical axis are measuring the voltage produced by the electrical activation of the heart. Each 1-mm square represents 0.1 millivolt (mv) of current being generated; 10-mm or two large 5-mm blocks represents 1 mv. Most ECG machines have a button labeled either "standardize," "calibrate," or "1 mv." Pushing this button will put a premeasured 1-mv current into the machine, and should cause a square 10-mm deflection if the machine is correctly calibrated. If the calibration is not accurate, interpretation of a standard 12-lead ECG run on that machine could be incorrect. Many machines also have control knobs that can alter the standardization. If the patient's PQRST complexes are too small to be easily seen, as in chronic obstructive pulmonary disease (COPD), the control can be placed at the double standard position, and when the 1-mv button is pushed, a 20-mm deflection should result. This will magnify all waveforms to twice their normal size. Some patients will have PQRST complexes that are too large to fit on the paper, as in ventricular hypertrophy, so the standard control can be turned to the one-half standard position. In this instance, a 1-mv current will produce a 5-mm deflection and shrink the complexes to one-half of their normal size, allowing them to fit on the paper. It is most important that the calibration marker is displayed for each of the 12 leads run, so that the physician reading the tracing knows which standard is used for each lead, and misinterpretation can thus be prevented.

Although the correct voltage is important in 12-lead ECG interpretation, the timing of cardiac events is the most important parameter in dysrhythmia interpretation.

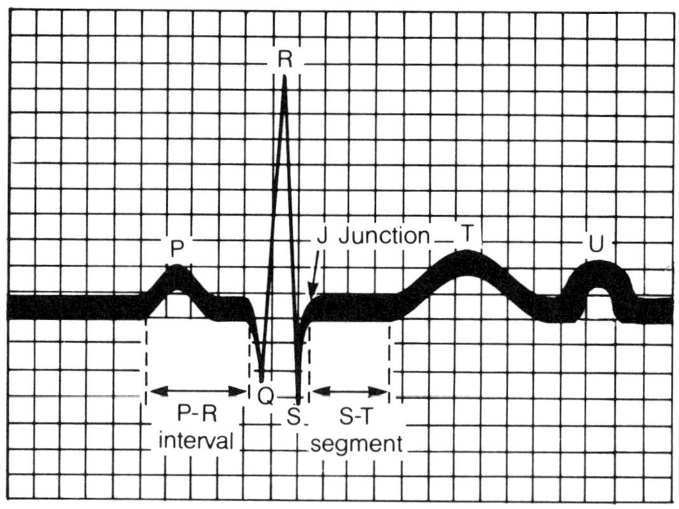

THE NORMAL COMPLEX

Although the shape of the normal PQRST will change from lead to lead and from person to person, normal parameters have been set for each of these waveforms. The range of measurements have been determined by combining the known conduction velocity in different areas of the heart with the amount of tissue to be depolarized.

The P Wave

The P Wave is produced by SA node firing and the resulting depolarization of the atrial myocardium. Although it can differ in shape, it should be no wider than 0.11 second or 2¾ small squares in duration. It is measured from the point that the rounded deflection first leaves the isoelectric line, to the place it returns to the baseline.

The PR Interval

The measurement of the PR interval includes all deflections from the start of the P wave to the initial deflection of the QRS complex. The PR interval measures the time it takes for the SA node to fire, atrial depolarization, AV node delay, and conduction through the His bundle, bundle branches, and Purkinje fibers. Normally, the PR interval should be no shorter than 0.12 second or three small squares, and no longer than 0.20 second or five small squares in duration. The PR interval may well be shorter or longer than the normal parameters, but if it is, a dysrhythmia is present. Because the PR interval represents the activation of virtually the whole conduction system, from SA node to Purkinje fibers, it is an important parameter to consider when interpreting dysrhythmias.

The QRS Complex

The QRS complex is formed by depolarization of the ventricular muscle. It will normally be no less than 0.06 second or 1½ small squares, and no wider than 0.12 second or three small squares in duration. Some references give the upper limit as 0.10 second, with a gray area between 0.10 and 0.12 second that may or may not be normal. This must, by necessity, call for a value judgment. To simplify matters we will use 0.12 second as top normal for our purposes.

The labeling of the waveforms in the QRS complex can be complicated, but if you remember the definition for each wave, it will be easier to understand. The Q wave is defined as the first negative deflection after the P wave. The R wave is the first *positive* deflection after the P wave. The S wave is the first negative deflection after the *R wave.* As you are well aware, not all QRSs look alike; they don't necessarily have all three waves present, and not all the waves are the same size. A quick exercise in naming these waves will be beneficial. One important point to remember is that big waves are denoted by capital letters, and small waves by lower-case letters.

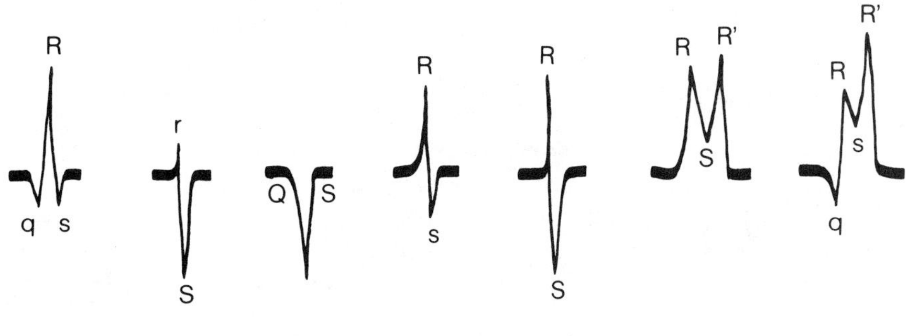

The QRS duration is measured from the start of the initial deflection off the isoelectric line, where you stopped measuring the PR interval, to the point where the S wave stops and the ST segment begins. The point where you stop measuring the QRS complex is termed the J Junction (see diagram on p. 44).

The ST Segment

The ST segment begins at the J junction and ends at the start of the T wave. The ST segment should run right along the isoelectric line. Finding the J junction is usually not a problem when the ST segment is isoelectric. But, unfortunately, a person with cardiac disease will have ST segments that are either depressed because of drugs or ischemia, or elevated because of injury to the myocardium. When the ST segment is displaced, so is the J junction, and measurement of the QRS duration may well become difficult. The ST segment corresponds to the absolute refractory period of the ventricular muscle.

The T Wave

The T wave represents the repolarization currents of the ventricles. The atrium must also repolarize, so there is a T wave for the P wave as well; however, the atrial T wave (T_p) is occurring during ventricular depolarization, so the wave is usually masked by the QRS complex.

The ventricular T wave is usually an upward rounded deflection in most leads. The upslope of the T wave is likely to still be a part of the absolute refractory period. The peak of the T wave is known as the vulnerable period of the cardiac cycle. The ventricular myocardium is at its most unstable point, and if a stray impulse should occur at this time, repetitive or chaotic firing of the ventricles could result, and produce ventricular tachycardia or fibrillation. A stray impulse appearing at this point in the cardiac cycle is known as the R on T phenomenon. The downslope of the T wave corresponds to the partial refractory period.

The U Wave

Sometimes there is another waveform after the T wave that is known as the U wave. The exact electrical activity that produces U waves is not known. There are theories that propose the origin of the U wave as after potentials from the papillary muscles, or perhaps the Purkinje fibers, but nothing has been proven. U waves will commonly be seen in the presence of a bradycardia, hyperkalemia, or ventricular hypertrophy.

THE 12-LEAD ELECTROCARDIOGRAM

The usual method of recording the electrical activity of the heart is the 12-lead ECG. The standard ECG looks at the depolarization and repolarization of the myocardium from 12 slightly different angles.

The standard 12-lead ECG is taken by applying five silver electrodes to the body's surface. Four of these are limb electrodes placed one on each extremity. One floating electrode is called the chest or precordial electrode, and is moved from place to place on the chest wall. The ECG is taken from different combinations of these five electrodes.

The first ECG machine was developed in the early 1900s by Einthoven, who used a string galvanometer to record the electrical activity of the heart. The subject sat with his extremities in buckets of electrolyte solution, and recordings were made of the difference in potentials between pairs of buckets. The leads that were used are what are known today as limb leads I, II, and III.

The Limb Leads

The first six leads of a 12-lead ECG are the limb leads I, II, III, aVr, aVl, and aVf. They are taken from combinations of electrodes placed on the right arm (RA), left arm (LA), right leg (RL), and left leg (LL). The active electrodes that provide the information on cardiac electrical activity are the RA, LA, and LL. The RL electrode is a ground or reference electrode that does not play a part in providing information. Every time you breathe, blink, swallow, and so forth, skeletal or smooth muscle is depolarizing. This produces electrical activity that is picked up by the electrodes, and would obscure the activity generated by cardiac muscle. However, the RL electrode carries away these unwanted muscle potentials so that only the activity of the heart is seen and recorded.

Limb leads I, II, and III are different from any of the other nine leads in that they are bipolar. This means that they are looking at the difference in potentials between two of the three active electrodes, one of which is positive, the other negative. Lead I is looking at the activity of the heart between the RA and LA electrodes. Lead II is looking from the RA to the LL electrodes. Lead III is looking from the LA to the LL. In lead I, the RA is negative and the LA is positive. In lead II, the RA is negative and the LL is positive. In lead III, the LA is negative and the LL is positive. These first three leads have been diagrammed as Einthoven's Triangle.

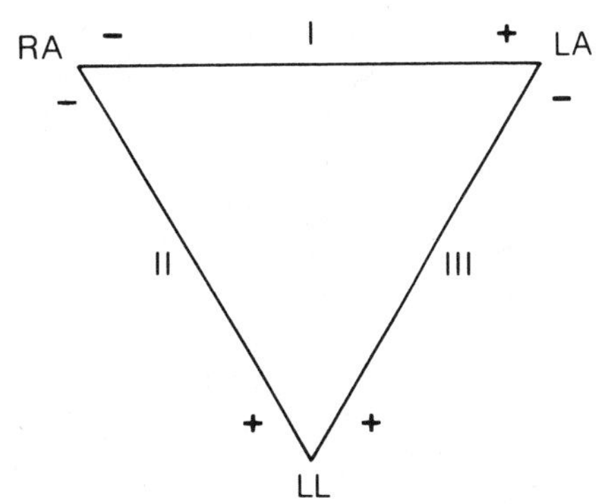

When you are running a tracing of these leads, you merely turn the lead selector dial on the ECG machine to the positions for each lead. The machine turns on the active electrodes for each lead and provides the appropriate polarity as well.

The last three limb leads are the augmented leads aVr, aVl, and aVf. They differ from the first three leads because they are unipolar rather than bipolar. This simply means that there is only one active electrode, and it is positive. The machine actually takes the other two active electrodes, makes them both negative, and sums them up against the one positive electrode, but it may be simpler to consider these leads to have only one positive electrode active. aVr is a single positive electrode at the RA. aVl is a single positive electrode at the LA. aVf is a single positive electrode at the LL or foot.

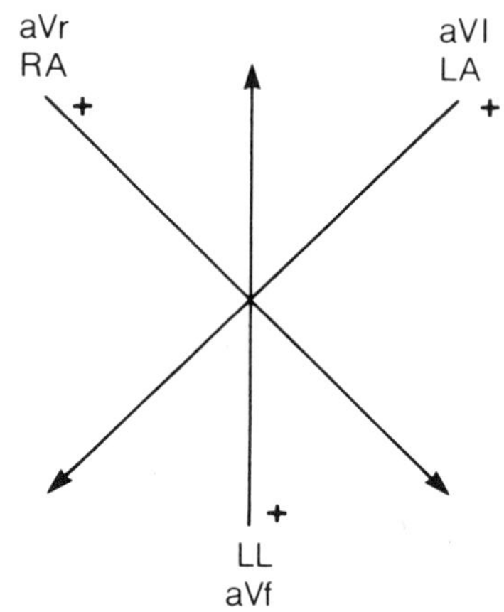

The limb leads are frontal leads that are looking at the activity of the heart on a two-dimensional plane, right and left, and up and down.

The Precordial Leads

The last six leads of the 12-lead ECG are the V leads 1 through 6. They are also called the chest or precordial leads. The V leads are looking at the heart on a sagittal plane, rather than the frontal plane of the limb leads. They view the electrical activity in a cross-section through the chest, from right to left, and from front to back. The V Leads are unipolar in that a single positive electrode is moved to different positions on the chest wall. The machine makes all three active limb electrodes negative, and sums them up against the single positive chest electrode. There are six definite positions on the chest where the positive floating electrode is to be placed.

V_1 is at the fourth intercostal space at the right sternal border.
V_2 is at the fourth intercostal space at the left sternal border.
V_3 is placed mid-way between V_2 and V_4.
V_4 is at the fifth intercostal space on the midclavicular line.
V_5 is on the plane of V_4 at the anterior axillary line.
V_6 is on the plane of V_4 and V_5 at the midaxillary line.

There are three more left chest leads, V_7, V_8, and V_9, but they are not part of the standard 12-lead ECG. V_7 remains in a line with V_{4-6} at

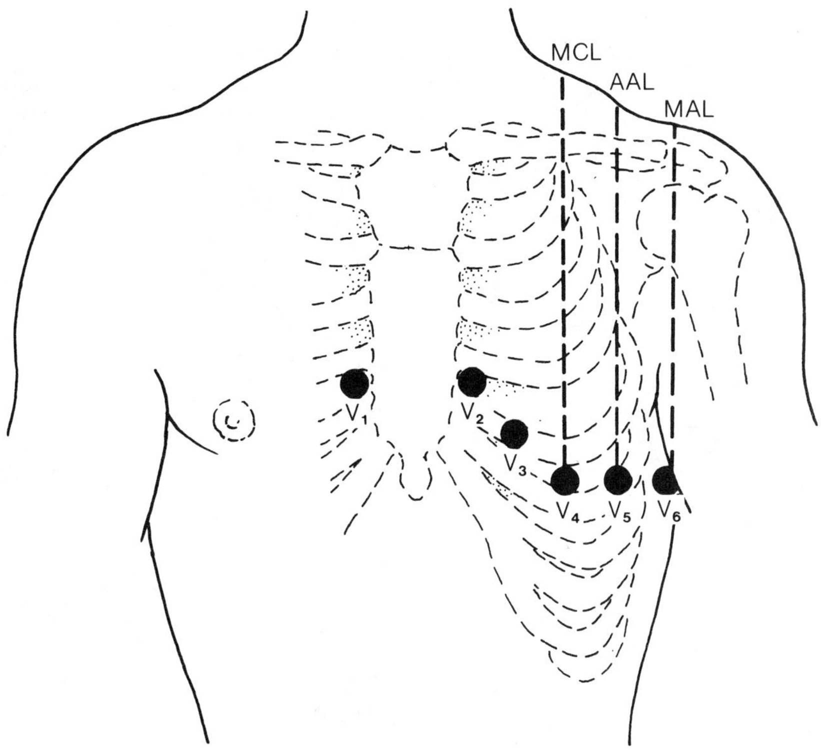

the posterior axillary line. V_8 is at the midscapular line in a line with V_7. V_9 is in the same plane at the left vertebral border. There are also nine more V leads as well. They are positioned at the same anatomic landmarks as the left precordial leads, but they run to the right of the chest instead. They are numbered V_1, V_2, V_{3R}, V_{4R}, V_{5R}, V_{6R}, V_{7R}, V_{8R}, and V_{9R}.

These 12 leads are looking at the heart from different angles; each lead views the surfaces of the heart differently than the others. Limb leads II, III, and aVf see the inferior or diaphragmatic surfaces the best.

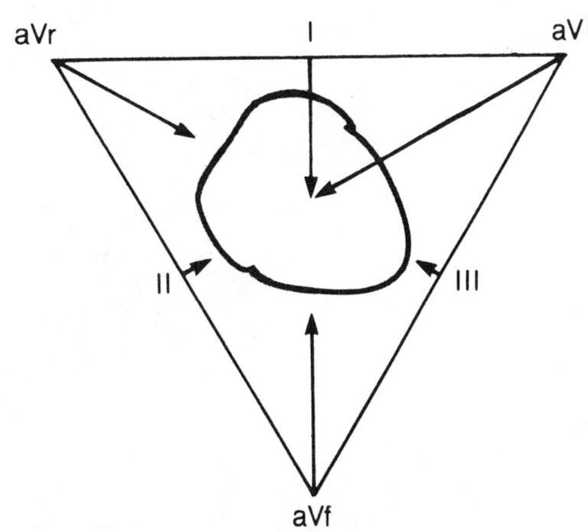

I and aVl look at the lateral surface. aVr sees only the base of the heart, which is mainly the atria and the great vessels.

The V leads ring the heart, looking at the anterior surface. V_1 through V_3 are positioned over the intraventricular septum. V_4 through V_6 are over the lateral surface. V_7 through V_9 are looking at the posterior surface.

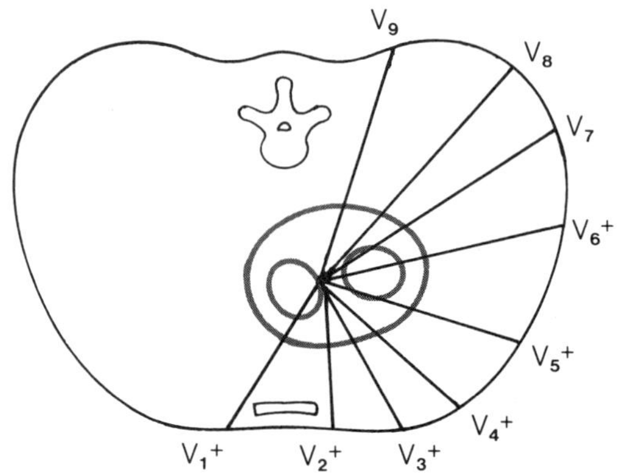

THE NORMAL 12-LEAD ELECTROCARDIOGRAPHIC DEFLECTIONS

Since each of the 12 leads are looking at the heart at a slightly different angle, even though the electrical activity remains unchanged, the deflections produced will vary from lead to lead. Let's take a look at what the normal deflection should be in each lead. Remember, if the wave of depolarization is heading toward the positive electrode, the deflection will be upward. Also, the direction of the wave of depolarization through the heart is normally oriented downward and to the left.

Lead I is looking from the RA to the LA, with the positive electrode

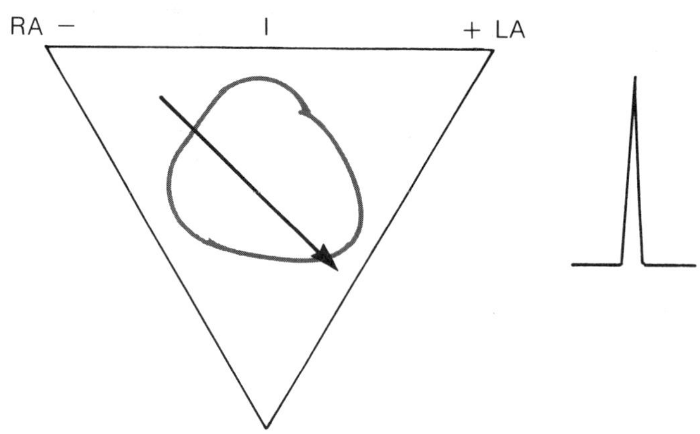

at the LA. The wave of depolarization is directed downward and to the left, toward the positive and away from the negative poles of lead I, so the QRS will have a positive or upward deflection.

Lead II is looking from the RA to the LL, with the positive electrode on the LL. The wave of depolarization heads directly toward the

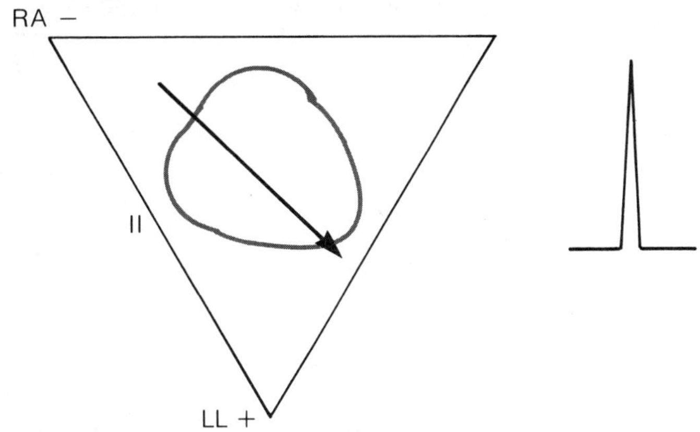

LL electrode, so the deflection in Lead II will also be upward.

Lead III is looking from the LA to the LL, the LL being positive. The wave is again directed toward the positive LL electrode, so the

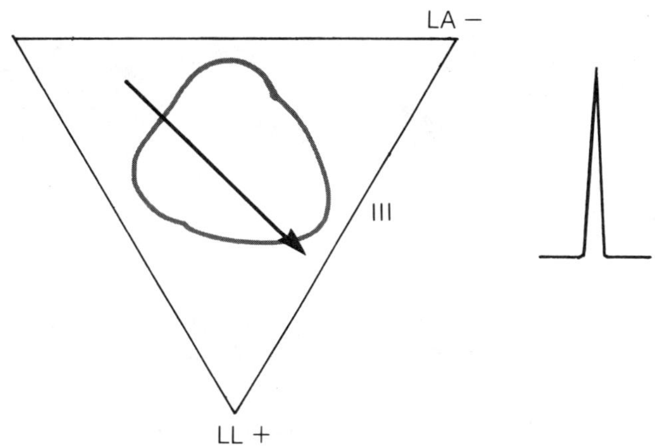

QRS continues to have an upward deflection.

aVr is a single positive electrode on the RA. The wave is moving

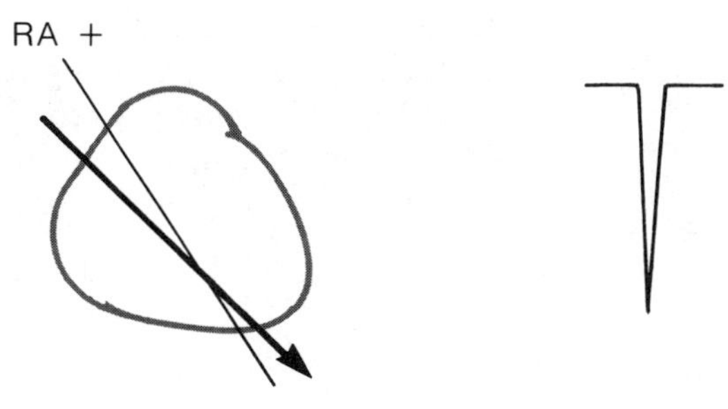

directly away from aVr, so the QRS deflection will normally be downward or negative in direction as will the P and T waves.

aVl is a single positive electrode at the LA. The wave first approaches the line of aVl, and then recedes away from it. This produces

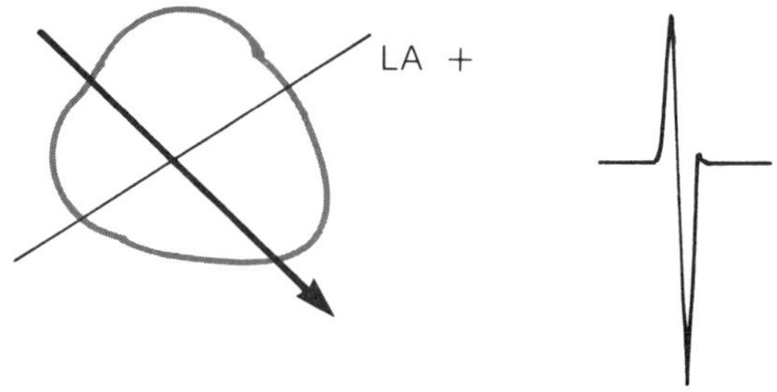

a biphasic deflection, first upward as the wave moves toward aVl and then downward as it moves away.

aVf is a single positive electrode position at the LL. The wave is

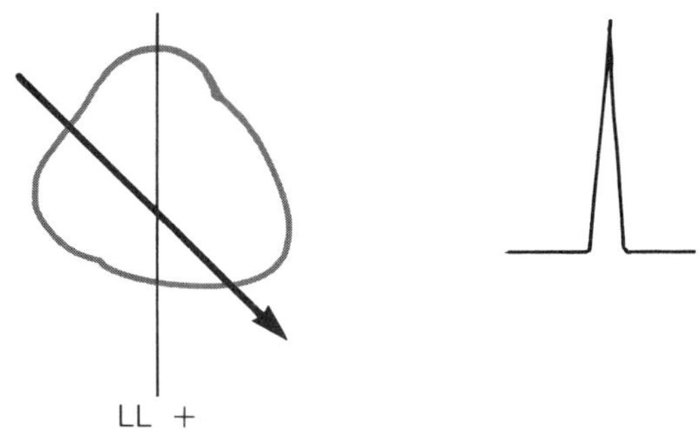

directed toward aVl so the QRS deflection will be upward.

The deflections in the precordial leads change as the electrode moves from right to left around the chest wall. Since the V leads are single positive electrodes looking at the heart in the sagittal plane, the way the deflections are produced is slightly different. Remember, the first part of the ventricles to depolarize is the intraventricular septum, from left to right, and then the wave moves down the septum to both ventricles, but only left ventricular forces are seen.

V_1 and V_2 will have similar appearances because they are positioned close together. They see the initial wave through the septum, from left to right, coming toward them, and produce a small positive deflection or r wave. Then the wave proceeds through the left ventricle, away from them, producing a deep negative S wave. V_1 and V_2 will normally have mainly negative QRS complexes.

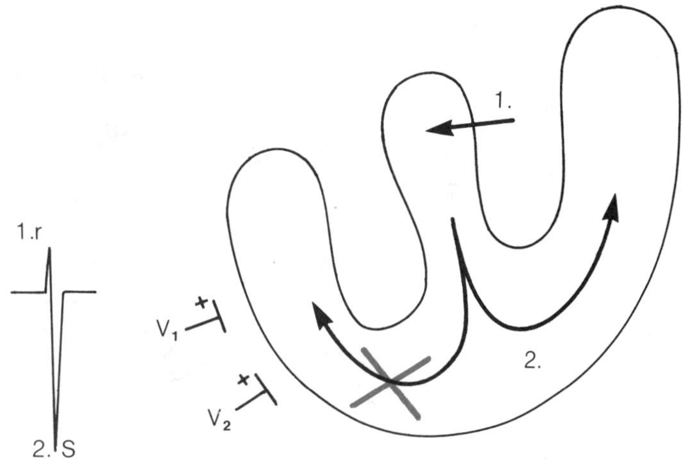

V_3 and V_4 also may be similar in configuration. Because of their location, they don't see the initial septal wave from left to right, but they do see the wave as it comes down the septum straight toward

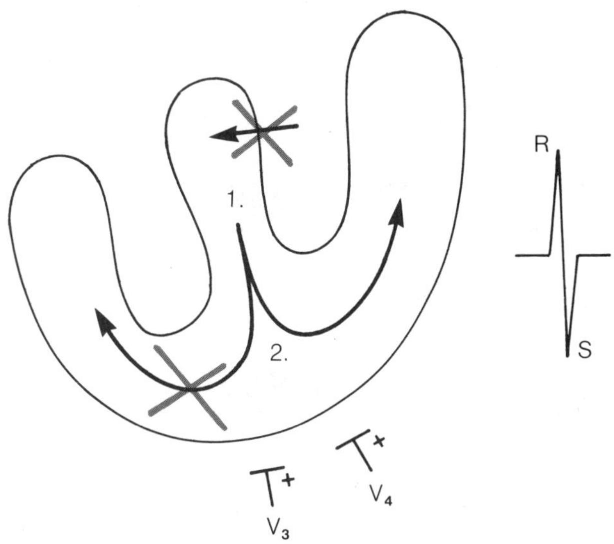

them, which produces a large positive R wave. Then the wave moves up through the left ventricular wall, away from V_3 and V_4, producing a deep negative S wave. Thus, V_3 and V_4 will have a biphasic QRS complex, first positive, then negative.

V_5 and V_6 are located laterally, and see the initial wave through the intraventricular septum moving from left to right away from them, and produce a small negative deflection, or q wave. Then the wave

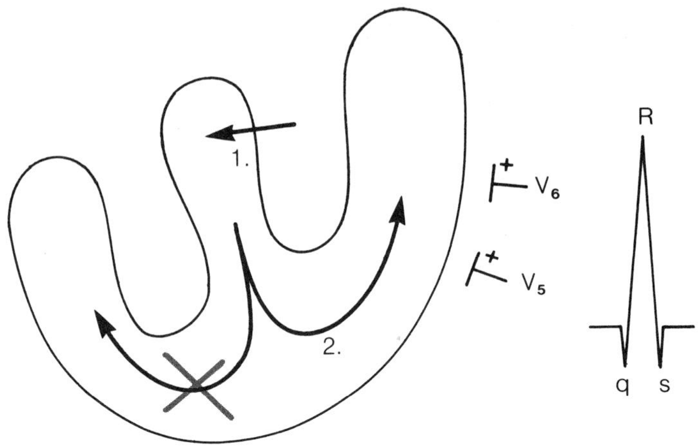

comes down the septum and begins to move toward V_5 and V_6, producing a large positive R wave. V_5 and V_6 will normally have exactly the opposite configuration as V_1 and V_2.

3

MONITORING

Although the knowledge and technique of recording the electrical activity generated by depolarization and repolarization of the heart have been available since early in this century, the ability to constantly monitor a patient was not developed until the late 1960s. Research completed for the space program provided the technology needed to produce a practical method of continuous cardiac monitoring that would be useful in the hospital setting. These developments made the concept of intensive coronary care possible.

Continuous ECG monitoring of any patient, but particularly those with cardiac disease, has prevented many deaths. It has been well documented that lethal cardiac dysrhythmias usually don't appear suddenly, but most always have been preceded by warning dysrhythmias that have occurred as precursors to the catastrophic rhythms. If warning dysrhythmias are recognized and the proper treatment instituted, lethal dysrhythmias don't occur.

The monitors are an important component in the care of cardiac patients, but they are merely a tool providing the information essential for a complete assessment of the patient. It is too easy to forget that there is a patient on the other end of the circuitry. This attitude sometimes leads to the pitfall of treating the monitor and not the patient. It is important to know which dysrhythmia the patient is having, but it is of paramount importance to observe how the patient is responding

Chapter reprinted from Hammond (Hurst), CE: Plain talk about cardiac monitors. *RN Magazine* 42(9):34–43, 1979; with permission.

hemodynamically to that particular dysrhythmia. As long as you can remember that the monitor is just a tool, this pitfall can be avoided, and both you and your patient will benefit.

MONITORING SYSTEMS

The sophisticated monitoring systems used today have really changed very little in basic components and mechanics from the first generation of equipment. Because of technologic improvements in the electronics field, the equipment is now more reliable and has many convenient new features that are useful to the nurse and beneficial for the patient.

The basic components included in a monitoring system consist of electrodes attached to the patient to pick up the ebb and flow of currents produced by the heart's electrical activity, wires and cables to transmit these electrical impulses to the monitor, and the monitor itself, which amplifies the small currents and displays them as waveforms on an oscilloscope (Fig. 3-1). The monitors have features such as rate meters, alarm systems, and recorders to provide a permanent copy of the patient's rhythm for studying or charting. Although different manufacturers' monitoring systems vary in display, styling, and controls, they all have the basic components of electrodes, cables, and monitors with oscilloscope, rate meter, and alarm systems.

ELECTRODE SYSTEMS

The monitoring equipment found in critical care units may be designed as two-, three-, or five-electrode systems, depending on how many electrodes are to be placed on the patient's chest. All of these systems are able to display the different leads of a 12-lead ECG. The method of obtaining different monitoring leads depends on the electrode system in use.

Two Electrodes

The two-electrode system is usually seen in telemetry monitors. Two electrodes, one positive and one negative, are placed on the patient's chest. The indifferent or reference electrode is built into the circuitry of the monitoring system. The different monitoring leads are obtained by changing the placement of the electrodes on the chest wall.

Three Electrodes

The three-electrode system is probably the most common type seen since it is less costly than the other two types. Three electrodes are placed on the patient's chest, one positive, one negative, and one ground or reference. Some of these three-electrode systems are set up in a lead-I configuration (RA−, LA+, and RL ground), some in a lead-II configuration (RA−, LL+, and RL ground), and some in a lead-III configuration (LA−, LL+, and RL ground), depending on the manufacturer. Again, the different monitoring leads are obtained by moving the electrodes to the appropriate positions on the chest wall. There are some three-electrode systems that have RA, LA, and LL electrodes on the chest and a lead selector switch on the monitor that allows display of limb leads I, II, and II by turning the dial to the appropriate position. The circuitry in the monitor changes the polarity of the electrodes to correspond to the lead chosen.

Five Electrodes

The five-electrode system is the most versatile, but it is also the most expensive. Four electrodes are placed on the chest in the RA, LA, RL, and LL positions, and any limb lead can be monitored by merely turning the lead selector switch on the monitor. A fifth electrode can be placed in any of the precordial lead positions, V_1 through V_6, and the lead selector switch is set at the V position.

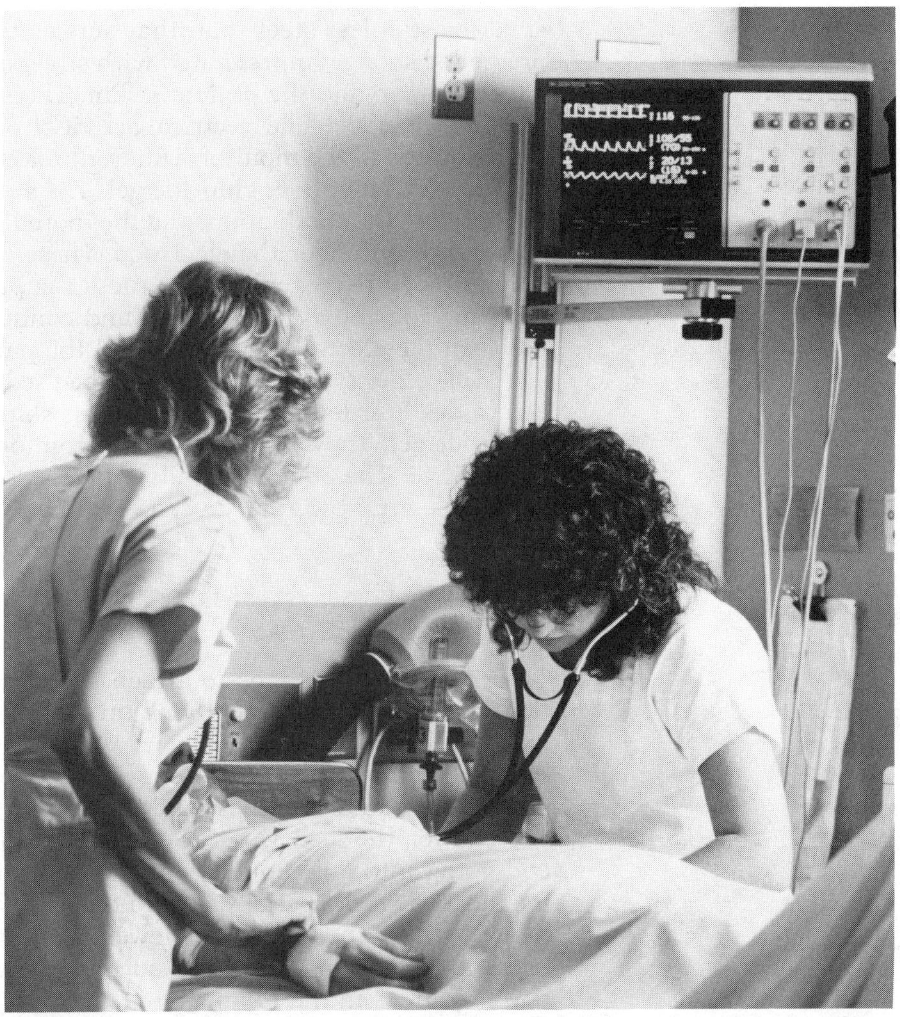

Figure 3-1 Monitoring systems are frequently in place at the patient's bedside. (Courtesy of Hewlett-Packard)

ELECTRODES

Basically, there are two types of electrodes, the silver plate and the floating disc. The silver plate electrode is the type used on the extremities when running a 12-lead ECG. A variation of this type of electrode is available for placement on the chest wall for continuous ECG monitoring. Use of this electrode requires the application of a conductive jelly between the patient's skin and the silver plate. If the chest electrode is used, it must be taped to the patient's skin. There are two disadvantages in the use of these electrodes. (1) The jelly can dry out, causing a loss of conduction from the patient with the resulting poor trace on the monitor. (2) The electrode must be taped, which can cause skin irritation and a loss of stability of the plate on the skin.

The floating disc electrode is the type most commonly used today. These electrodes are commercially available from many different manufacturers as a prepackaged, disposable product. These electrodes consist of a self-adhering foam, paper, or fabric disc that surrounds a silver or stainless steel snap that acts as the disc electrode. There is a pre-gelled sponge impregnated with silver chloride gel that is in contact with the snap and the patient's skin. The silver chloride gel is the medium that conducts the electrical activity from the patient's heart through the electrode to the monitor. Different manufacturers will vary the concentration of the silver chloride gel. The stronger the gel concentration, the better is the conduction, and the more likely the patient will develop skin irritation under the electrode. These self-adhering electrodes may stay in place for several days unless the patient is extremely diaphoretic, and the gel will stay moist and conductive if there is a good seal between the electrode adhesive and the patient's skin.

One other type of electrode can be used, the needle electrode. Needle electrodes inserted under the patient's skin and taped in place need no electrode gel. They are extremely uncomfortable and also very difficult to stabilize. The obvious disadvantages of these electrodes are the reasons they are now rarely used; ordinarily they were found on crash carts.

PATIENT CONNECTORS

There are three methods to attach the patient to the monitor: the patient cable or "hard wire" hook up, telemetry monitoring, and quick-look paddles.

Hard wire connections consist of two parts: the lead wires that snap to the skin electrodes; and the patient cable that has terminals at one end for the lead wires to plug into, and a connector on the other end going into a receptacle on the monitor. In most acute care areas the hard wire connection is commonly used, particularly while the patient is still on bed rest. The newer, well-shielded cables prevent electrical artifact from being picked up by induction current from other power sources in the room.

When the patient is past the acute phase and begins ambulating, the hard wire connections become too confining. Many hospitals now have telemetry monitors in their step-down units that allow continuous monitoring and permit ambulation as well. Telemetry monitoring systems consist of patient electrodes attached to a small radio transmitter worn on a belt or halter. The transmitter changes the electrical impulses from the heart into radio waves, and sends these waves to a receiver in the monitor. The monitor converts the radio signal back into the waveforms usually seen on the ECG and displays them on the oscilloscope. The patient can ambulate as much as his physical condition permits, and, as long as he stays within a certain number of feet from an antenna, he can be monitored. These antennas are installed throughout the step-down unit. Telemetry monitoring is also useful in stress testing when the patient is exercising on a treadmill or bicycle. Vigorous movement can put tension on the patient cable and lead wires that will pull the electrode. Any movement of the electrode on the skin produces artifact on the monitor that may obscure the pattern of the patient's ECG tracing. Telemetry is also useful in the operating room because it eliminates the wires from the patient to the monitor.

The quick-look paddles found on many crash carts are the third type of patient connector. In this instance, the defibrillator paddles act as the electrodes, and when placed on the patient's chest they transmit the ECG pattern to the monitor for instant display. These paddles are extremely useful in the "Code Blue" situation, particularly when the patient had not been on a monitor before the arrest situation. The quick-look paddles give instant access to the patient's rhythm without the delay necessary to apply electrodes and hook up to the monitor. The same paddles can also deliver a countershock to the patient if necessary.

THE MONITOR

The final component of any monitoring system is the monitor itself. Monitoring systems in acute care areas generally have small monitors at each patient's bedside that allow observation of the patient's rhythm while the nurse is with the patient. Most intensive care units have a central bank of monitors at the nurse's station to permit constant observation of the rhythms of all the patients in the area at one time. The central monitors usually have a module that can record the trace of any patient. The recorder allows the nurse to obtain hard copy or any dysrhythmia for closer study or for documentation on the patient's chart. Most recorders can be activated manually or they can be triggered automatically when an alarm situation occurs.

Oscilloscope

The monitor is basically an oscilloscope that displays the patient's ECG waveforms as a beam of light. The beam of light is analogous to the stylus on an ECG machine. Older monitoring systems have a display known as a "bouncing ball" trace. In this display, a dot of light moves across the scope, leaving a glowing trace behind it. Unfortunately, this trace fades quickly and only a few complexes are visible at any one time.

The newer monitor models have a type of display known as a "non-fade" trace. In this case, the complex that is being generated by the patient appears on one side of the monitor scope and moves across the screen, followed by each succeeding complex. It appears much as a stylus writing on recording paper. With this type of display, 6 to 10 seconds of a patient's ECG pattern can be clearly observed at one time. Another mode of display in the non-fade trace features a blanking or erasing bar that sweeps across the screen obliterating the old information and putting the new pattern on the scope behind it. This also provides 6 to 10 seconds of trace clearly visible at one time. Many monitors with a non-fade trace have an option called the freeze mode that takes the patient's real-time trace, and freezes it or holds it in place. Some systems will drop the frozen trace to a lower channel while the current information is still being displaced on the patient's channel.

Many monitors have the ability to display information from more than one source, with the addition of two to four channels on each scope. For example, the ECG trace may be displayed on Channel 1, while the pressure waveform from an arterial line occupies Channel 2. Additional parameters that can be monitored include Swan-Ganz pressures, respirations, temperatures, intracranial pressures, cardiac outputs, and others.

Some multichannel monitors have a special feature, known as the cascade mode, which takes the real-time information from the patient's trace and moves it down to the next lower channel, so there will be two or more lines displaying the parameter being monitored.

Controls

Although the appearance of monitoring equipment seems to vary from one manufacturer to another, all systems must have certain basic controls that remain the same because they are essential components (Fig. 3-2). Different systems do vary in the placement and labeling of the different controls. To use your equipment effectively, read the manuals provided by the manufacturer of your own system. The controls basic to any system include the rate meter, gain control, alarm system, and the lead selector switch.

RATE METER The rate meter is a vital part of any monitoring system. It has the obvious function of showing the patient's rate at any point in time, but it also is the heart of the alarm system as well. The constant display of the patient's heart rate is accomplished by a small computer that counts R waves. The rate displayed is really an average of a certain number of beats, so when the rate changes abruptly, the rate meter will lag slightly behind the actual heart rate. The rate display on older models is an analog type of rate meter with needle and rate gauge. Newer models display the rate as a digital readout.

SENSITIVITY CONTROL The sensitivity control is also called the gain control on some equipment. It controls the size of the PQRST complexes, making them larger or smaller as required. The QRS complexes must be a certain size in order to trigger the rate meter or to be sensed by

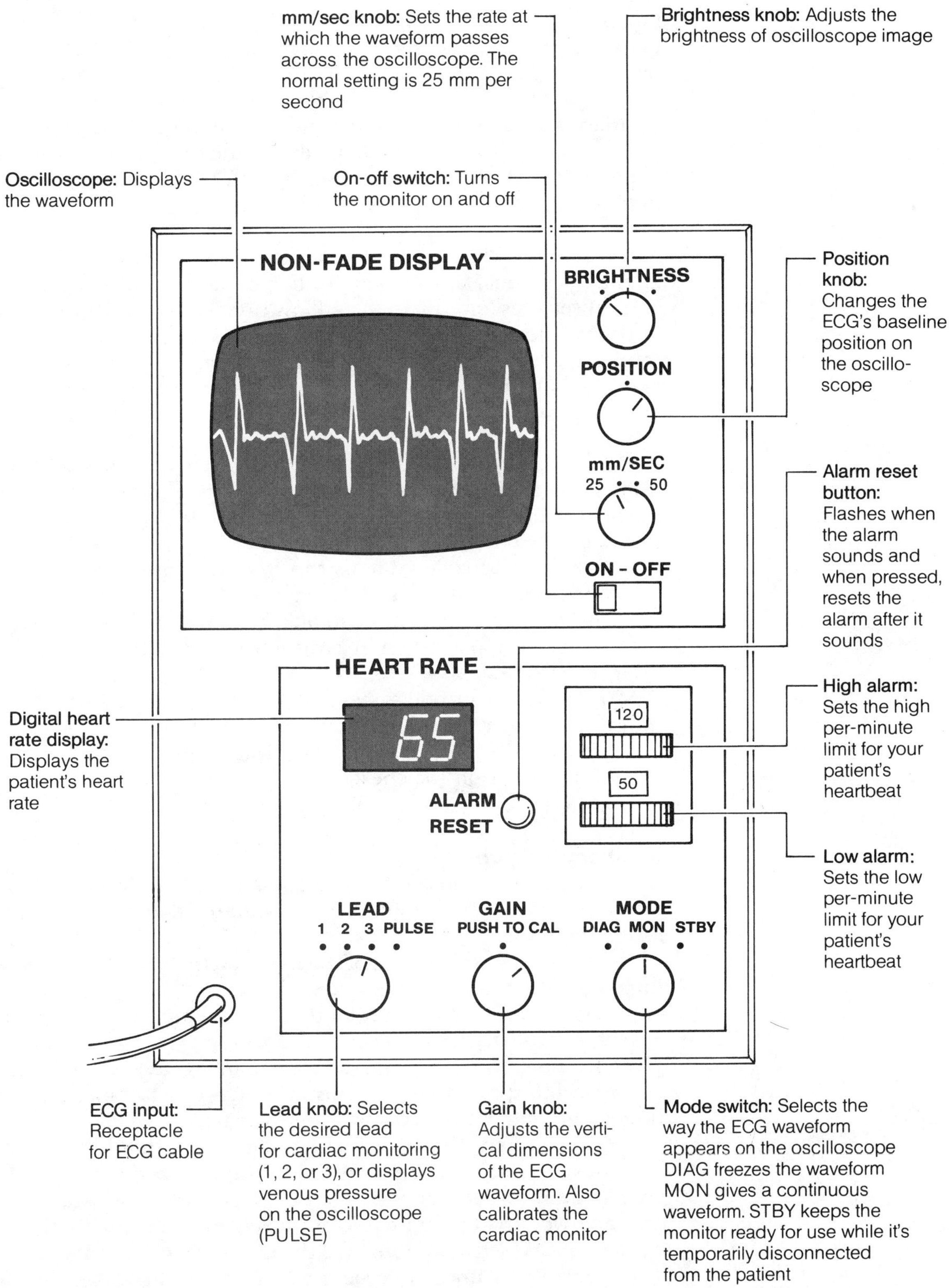

Figure 3-2 Diagram showing major parts of cardiac monitor.

the cardioverter if a countershock is to be delivered. If the R wave is too small, it won't be sensed by the rate meter, so the gain must be increased and the complexes enlarged. If the PQRSTs are too large to be accurately seen on the scope, the gain must be turned down and the complexes reduced in size so that they fit on the oscilloscope, are clearly seen, and are displayed without distortion. The newest generation of monitors has a sensitivity control built into the microprocessor chips that adjusts the gain automatically.

ALARM SYSTEM The alarm system is the heart of the monitor that alerts nursing personnel to a change in the patient's rate. The alarm consists of limit settings for both high and low rates. If the patient's rate exceeds or drops below the preset limits, it triggers an alarm and activates the recorder at the central station. Unfortunately, this type of system will not warn of premature beats or any other dysrhythmia that doesn't alter the rate.

LEAD SELECTOR SWITCH All five-electrode systems and some three-electrode systems have a lead selector switch that allows the nurse to change the lead being monitored without changing the placement of the electrodes on the chest.

The five-electrode systems can monitor any of the six limb leads by merely turning the lead selector switch to the desired lead. Any of the chest or precordial leads can also be monitored by turning the lead selector to the V position and putting the fifth electrode on the appropriate area of the chest wall.

The three-electrode systems with a lead selector switch allow the nurse to monitor limb leads I, II, and III by turning the knob to the appropriate position. However, the electrodes must be in the RA, LA, and LL positions on the chest.

Additional Features

The newest generation of monitors has many additional features that increase the amount of information available and also make life easier for the nurse.

Computers added to monitoring systems can do just about anything you want them to. They can add memory, which allows retrieval of previous dysrhythmic events; they can be programmed to alarm for nearly any dysrhythmia you want; and they can store information to give you the number of premature beats in a given period of time; they can even interpret rhythm strips and give you the measurements for the PR interval, QRS duration, and the rate.

Some systems have a short-term memory that allows reprints of alarm events. Older equipment had a tape-loop memory system that constantly recorded the patient's ECG trace. When an alarm occurred, the tape would stop and could be keyed to print out the information on the tape, which would include the events before the alarm situation. This system was unreliable because of constant mechanical malfunctions. Newer equipment has small computers accomplishing the same function as the tape-loop, but the information is stored electronically. Monitors with non-fade traces automatically have 5 to 10 seconds of information on the scope at any one time. With the addition of the freeze mode and cascade capability, the amount of memory is increased.

A monitoring system may also have a trend recorder that records and displays the patient's ECG for an extended period of time. A computer can do this, but for systems without a computer, trend recording can be obtained with the help of a special recorder that prints out at the rate of 1 mm per second, rather than the normal rate of 25 mm per second. Since the paper is moving slowly, each beat is recorded almost on top of the preceding beat. Abnormal beats and irregular rhythms show up very clearly against the background of the regular rhythm.

MONITORING PROCEDURE

Attaching a monitor can be a frightening procedure to a patient who is already anxious and possibly in pain. Although most people today are aware of monitors and their uses because of the number of medically oriented programs on television, it is difficult to know how many misconceptions the general public has acquired. Some people may think the monitor is like a pacemaker and thus is keeping their heart beating. The cardiac patient really doesn't need anything to increase his anxiety level, so a simple, nontechnical explanation of what is being done and the function of the monitor can be very reassuring to even the most anxious patient.

SKIN PREPARATION

The importance of a good skin prep cannot be emphasized enough!

The first and most important step in hooking a patient to the monitor is a thorough preparation of the skin before applying the electrodes. The areas where the electrodes are to be placed should be thoroughly cleansed with alcohol or acetone to remove any body oils or dirt. If the patient has a heavy growth of body hair at electrode sites, they should be shaved. The skin should be rubbed briskly, with a dry 4×4 or with the special abrasive material that comes on the cap of some electrodes, until the skin is slightly reddened. Skin abrasion removes the dead surface cells that prevent good skin contact with the electrode. The dead cells have a large amount of resistance to the flow of electrical current from patient to electrode. Removing these cells allows a good, clear ECG trace on the monitor (Fig. 3-3).

Many patients are diaphoretic because of pain or fear. Use of a spray antiperspirant or tincture of benzoin under the adhesive material of the electrode will prevent the electrode from falling off. There are also some special diaphoretic electrodes available from certain manufacturers.

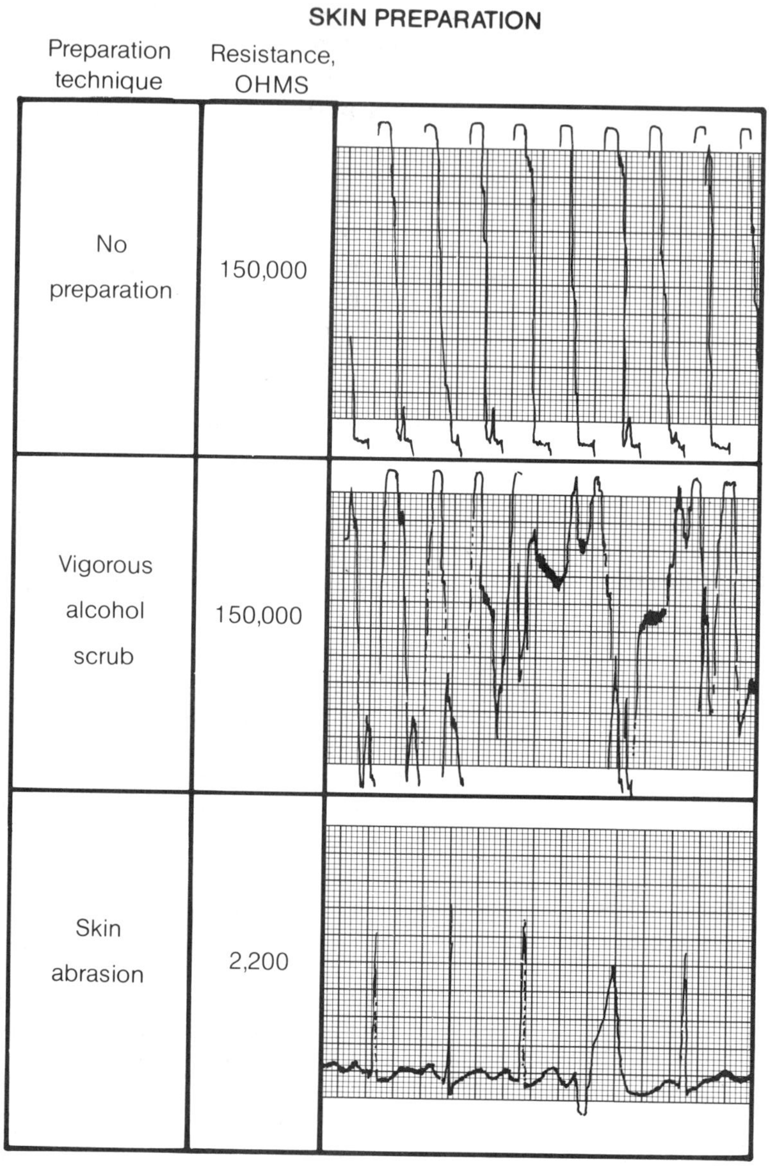

Figure 3-3 Effect of skin preparation on the ECG.

ELECTRODE PLACEMENT

After the skin is adequately prepared, apply the electrodes. The positions of the electrodes will depend on the lead to be monitored and the electrode system of the equipment being used. Electrode positions for different leads and lead systems will be discussed in detail later in this chapter. There are, however, some general considerations of electrode placement that are relevant no matter what lead or system is used.

Positioning the electrode away from large muscle masses is important because it will reduce the amount of artifact produced by skeletal muscle "noise" that interferes with a clear trace on the scope.

The electrodes should also be positioned where they are most stable. The RL and LL electrodes in particular can be in areas that are constantly moving because of inhalation and exhalation. If the patient is breathing normally, with the rib cage moving, the electrodes can be placed on the upper abdomen where they will be more stable. If, on the other hand, the patient is an abdominal breather, these lower electrodes will be more stable if placed on the lower rib cage.

Another factor to consider in electrode placement is mechanical convenience; leave the precordium clear for auscultation, serial 12-lead ECGs, countershock, or cardiopulmonary resuscitation (CPR) if the necessity should arise. Check the electrodes before applying them, to be sure the silver chloride gel is moist, since dried gel is not a good conductor of electrical activity from the patient to the monitor. Some newer electrodes are on the market now that are "dry-gel" electrodes. These are not very moist to the touch as are the older electrodes.

HARD WIRE ATTACHMENT

After the electrodes are in position, attach the lead wire snaps and insert the pins into the patient cable connector. Arrange the lead wires so there is no tension between the cable connector and the electrode. Tension on the lead wires causes movement of the electrode on the chest wall, which produces artifact on the monitor. Putting a stress loop in the lead wire around the electrode can help alleviate this problem. The patient cable connector should be secured to the patient's gown at the shoulder to prevent the lead wires or electrodes from becoming dislodged. Support the patient cable so that it isn't dangling, and position it so it doesn't become entangled in the bed rails or so the patient isn't lying on it.

If these steps are followed, there should be few difficulties in the continuous monitoring of patients.

MONITORING LEADS

When choosing a lead to use for monitoring a patient, there are several principles to consider. First, most units usually have one lead that is routinely used to monitor all patients, but this practice is ill-advised at best. Not all patients will have the best complexes in only one lead, for example lead II. The lead chosen must give you the maximum amount of information from the individual patient being monitored and that might not be lead II. Many things will alter the electrical patterns and make one lead better than another to give the most information. Some things that affect lead selection include axis deviation, abnormal ventricular conduction, chest shape and size, and some medical conditions such as COPD. So, remember that one lead isn't enough for monitoring. Be aware that other monitoring leads are available; know what the other leads are; and know in which situations these other leads are most helpful. The method used to obtain the different monitoring leads changes with different types of monitoring systems. The discussion for electrode placement will show the electrode configuration used for two-electrode, three-electrode, or five-electrode systems.

LEAD II

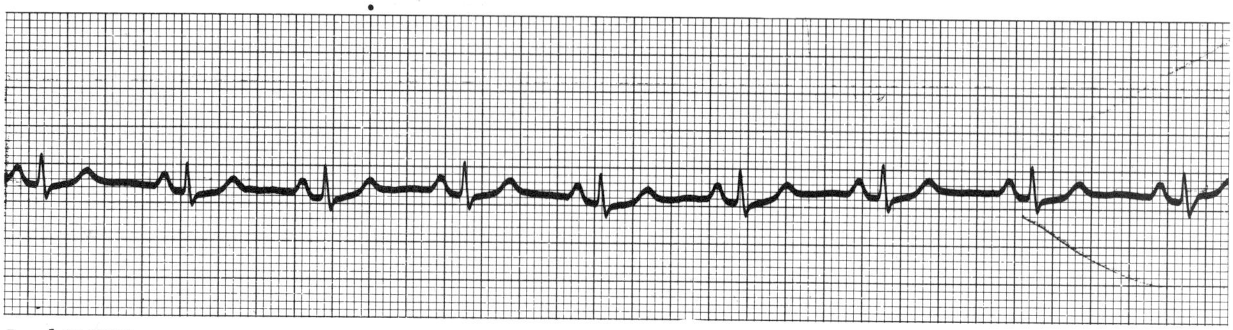

Lead II ECG

Limb lead II has been the traditional lead in use since the advent of continuous monitoring in the intensive care setting. It was used for a number of reasons. The P wave definition in lead II is usually good, with a rounded upright configuration that is easily seen. The P wave made lead II a good one for dysrhythmia interpretation.

Lead II normally has an upright QRS complex, which was important because the rate meters and alarm systems of the first generation of monitors could only be triggered by positive QRS deflections. Newer equipment can count either positive or negative QRS complexes. Lead II is still a good lead to use for dysrhythmia detection and interpretation, but it is limited in the information it supplies on ventricular conduction patterns. It's easy to tell when there is delayed conduction through the ventricles (bundle branch block) because the QRS complex widens. However, in lead II you can't tell if the problem is in the right or left bundle branch.

LEAD II

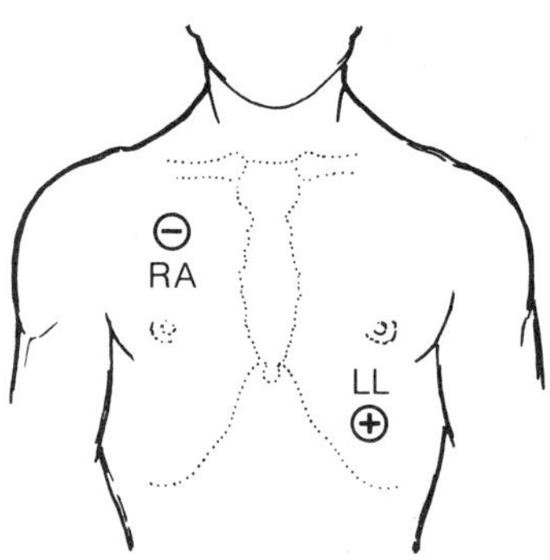

Two lead system

- Place the positive electrode in the LL position.
- Place the negative electrode in the RA position.

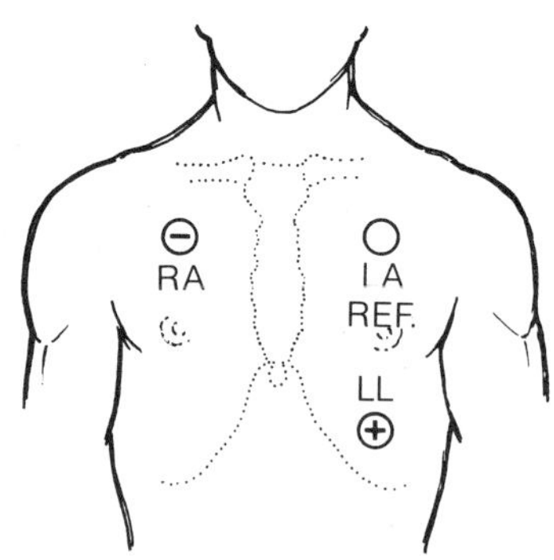

Three lead system

- Place the positive electrode in the LL position.
- Place the negative electrode in the RA position.
- Place the reference electrode anywhere, but in good contact.

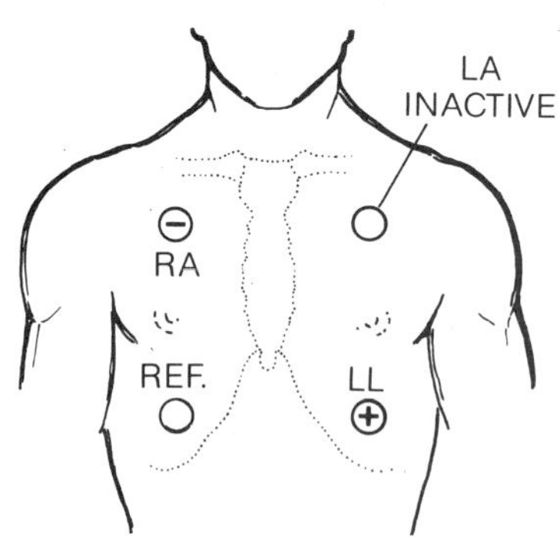

Five lead system

- Place the lead selector switch on Lead II.
- Place all four basic electrodes as indicated.
- The LA electrode is inactive in Lead II.

The electrode placement for lead II depends upon the type of monitoring system being used. However, the position of the positive and negative electrodes doesn't change, no matter what kind of equipment is being used. The positive electrode should be in the LL position, and the negative electrode at the RA position.

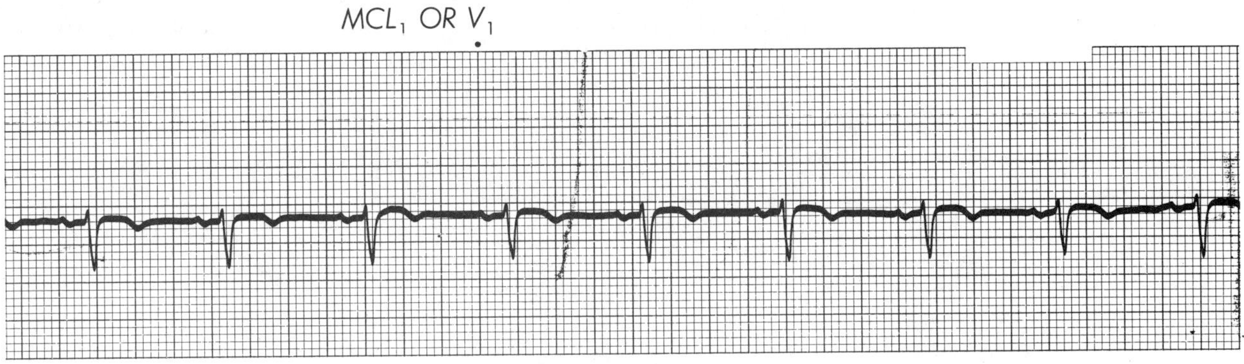

Lead MCL_1 or V_1

This V lead or its modification has now become the best lead to use in continuous monitoring. With a five-electrode system, a true V_1 will be monitored. The two- and three-electrode systems are using the MCL lead instead, but are still providing the same information given by V_1. MCL_1 means Modified Chest Left arm in the V_1 position. This lead is also referred to as the Marriott chest lead, because Dr. Marriott has been instrumental in promoting the use of this lead in units throughout the country.

MCL_1 or V_1 has a well-defined P wave that is easily seen, although its configuration is diphasic. This good P wave definition means that the MCL_1 gives you the information needed to accurately interpret dysrhythmias. The QRS in MCL_1 is usually a negative deflection. This lead gives very specific information about ventricular conduction. It's easy to see that bundle branch block is present when the QRS widens, but in MCL_1, the QRS configuration also tells whether it is right or left bundle branch block. The QRS configuration in MCL_1 can also help

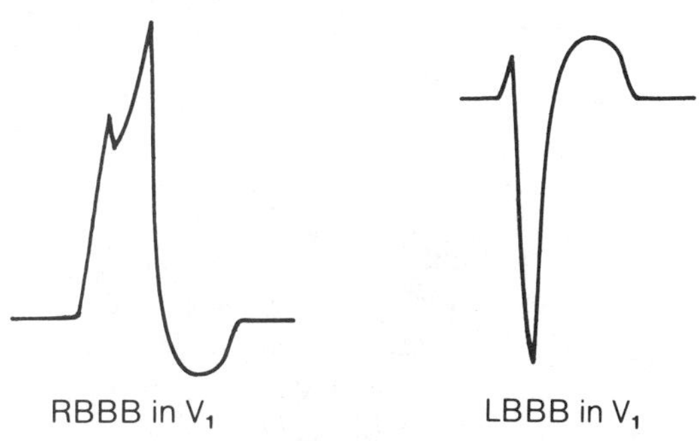

determine if an ectopic ventricular beat is coming from the right or left ventricle, and in certain instances can tell if the wide funny looking beat (FLB) seen is being produced by an ectopic pacing focus in the left ventricle or by aberrant conduction of a supraventricular impulse.

Electrode placement for V_1 or MCL_1 is diagrammed below. The positive electrode in MCL_1 is at the V_1 position, and the negative electrode is at the LA. In a true V_1, the positive electrode is again at V_1, and the limb electrodes are all negative with the exception of the RL electrode which is, of course, the ground or reference electrode.

MCL$_1$

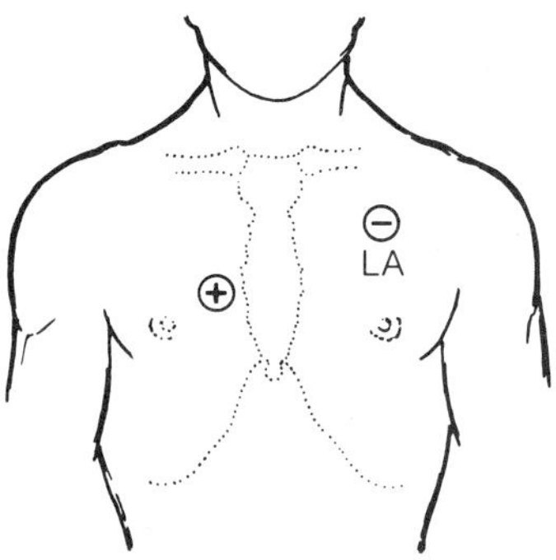

Two lead system

- Place the positive electrode at the fourth intercostal space on the right sternal border.
- Place the negative electrode in the LA position.

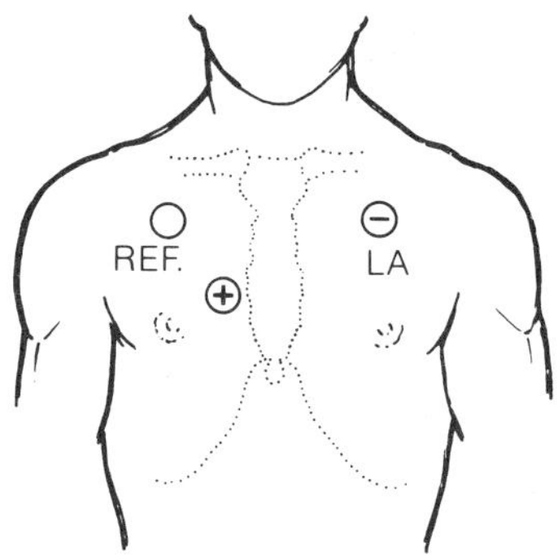

Three lead system

- Place the positive electrode at the fourth intercostal space on the right sternal border.
- Place the negative electrode in the LA position.
- Place the reference electrode anywhere, but in good contact.

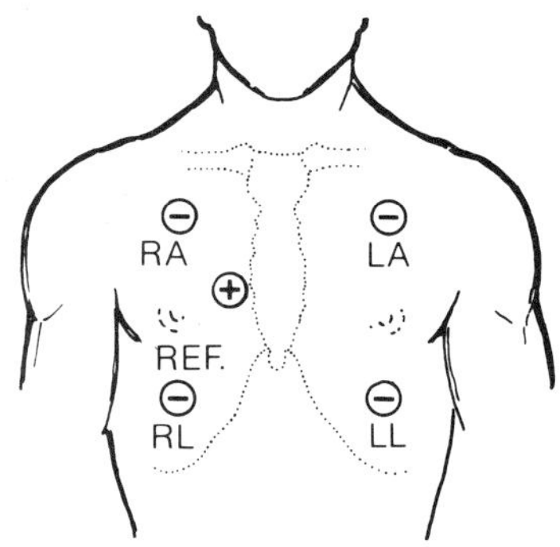

Five lead system

- With the five lead system, you don't have an MCL, but a true V_1.
- Put the lead selector switch on V.
- Attach the fifth electrode to the C slot in the patient connector.
- Place the fifth electrode at the fourth intercostal space on the right sternal border.
- The four basic electrodes must all remain in place.

Obviously, this lead gives much more important information than lead II can. If, for some reason, V_1 cannot be used, the same information is provided by MCL_6 or V_6. The complex configuration in V_6 will be the opposite of that seen in V_1, since the V_6 position is on the other side of the heart from V_1.

M_3

Modified lead III (M_3) is a lead that will show whether the P waves are sinus or retrograde in origin. The sinus P wave will be upright or positive in configuration. The retrograde P wave will be negative.

Electrode placement is that of lead III, with the positive electrode at the LL position, but moved down onto the abdomen just off the rib cage. The negative electrode is in the LA position.

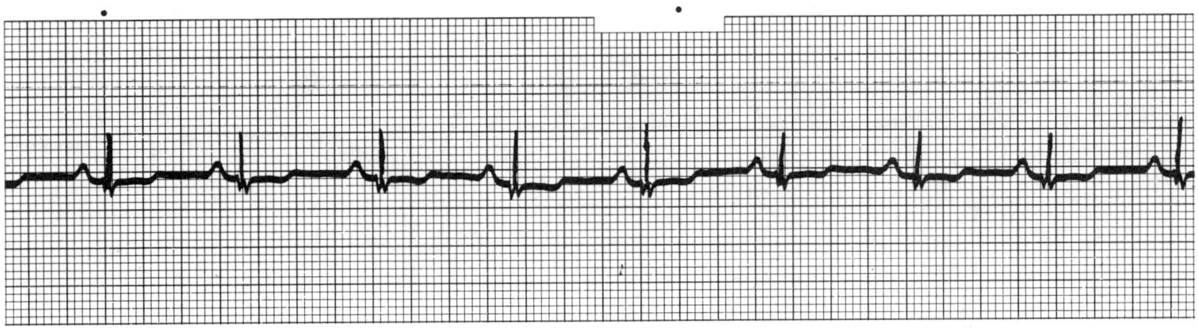

M_3 (modified lead III)

Modified lead III

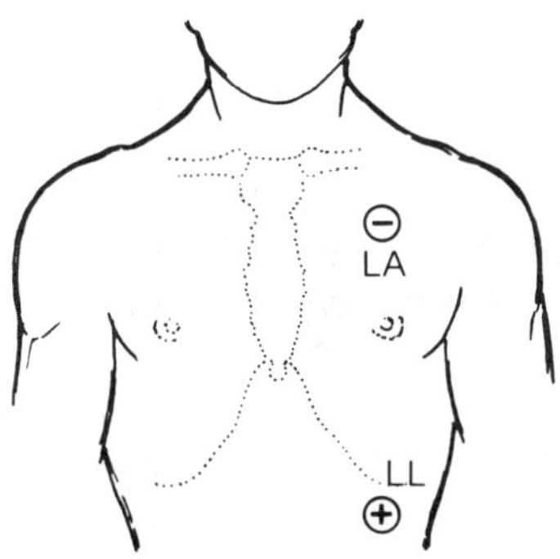

Two lead system

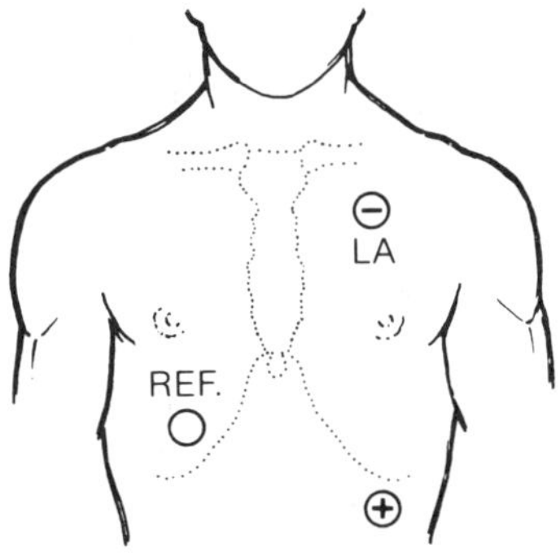

Three lead system

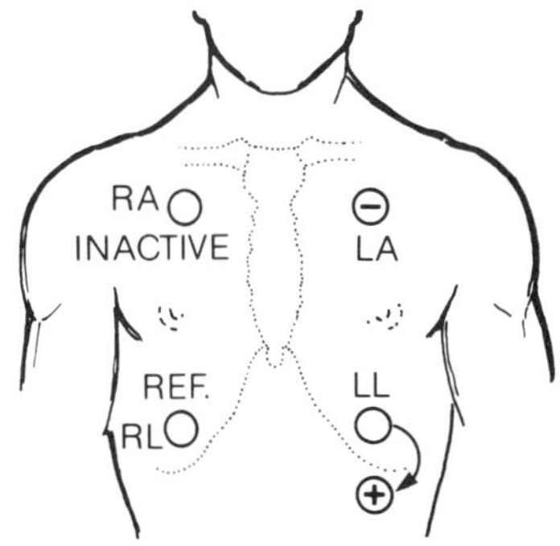

Five lead system

- ○ Place the positive electrode on the abdomen just off the rib cage on the left side.
- ○ Place the negative electrode in the LA position.

- ○ Place the positive electrode on the abdomen just off the rib cage on the left side.
- ○ Place the negative electrode in the LA position.
- ○ Place the reference electrode anywhere, but in good contact.

- ○ Put the lead selector switch on III.
- ○ Move the LL electrode, which is positive in lead III, to the abdomen just off the rib cage on the left side.
- ○ The other basic electrodes remain in the same position. The fifth, or chest, electrode is not used.

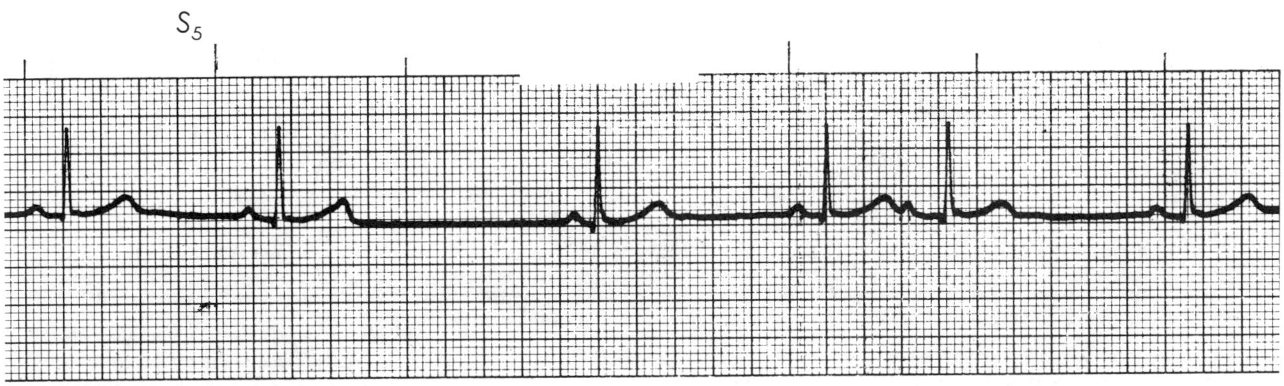

Patient's rhythm in Lead II. P waves are visible, but their shape is not well defined. Rhythm is hard to identify.

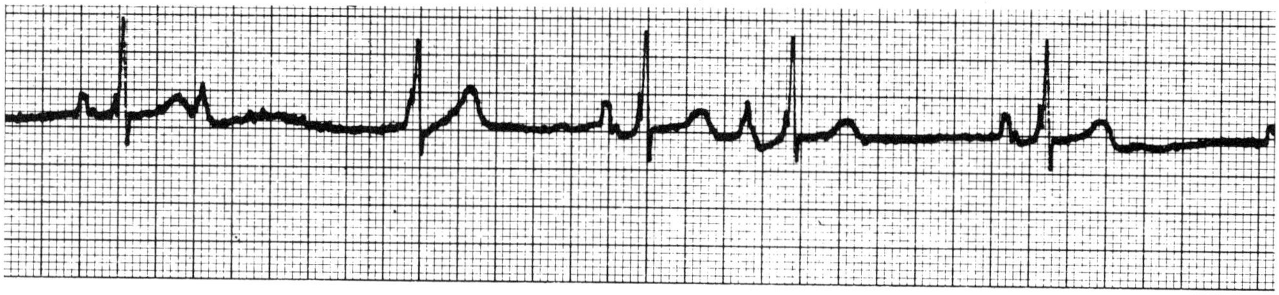

Same rhythm run in S_5. P waves differ markedly in early beats, and nonconducted early P waves are now visible in some T waves. This rhythm is NSR with frequent PACs.

S_5, a lead developed by French cardiologists, enhances atrial activity. It is especially useful when atrial activity is not readily visible, or when P wave configuration needs careful observation. It replaces an esophageal lead that obtained information about atrial activity by having the patient swallow a special catheter with an electrode in it. This invasive procedure was not very pleasant for the patient. It could also cause a drastic increase in vagal tone, which post-myocardial infarction (MI) patients certainly didn't need.

Electrode placement in S_5 puts the positive electrode on the fifth intercostal space at the right sternal border, one interspace below the V_1 position. The negative electrode is placed at the sternoclavicular notch.

Lead to enhance monitoring of atrial activity

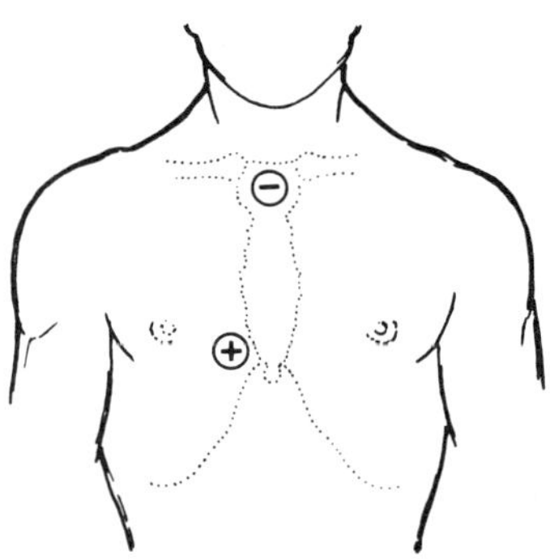

Two lead system

- Place the positive electrode at the fifth intercostal space on the right sternal border.
- Place the negative electrode just below the sternoclavicular notch.

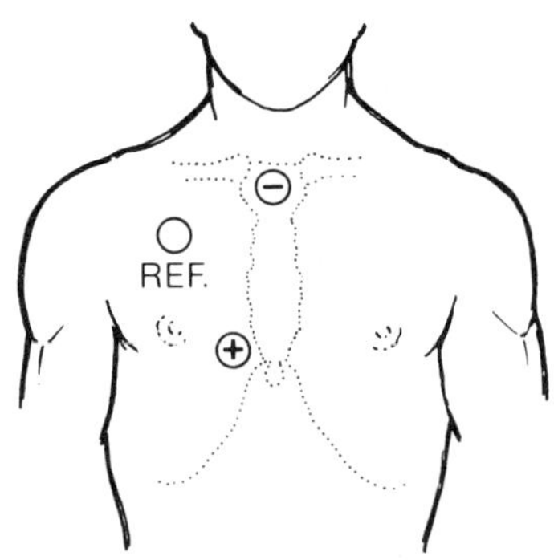

Three lead system

- Place the positive electrode at the fifth intercostal space on the right sternal border.
- Place the negative electrode just below the sternoclavicular notch.
- Place the reference electrode anywhere, but in good contact.

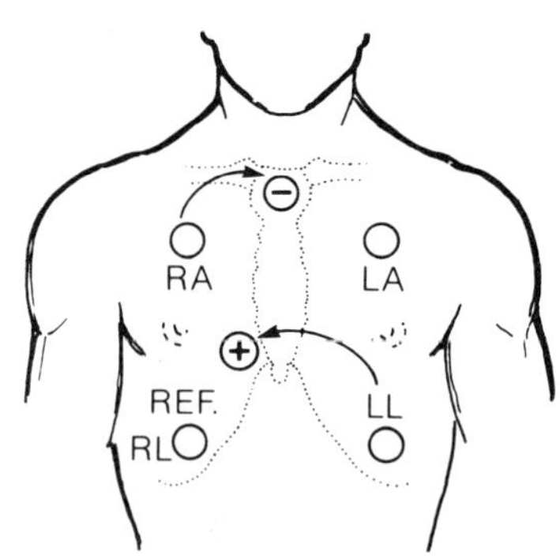

Five lead system

- Put the lead selector switch on II.
- Move the positive LL electrode to the fifth intercostal space in the right sternal border.
- Move the negative RA electrode to the sternoclavicular notch.

TROUBLESHOOTING THE MONITORS

With a careful skin prep and close attention to monitoring principles, there should be no major problems in attaching the patient to the monitor. If difficulties do occur while a patient is being monitored, the use of a systematic approach to define the problem and discover its probable cause will normally provide a simple solution. Problems generally arise in three basic areas: interference, false alarms, and mechanical failure.

INTERFERENCE

Interference is one of the most common problems occurring in the continuous monitoring of patients. Interference is exhibited by the appearance of large amounts of artifact on the oscilloscope, which obscures the ECG trace.

60-Cycle Interference

AC or 60-cycle interference is artifact produced by an outside electrical current source. It is characterized by a baseline widened by regularly occurring spikes at a rate of 60 per second.

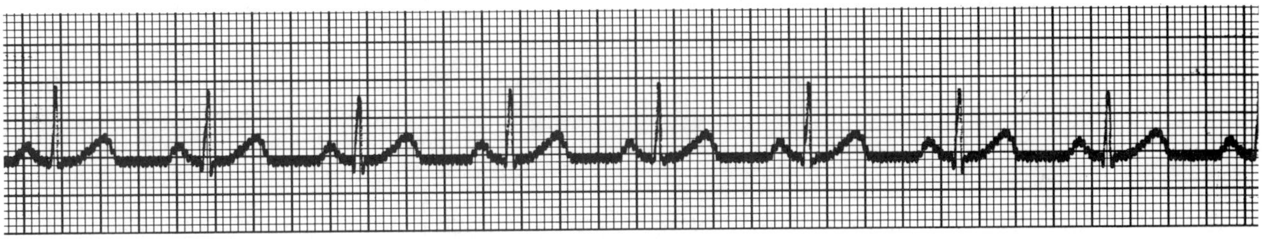

60-cycle interference

The above is a typical example of 60-cycle interference, but the baseline may be much wider and more distorted, and even the QRS complexes may be obscured.

AC interference is caused by leakage current from other electrical equipment in the room such as radios, electric razors, lamps, fluorescent light fixtures, or intravenous (IV) controlling devices. If leakage is the cause of interference, simply disconnecting the appliance from the power outlet will eliminate the problem. Another cause of 60-cycle interference is having the patient cable too close to the power cord of the monitor or any other piece of electrical equipment. By isolating the patient cable from the power cord, the interference should disappear. Newer monitoring systems have patient cables that are shielded so that an induction current cannot be produced by outside sources.

Tremor

Tremor, another type of interference, is caused by somatic or body tremor in the patient. It is exhibited by an irregular shaky baseline. The artifact produced by patient movement, which obscures the whole trace, is an exaggeration of somatic tremor. If a patient is tense or

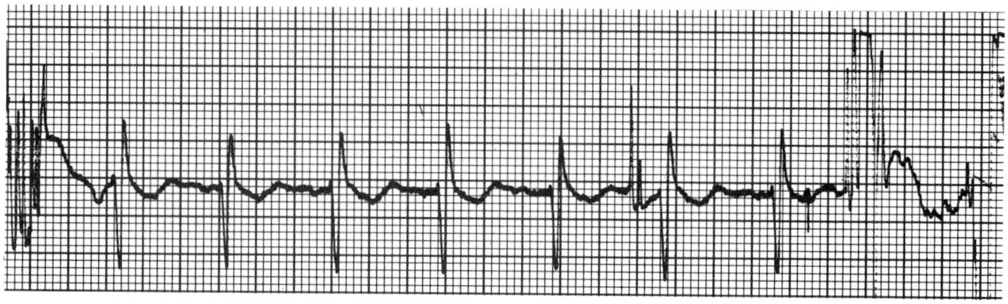

Tremor

anxious, cold, or chilling as a result of fever, fine skeletal muscle tremors occur that produce this pattern.

Tremor artifact can be eliminated in most cases by checking the electrode contact, making the patient more comfortable and relaxed, and removing the cause of the muscle tremor, if possible.

Wandering Baseline

Wandering of the baseline is another common problem. The trace may be clear, but the baseline undulates up and down the scope, distorting the position of the ST segment and changing the shapes of the complexes. Wandering baseline may be caused by loose electrodes, or by tension on the lead wire that causes the electrodes to move on the chest wall with respirations.

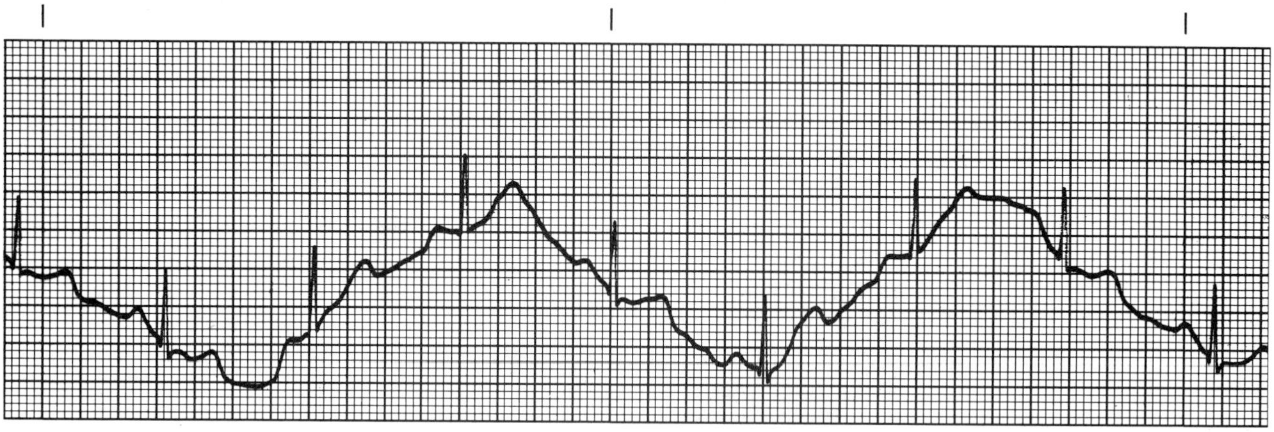

Wandering baseline

Wandering baseline can be corrected by checking the contact of the electrodes, and by supporting the patient cable connector so that no tension is placed on the lead wires. A stress loop in the lead wire may also be helpful in this situation.

Jitters

Jittering of the trace, which gives chaotic spikes and dips that resemble fibrillation waves and may obscure the entire ECG trace, is a third type

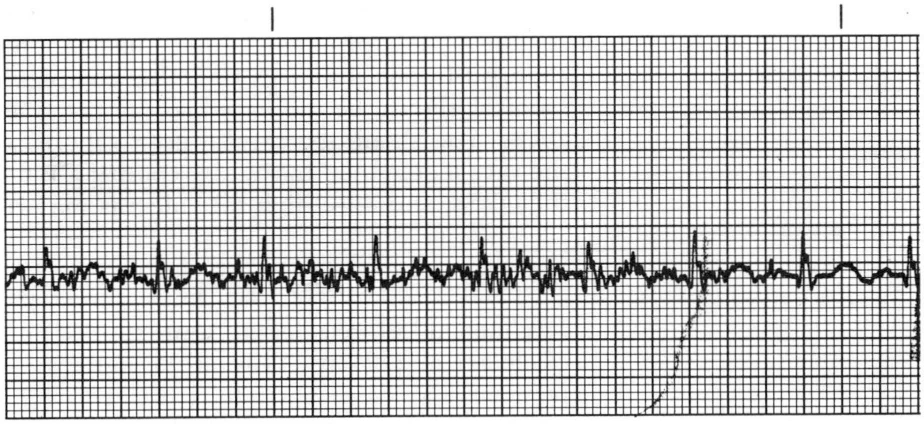

Jitters

of interference. This artifact is caused by poor electrode contact resulting from improper skin preparation, dry silver chloride gel, or poor connections along the lead wire or patient cable because of dirty or corroded connections. Jittering rarely will occur in a patient who has small particles of metal imbedded in his skin. Jittering artifact can be eliminated by checking the electrodes with an electrode tester, giving a proper skin preparation, and cleaning wire connections on the lead wires or patient cable.

FALSE ALARMS

False alarms are another frequent problem. Superficially, they seem to be only a minor irritation to the nurse, but they actually can prove to be a dangerous situation. When a patient's alarm system is activated repeatedly because of artifact in the trace, there is a tendency to move the rate limit setting higher or to respond less promptly to the alarm. If the patient should experience a true dysrhythmic event, and the rate alarm is either turned off or set too high, it could delay the nurse's immediate recognition and treatment of a life-threatening situation.

False High-Rate Alarms

The majority of false high-rate alarms are caused by artifact in the trace producing deflections counted as QRS complexes by the rate meter. The situations producing the artifact include AC interference, jittering trace, and tremor. The number of false high-rate alarms can be decreased by careful preparation of the skin and proper placement of the electrodes when the patient is attached to the monitor. Also, care should be taken when setting the high rate limit on the alarm system.

False Low-Rate Alarms

False low-rate alarms result from loss of signal from the patient. This loss of electrical conduction may be caused by improper electrode contact, wire or cable failure, or a QRS complex voltage that is too small to be counted by the rate meter. Again, checking the electrodes and a careful skin prep will prevent a loss of signal. If low QRS voltage is producing the problem, either the lead being monitored should be changed to one that sees the QRS complexes well, or the gain on the monitor should be increased so the rate meter starts counting all the QRSs. You should be careful not to increase the gain too much, since the rate meter then may start counting P waves or T waves as well as the QRSs, and false high-rate alarms may result.

MECHANICAL FAILURE

Mechanical failure refers to some type of physical failure in conduction of electrical activity between the patient and the monitor. In a small percentage of cases, the failure is due to a malfunction of the electronic circuitry of the monitor itself. However, today's monitoring systems are usually reliable, so the great majority of mechanical problems lie in the connections between the patient and the monitor.

The most common site of mechanical failure is at the electrode. Improper skin preparation is the chief offender. Another cause can be dried silver chloride gel, which is not a good conductor of electrical impulses. The manufacturer seals the package containing the electrode to prevent the gel from drying out, but if the seal is broken, the gel can dry. The condition of the gel pad should always be checked before the electrode is applied to the patient's chest. If problems arise after the electrode has been in place over a period of time, the electrode should be replaced.

The electrode may become dislodged due to loss of adhesion to the skin. If the patient is diaphoretic, keeping the electrode in place can become a real problem. There are special diaphoretic electrodes available that will maintain adhesion even when the patient is profusely diaphoretic.

Mechanical failure also can occur in the wires and cables connecting the patient to the monitor. The lead wires or patient cable may not be connected. The patient cable may not be securely connected to the monitor. Sometimes, there may be a wire fracture within the lead wire or the patient cable. The patient cable can be checked for integrity by pulling the lead wire attachment slightly loose from the patient cable connector, and laying a piece of metal such as a paper clip across the exposed ends of the lead wire pins. If the monitor displays a straight baseline, the patient cable is intact.

A simple procedure can also check the function of the monitor itself. Simply turn the lead selector switch to the calibrate position and push the 1-mv button. If a straight line appears on the oscilloscope with a square 10-mm deflection when the standard button is pushed, the problem is most likely not in the monitor.

SYSTEMATIC APPROACH TO TROUBLESHOOTING THE MONITOR

Now that we have explored common problems occurring in continuous ECG monitoring of the cardiac patient and how to prevent these problems, here is a check list to use in a systematic manner when a problem does occur.

1. *Check the patient!* Is he or she comfortable? Is he or she cold, anxious, or in pain? Tremor artifact may be caused by any of these things.
2. *Check the electrodes.* Is there an adequate skin prep? Is the electrode loose? Is the silver chloride gel dry or moist?
3. *Check the lead wires.* Are they snapped securely to the electrode? Is there any tension on the lead wire causing electrode movement on the chest wall?
4. *Check the patient connector.* Is it intact, with all lead pins clean and securely fastened? Is the connector pinned to the patient's gown to prevent pull on the lead wires?
5. *Check the patient cable.* Is it securely attached to the monitor? Is it supported so that it isn't dangling? Is it too close to an electrical power cord? Is there a wire fracture in the cable or is it intact?
6. *Check the monitor.* Is it turned on? Is the gain sufficient to produce readable complexes and trigger the rate meter and alarm system? Are the alarm limits appropriately set?
7. *Call electronics department.* If you are still unable to correct the problem, call for assistance.

4

THE DEVELOPMENT OF DYSRHYTHMIAS AND SYSTEMATIC INTERPRETATION OF NORMAL SINUS RHYTHMS

The control of the electrical activity that produces the heart's rhythms is a finely balanced composite of complexly interrelated neural and chemical forces. Many widely varied factors can subtly alter these forces and thus produce changes in the heart's cycles of depolarization and repolarization, causing the development of abnormal rhythms—the dysrhythmias.

Traditionally, these abnormal rhythms have been termed arrhythmias. But, if you break down this word, in medical terminology the prefix "a" usually means "an absence of." The prefix "dys," meaning "bad or difficult," more accurately describes what is happening to the rhythm, since we actually are dealing with an abnormality rather than an absence of activity in the heart. Thus, the term dysrhythmia is more correct.

There are really two general categories of dysrhythmias—those produced by suppression, and those produced by irritability. The presence of either irritability or suppression has an effect on the special properties inherent in myocardial tissue: automaticity and conductivity. Since these properties are the basis for all the electrical activity in the heart, any alteration in their function will generate changes in the rhythm. Some dysrhythmias may be benign, but many of them may alter the hemodynamics to such an extent that life can be threatened.

SUPPRESSION DYSRHYTHMIAS

If suppression is present, both automaticity and conductivity are affected. The automatic rate of depolarization, the spontaneous discharge cycle, of any pacing cell is decreased, and the conduction velocity is slowed throughout the heart. The dysrhythmias thus produced obviously would be slow rates, pauses, late beats, and alterations in conduction such as the AV blocks or bundle branch block.

THE CAUSES OF SUPPRESSION

The causes of suppression are numerous and include such varied factors as alterations in autonomic stimulation, drugs, fibrosis or necrosis of the myocardium, cold, and electrolyte imbalances.

The alterations in autonomic stimulation producing suppression are increases in parasympathetic tone and decreases in sympathetic tone. Whenever parasympathetic or vagal tone is increased, suppression results. Since the vagal fibers are located in the atria, mainly clustered around the sinoatrial (SA) and artrioventricular (AV) nodes, the rate of SA depolarization and AV conduction will be slowed. The reasons for an increase in vagal tone were covered in detail in Chapter 1; but in review, Valsalva maneuvers, carotid sinus massage, hypertension, nausea and vomiting, pain, or fright are a few factors that are likely to produce intense vagal firing.

If sympathetic tone is decreased, the main source of stimulation to the heart's electrical activity is lessened. Since sympathetic fibers are located throughout the heart, a generalized slowing of depolarization and conduction velocity may result. Of course, decreased sympathetic tone will also decrease contractility of the myocardium as well. The most common causes of decreased sympathetic tone are the drugs that produce beta blockade (*i.e.*, propranolol, metaprolol, nadolol, atenolol, or timolol).

Drugs other than the beta blockers can also produce suppression of the myocardium. Some of the chief offenders are the very same pharmacologic preparations used to treat irritability. Digitalis is, of course, a drug that will produce suppression, as will quinidine, procainamide, or disopyramide. The calcium antagonists also have a suppressive effect. In this relatively new (in the U.S.) category of drugs, verapamil and diltiazem are the only ones with significant suppressive effects.

Noncardiac drugs that may cause suppression include the barbiturates, morphine and Demerol, and reserpine.

Suppression is frequently produced by coronary artery disease and the accompanying myocardial ischemia it causes. If the ischemia is chronic, fibrosis of the structures of the conduction system may result, thus decreasing conduction velocity and spontaneous discharge cycle rates. On the other hand, the ischemia may be an acute event that proceeds to myocardial infarction (MI) and tissue necrosis, with the same resultant suppression of automaticity and conductivity.

Other causes of suppression include decreased body temperature, hyperkalemia, hypocalcemia, and increased intracranial pressure.

SUPPRESSION-PRODUCED DYSRHYTHMIAS

No matter what the causative factors, the dysrhythmias produced will have very specific characteristics that result from alteration of automaticity or conductivity. Everything slows and may even stop. If the automaticity of the SA node is decreased, sinus bradycardia will result. If the SA node is further suppressed, it may stop completely for brief periods—a sinus arrest. Sinus node suppression may be great enough that lower pacemakers are allowed to complete their spontaneous discharge cycles and depolarize, either for a single complex, an escape beat that arrives after the next sinus beat is expected, or as the predominent pacemaker, an escape rhythm. If the lower pacemaker is in the atria, atrial escape beats or wandering atrial pacemaker will be seen. If the lower pacing activity arises in the AV junction, junctional escape beats or junctional rhythm will occur. If all higher pacemakers are either blocked or suppressed, the ventricles must come to the rescue in the form of a ventricular escape beat or idioventricular rhythm. These dysrhythmias produced by suppressed automaticity will characteristically appear as slowed rates, late beats, and pauses in the rhythm.

Suppressive alteration in the form of slowed conduction velocity will have the characteristics of decreased conduction through the SA junction and the AV node—the three degrees of AV block—or through the bundle branches producing either right or left bundle branch block or the hemiblocks. Thus, these dysrhythmias produced by suppressed conductivity will appear as prolonged PR intervals, widened QRS complexes, or P waves without QRSs.

THERAPY OF SUPPRESSION DYSRHYTHMIAS

Therapy for symptomatic suppression dysrhythmias consists of drugs to counteract the autonomic imbalances. Atropine decreases suppression by blocking vagal tone, thus allowing the sympathetic system to dominate. If the dysrhythmia does not respond to atropine, isoproterenol is the next drug of choice. Isoproterenol increases stimulation of the $beta_1$ receptors in the heart, and it relieves the suppression by increasing sympathetic tone. If drugs are ineffective, or the suppression becomes chronic, electrical pacing with either a temporary or a permanent cardiac pacemaker will be used.

IRRITABILITY DYSRHYTHMIAS

When irritability is present, automaticity and conductivity again are affected, but the alterations are the opposite of those produced by suppression. The spontaneous discharge cycle of any pacing cell can be accelerated and, in certain cases, the conduction velocity is either increased or becomes abnormal. The resulting dysrhythmias will have the characteristics of fast rates and early beats; or flutter or fibrillation may become the predominant rhythm.

THE CAUSES OF IRRITABILITY

Many of the causes of irritability are the direct opposite of the factors that produced suppression. These causative factors are increased sympathetic stimulation, decreased vagal tone, drugs, ischemia or injury of the myocardium, heat, electrolyte imbalances, myocardial stretch, and hypoxemia and acidosis.

Obviously, to produce irritability, the autonomic alterations would have to have the opposite effects of those causing suppression. Instead of decreased sympathetic tone, increased $beta_1$ stimulation is one of the most common reasons for increased irritability. Again, the factors causing increased sympathetic tone were well covered in Chapter 1 but, briefly, a few are hypotension, decreased circulating volume resulting from hemorrhage or dehydration, exercise, fright, stress, fever, or drugs. Increased sympathetic tone increases the automaticity and conductivity of the heart, and also increases myocardial contractility.

Many drugs may increase irritability. Isoproterenol increases beta stimulation, which is the reason it is used to treat suppression. Digitalis toxicity will also greatly increase irritability, and is one of the most common causes of irritability dysrhythmias in cardiac patients. Epinephrine will increase irritability since it causes both alpha and beta stimulation. Two noncardiac drugs that commonly produce irritability, even in a normal heart, are nicotine and caffeine.

Decreased vagal tone removes the inhibitory influence of the parasympathetic system on the heart and allows sympathetic effects to dominate. Atropine, of course, blocks vagal tone pharmacologically.

The injury and ischemia found in the myocardium of the infarcted heart produces irritability frequently seen in patients with acute MIs. When a coronary artery occludes and infarction results, there is an area of cells that are dying or dead. However, this zone of necrotic tissue is surrounded by an area of injured cells. The injured cells are surrounded by another area of cells that are ischemic. The zones of injury and ischemia have different electrical potentials, and where these areas in-

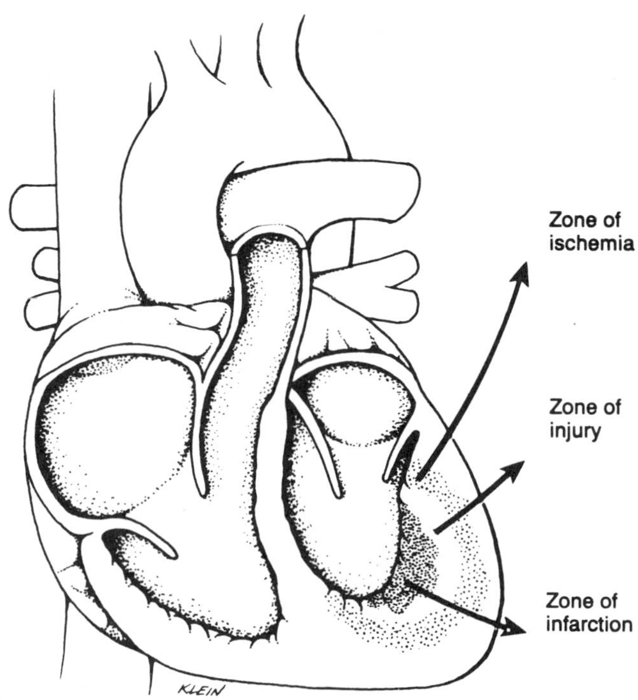

terface the possibility of current flow exists that may produce irritability.

Electrolyte imbalances, particularly hypokalemia, make the myocardium extremely irritable. This seems reasonable since the flow of potassium ions, along with sodium, back and forth across the cell membrane is the mechanism that changes the polarity of cellular electrical potentials, thus allowing depolarization and repolarization of the heart.

Congestive heart failure causes a triple threat to the myocardium. As the left ventricle fails, there is an increase in hemodynamic pressures and volumes in the chamber because the ventricle cannot eject all the blood with each contraction. The increasing pressures and volumes put stretch on the ventricular and atrial myocardium which, in turn, increases irritability. Along with the increasing pressures, there eventually will be decreased oxygenation of the blood as the lungs become filled with fluid. Hypoxemia, coupled with a decreasing cardiac output, causes decreased perfusion of the coronary arteries. As the oxygenation of the myocardium decreases, acidosis will occur. Both hypoxemia and acidosis will produce increased irritability. Other factors that produce irritability include increased body temperature and stress.

IRRITABILITY-PRODUCED DYSRHYTHMIAS

Irritability also affects both the automaticity and conductivity of the heart. Both will be increased.

If the automaticity of the SA node is increased, the spontaneous discharge cycle is accelerated, and sinus tachycardia results. If irritability increases the automaticity of a pacemaker outside the SA node, the ectopic focus will develop a spontaneous discharge cycle faster than that of the SA node and usurp the pacing function. When the ectopic focus has enough irritability that it will fire itself off before the SA node is due to depolarize, a premature beat occurs. The location of this irritable focus in the heart determines whether the premature beat will be a premature atrial contraction, premature junctional contraction, or a premature ventricular contraction. If the focus becomes even more irritable, it may become the dominant pacemaker, in which case a tachycardia results. Again, depending upon the location of the irritable focus, there will be either atrial tachycardia, junctional tachycardia, or ventricular tachycardia.

If irritability continues to increase, the method of depolarization changes and that, coupled with increased conductivity, allows the mechanism of flutter to occur. Flutter is described as a "circus movement" of electrical activity. A wave of depolarization travels in a circle around the chamber that is fluttering. This wave of depolarization is followed by a wave of repolarization, which perpetuates this rhythm. Flutter, which appears on the ECG as a regular saw-tooth waveform, can occur in either the atria or the ventricles.

If irritability increases even further, the method of depolarization changes again, and fibrillation results. Fibrillation is continuous chaotic depolarization of all the muscle fibers in a chamber. There is no pattern to this random depolarization and repolarization, and the muscle is actually twitching and squirming. Fibrillation, which appears on the ECG as totally irregular wiggles and spikes on the baseline, can also occur in either the atria or the ventricles.

The characteristics of dysrhythmias produced by increased irritability thus will be early beats, tachycardias, flutter, or fibrillation.

THERAPY OF IRRITABILITY DYSRHYTHMIAS

The drug therapy for irritability dysrhythmias includes all of the drugs that cause suppression. Digitalis, quinidine, procainamide, and disopyramide have their main effect by causing decreased automaticity and/or conductivity. The calcium antagonists (*i.e.*, verapamil) slow AV conduction by blocking calcium entry into the cell through the slow channels. Xylocaine, bretylium, and mexiletine work on the cell level in the ventricles to slow sodium entry into the cell through the fast channel, which increases the threshold level and thus decreases irritability.

The beta-blockers that decrease $beta_1$ stimulation to the heart and suppress automaticity and conductivity are also used to treat irritability. Propranolol is the best-known example of this class of drugs.

Two other drugs used to treat irritability are phenytoin and potassium. Phenytoin is used mainly to soothe the type of irritability produced by digitalis toxicity. Potassium, of course, is used when hypokalemia is the cause of irritability.

If drug therapy proves ineffective, or if the patient's hemodynamic status is being compromised by the dysrhythmia, the electrical therapy for irritability is countershock in the form of cardioversion or defibrillation.

BEAT CONFIGURATION

You have now been introduced to the various mechanisms of dysrhythmia development and the characteristics of the rhythms produced (See Table 4-1). You know that a late beat that arrives after the next sinus beat is expected is called an escape beat. You also know that the early beat arriving before the next sinus beat is expected is called a premature beat. The tricky part comes when a decision must be made as to where the escape beat is being generated: The atria? The AV junction? The ventricles? Is the tachycardia arising in thc SA node, atria, junction, or ventricles? In order to make this decision, first determine what the patient's normal PQRST complex looks like in the lead being monitored. The characteristic changes in beat configuration that occur when the pacing site moves away from the SA node then should be ascertained. By comparing the abnormal beat with what is known to be normal, it is not only possible, but actually easy to determine where the funny-looking beat (FLB) is coming from.

There may be a problem, however, in determining what is normal. The normal PQRST differs in shape from person to person, and changes shape from lead-to-lead in the same person. Knowing what is normal for that patient in that lead is essential! Let's take a look at what the

TABLE 4-1. CHARACTERISTICS OF DYSRHYTHMIAS

DYSRHYTHMIA	ECG CHARACTERISTICS
Suppression Dysrhythmias	
Sinus bradycardia	Normal beats at a slow rate of less than 60
Arrests	Pauses in the rhythm
Escape beats	Late beat arriving after the next sinus beat is due
Escape rhythms	Slow rhythms differing in shape from the sinus
AV blocks	Long PR intervals; P waves without QRS complexes; P waves and QRS complexes not related
Bundle branch block	Wide, bizarre QRS complexes
Irritability Dysrhythmias	
Premature beats	Early beats arriving before next sinus beat is due
Tachycardias	Fast rate of greater than 100
Flutter	Regular saw-tooth waveforms
Fibrillation	Irregular, chaotic wiggles and dips of the baseline

normal beat should look like, and what changes occur when the beat arises somewhere other than the SA node.

THE SINUS BEAT

The first, and most important, criterion for identifying a beat arising from the SA node is the presence of a normal P wave. As was just mentioned, a normal P wave may differ from person to person, and it will differ in the same person from one lead to another. The P wave in lead II may have this shape:

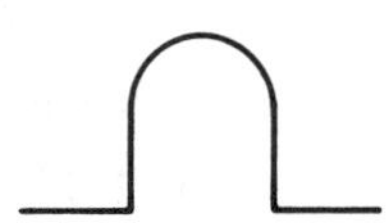

But it may look like this in V_1 or MCL_1:

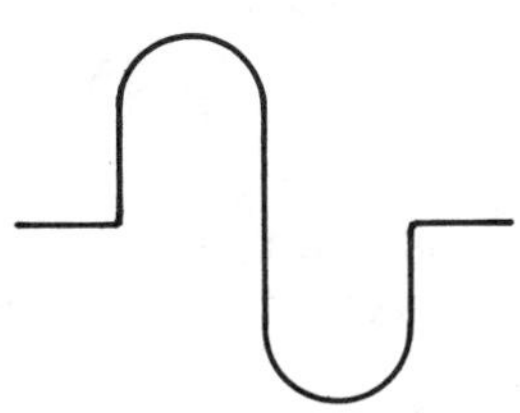

For the purpose of this discussion, we will designate the normal P wave as being shaped as the following:

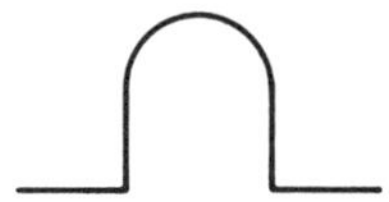

The normal QRS complex will also vary from lead to lead, and from person to person, so we will denote the normal QRS as having this shape:

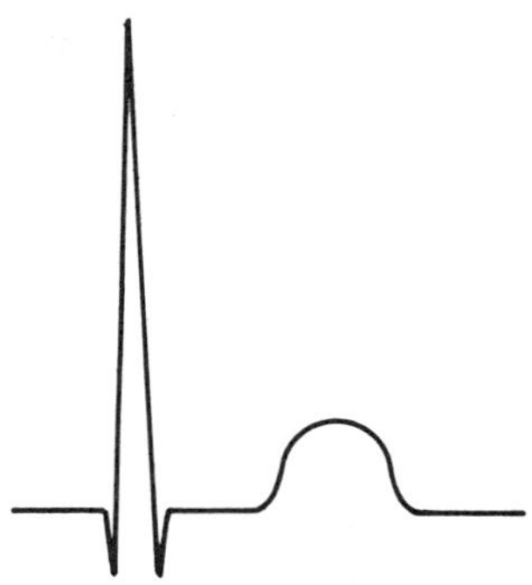

Thus, any beat coming from the SA node will have this normal configuration:

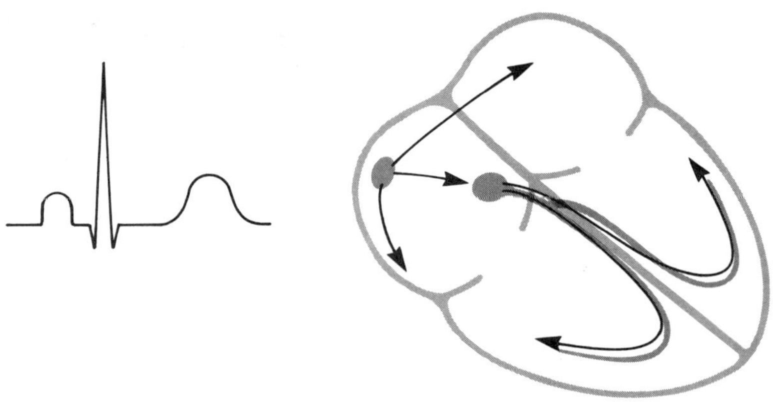

Assuming that this impulse from the SA node is conducted normally through the rest of the heart, the sinus beat will have a PR interval in the normal range of 0.12 to 0.20 second, and a QRS duration of 0.06 to 0.12 second. Every beat arising from the SA node will be identical in configuration.

THE ATRIAL BEAT

The beat that arises in the atrial myocardium also will begin with a P wave, but the P wave will be abnormal in configuration and will differ from the shape of the sinus P wave. The ectopic pacing focus producing the atrial beat is located somewhere in the atrial myocardium. The wave of depolarization does not move through the normal atrial pathways, but flows in an abnormal way through the atria; thus, the shape of the P wave changes. Each time a different ectopic focus in the atria fires, the shape of the P wave will change. The PR interval of the atrial beat may differ from the PR measurement of the sinus beat, but it will probably still be within the normal limits of 0.12 to 0.20 second. The change in the PR measurement is not a reflection of a change in AV conduction, but rather is a function of the location of the ectopic focus in relation to the AV node and the time required for the impulse to reach the AV node. If, again, we assume that transmission of the impulse through the rest of the conduction system proceeds in the normal fashion, the rest of the beat should have the same configuration as the sinus beat with a normal QRS duration. Thus, a beat arising in the atria will have the following configuration.

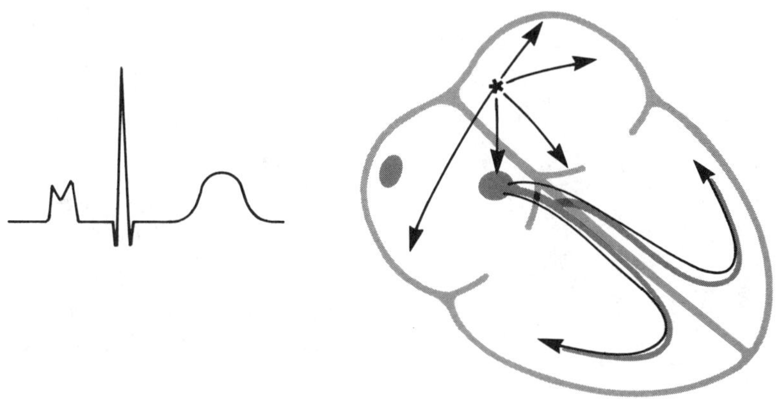

THE JUNCTIONAL BEAT

When the AV junction initiates the PQRST complex, the ectopic pacing focus will be located in the His Bundle, in the nodal-His (NH) region or the atrionodal (AN) region above the node, not in the AV node itself, which is the only place in the heart devoid of pacing cells.

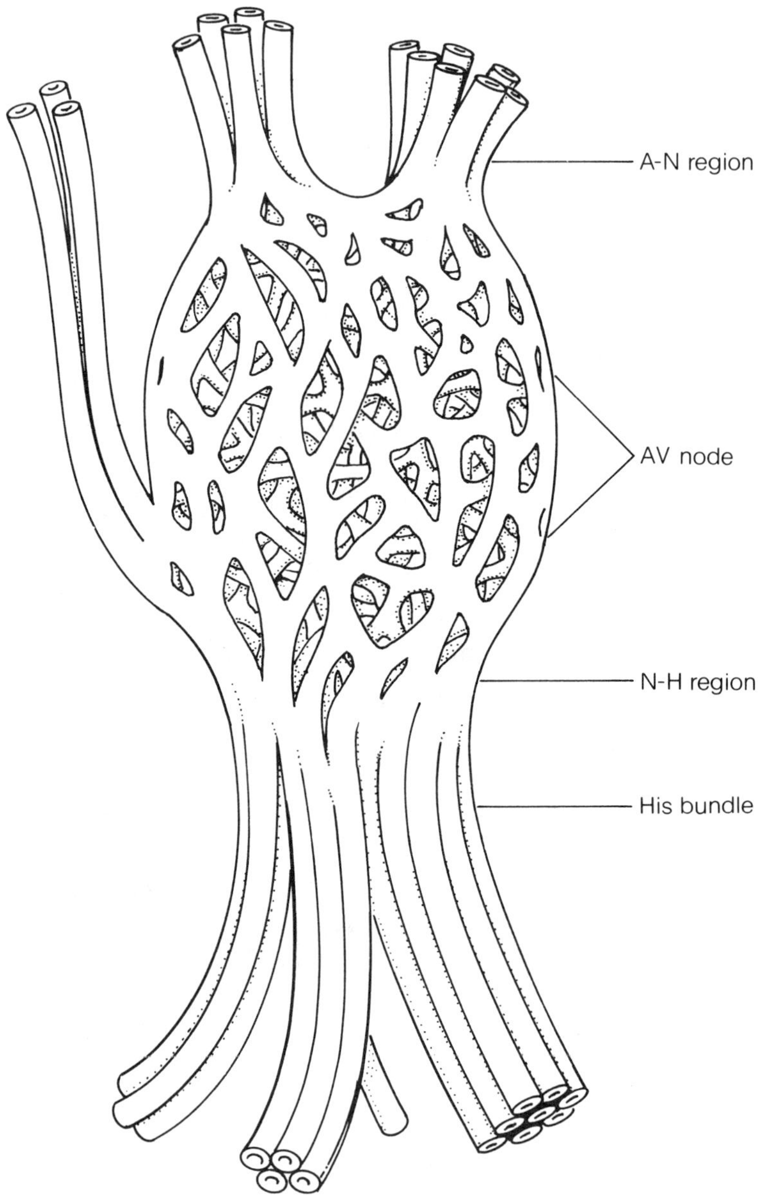

The impulse arising in the AV junction goes through the ventricular conduction system in the normal way, producing a normal QRS complex. The presence of a normal QRS is one of the main factors in the identification of a junctional beat.

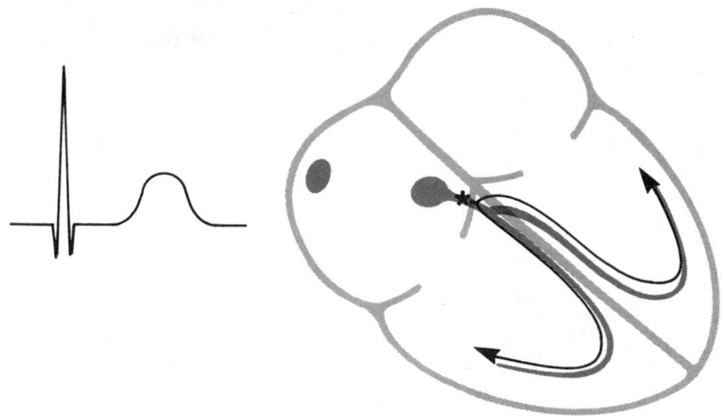

The atrial activity initiated by a junctional focus is altered in a characteristic manner that also helps in identifying these beats. The atria are depolarized from below by the impulse proceeding back up through the AV node. This type of backward activation is called retrograde conduction. Normal forward conduction of the sinus impulse is termed orthograde or antegrade conduction.

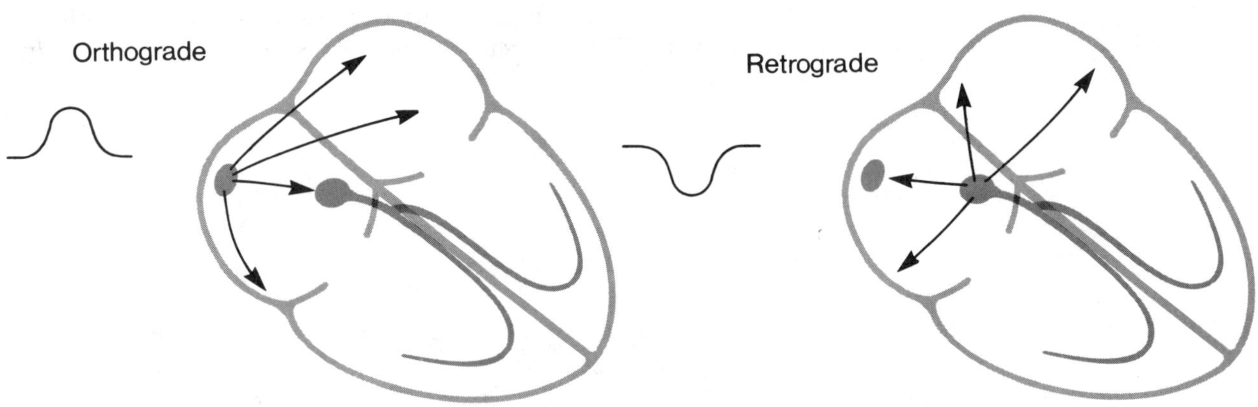

Since the wave of depolarization is moving from below up through the atrial myocardium, the P wave will have the opposite deflection from the sinus P wave. If the sinus P wave is upright, the retrograde P wave will be inverted.

The position of the P wave, in relation to the QRS complex, can vary, depending entirely upon the amount of retrograde delay in transmission of the impulse back through the AV node.

If the impulse moves back through the AV node and stimulates the atria at the same time the ventricles are depolarizing, the retrograde P wave will be positioned in the middle of the QRS complex and will be masked by the larger QRS deflection. If there is no retrograde conduction and no P wave, all that is seen is the normal QRS.

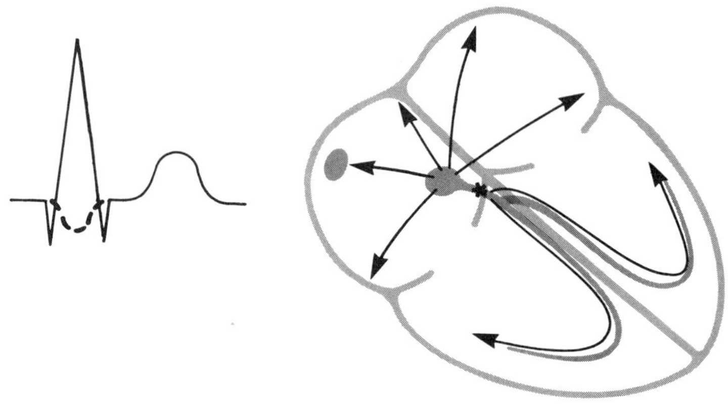

If the AV node provides no delay with retrograde conduction, or if the pacing focus is located in the AN region, the atria will be stimulated before the ventricles. This positions the retrograde P wave in front of the normal QRS complex, but because of the close timing of these two events, the PR interval will be very short, and will measure less than 0.12 second.

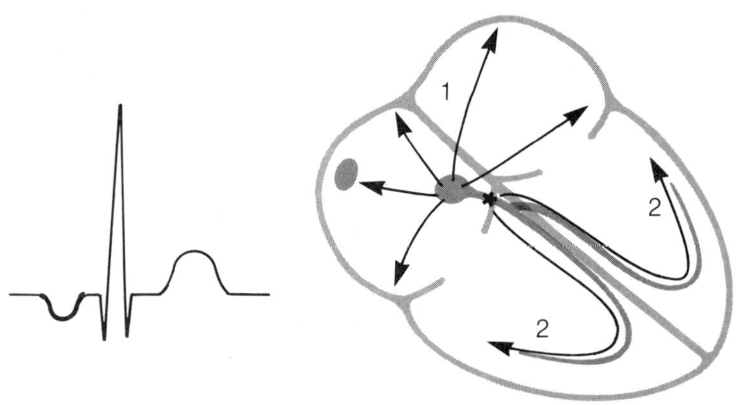

If the AV node does cause delay in retrograde conduction of the impulse, the atria are stimulated after the ventricles are activated. This will position the retrograde P wave after the QRS complex, somewhere on the ST segment or T wave.

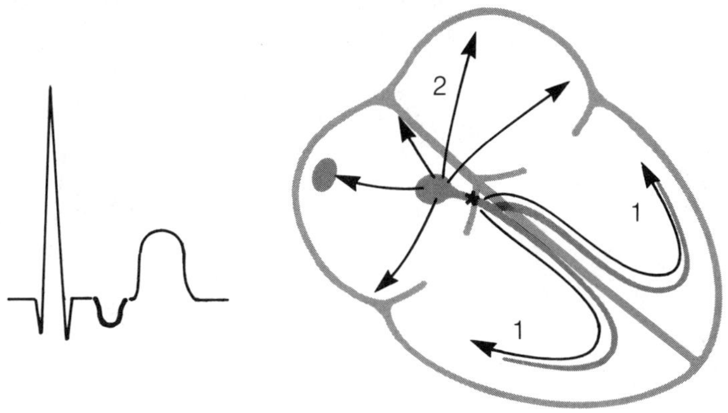

THE VENTRICULAR BEAT

When the ectopic focus acting as the pacemaker is located in the ventricles, the complex becomes very distorted. First, retrograde conduction to the atria doesn't occur very often, so the ventricular beat characteristically has no P wave associated with it. Second, conduction of the wave of depolarization through the ventricles is not accomplished through the bundle branches and Purkinje fibers. The wave of depolarization must travel through the ventricular myocardium in a cell-to-cell, fiber-to-fiber fashion, which takes longer than normal transmission through the conduction system. The wave of depolarization also moves through the ventricular myocardium in an abnormal direction, which alters the shape of the QRS complex. Thus, the ventricular beat will have a bizarre configuration that measures greater than 0.12 second in duration. Each time a different ectopic ventricular focus fires, the QRS complex will change in configuration.

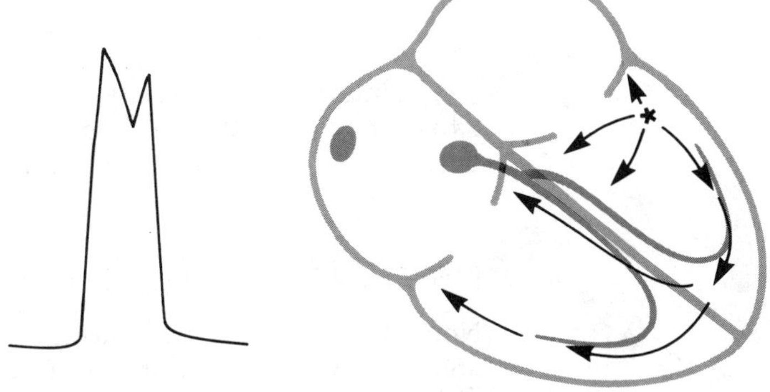

The wide bizarre ventricular QRS complex has certain characteristics that will help in identifying these beats. Since depolarization is altered, so is repolarization. If the main QRS deflection is upward or positive, the ST segment will slope downward and T wave will be inverted.

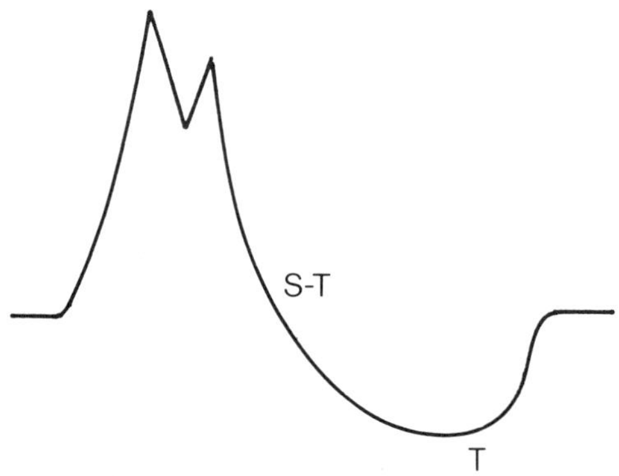

If the main QRS deflection is downward or negative, then the ST segment will slope upward, and the T wave will have a positive deflection.

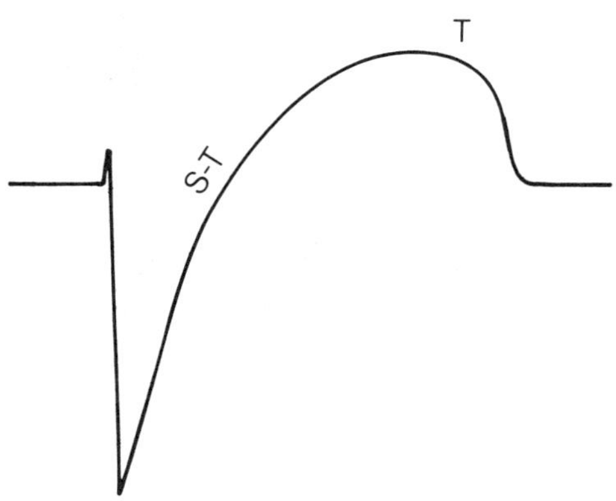

Thus, the ST segment and T wave will go in the opposite direction from the main QRS deflection. These "footprints" of ventricular ectopic activity are a great help in making identification of these beats easier.

IDENTIFICATION OF BEATS

Now, let's combine the information about dysrhythmia development and its ECG characteristics (Table 4-1), with the typical characteristics of beat configuration (Table 4-2), and try to interpret some common dysrhythmias.

TABLE 4-2. BEAT CONFIGURATION

Sinus

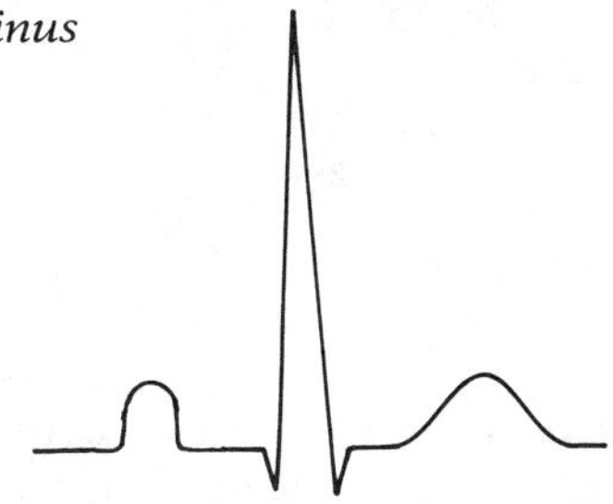

A

Normal P wave
Normal PR interval (0.12–0.20 sec)
Normal QRS duration (0.06–0.12 sec)

Atrial

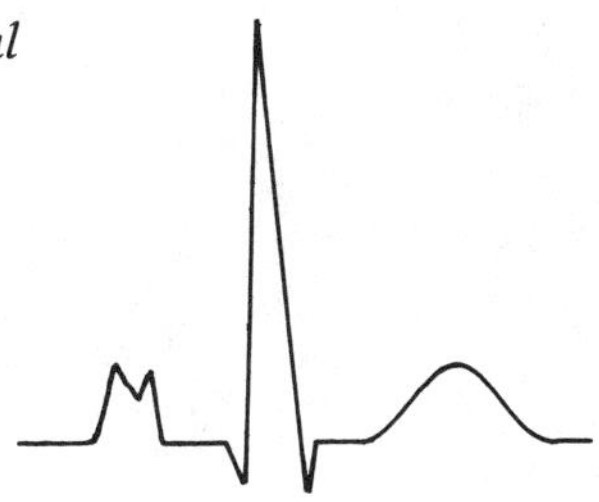

B

Abnormal P wave
Normal PR interval (differs from sinus)
Normal QRS complex

Junctional

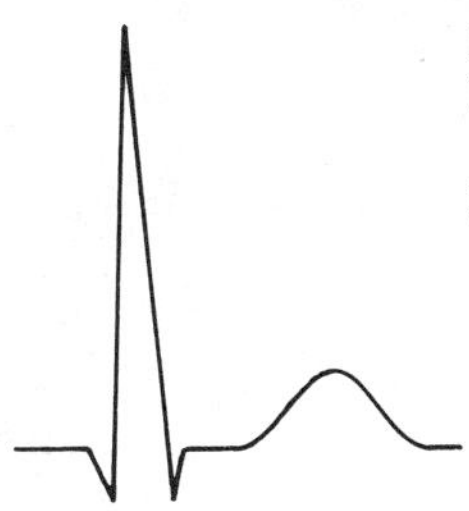

C

Normal QRS complex
No visible P wave, or retrograde P wave before or after QRS complex
PR interval less than 0.12 sec if retrograde P wave in front of QRS

Ventricular

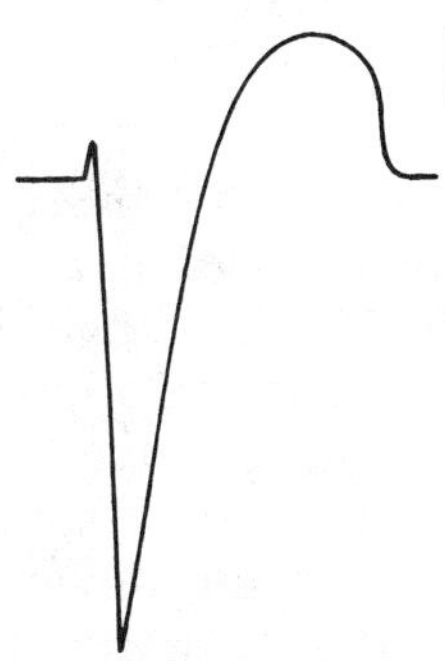

D

No P wave
Wide (greater than 0.12 sec); bizarre QRS complex, with ST segment and T wave going in opposite direction of main QRS deflection

INTERPRETATIONS

1.

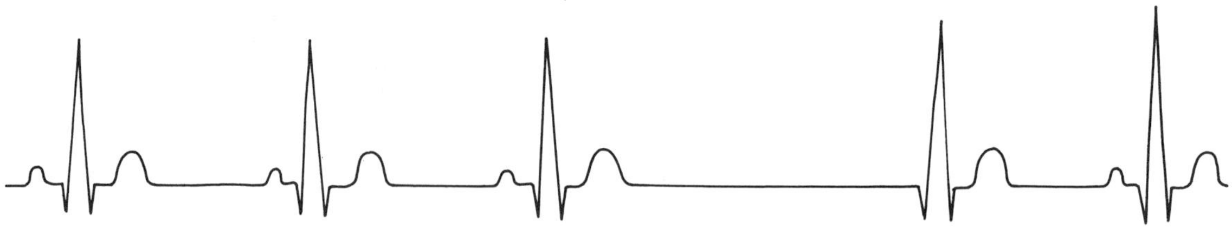

This example shows normal sinus beats in a regular rhythm, but then there is a pause in the rhythm with no sinus complex. The pause is ended by a late beat that has a normal QRS complex but no visible P wave. The last beat is normal. This strip would be interpreted as normal sinus rhythm (NSR) with a sinus arrest and a junctional escape beat.

2.

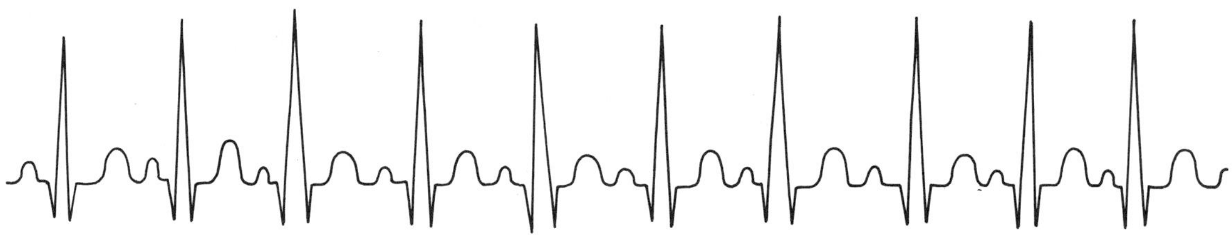

This strip shows one sinus beat after the other, at a rapid rate, and would be interpreted as a sinus tachycardia.

3.

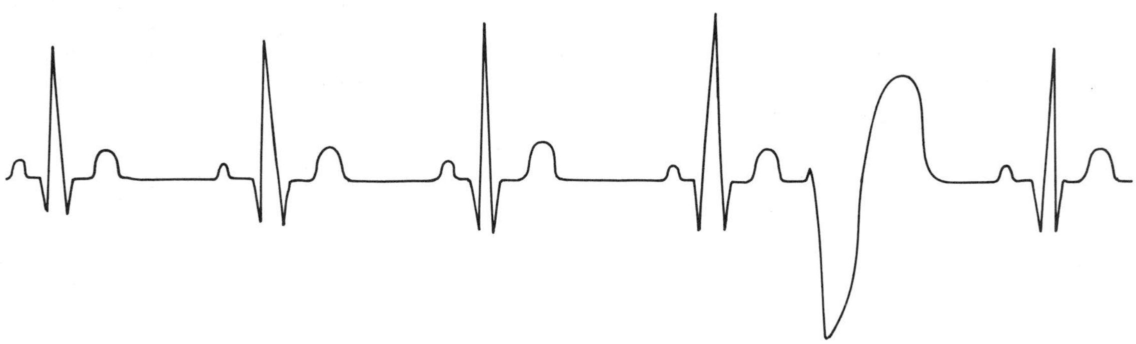

This third example shows sinus beats that are occurring in a regular rhythm at a normal rate, but suddenly an early beat interrupts the sinus beats. The early beat is wide and bizarre, with the ST segment and T wave going in the opposite direction from the main QRS deflection, and it has no P wave. This strip should be interpreted as NSR with one premature ventricular contraction (PVC).

Perhaps these simplified examples of the way dysrhythmias appear will show that watching for the changes in beat configuration can help in making an interpretation easier. Naturally, a real ECG rhythm strip is not quite as simple to read. Real rhythm strips have artifact, and a normal beat may not be all that easy to find. There is, however, a five-step approach to dysrhythmia interpretation that can make things a little easier when faced with rhythm strip to interpret.

THE SYSTEMATIC APPROACH TO DYSRHYTHMIA INTERPRETATION

Combining knowledge of the development of dysrhythmias and the configuration of beats arising from different areas in the heart with a logical and systematic five-step approach to any rhythm strip, it's possible to come up with a correct and complete interpretation of dysrhythmias. The importance of proceeding in this structured search of the ECG strip cannot be stressed enough. Thorough examination of each of the five parameters will ensure that no abnormalities are overlooked. A quick glance at a dysrhythmia may uncover some obvious abnormalities, but some more subtle changes may be missed. The less obvious problems may be more serious than the blatant abnormalities that are readily observed. In order to ensure the correct treatment, all abnormalities must be found and identified.

The five parameters to be investigated are the rhythm, rate, P waves, PR interval, and QRS duration.

THE RHYTHM

When looking at the rhythm, it is helpful to know the different ways it can vary. It may be regular, irregular, or regularly irregular.

A regular rhythm means just that. All the beats are equally distant from each other. However, human beings are somewhat unpredictable in many ways, and their ECGs are no exception. If the rate is within a normal range of 60 to 100 beats per minute, the beats may be slightly irregular and still be considered regular. If there is no more than three small, 1-mm squares of variation between beats, the rhythm may still be called regular. At tachycardic rates over 100 beats per minute, the 3-mm leeway in the regularity of rhythm does not apply.

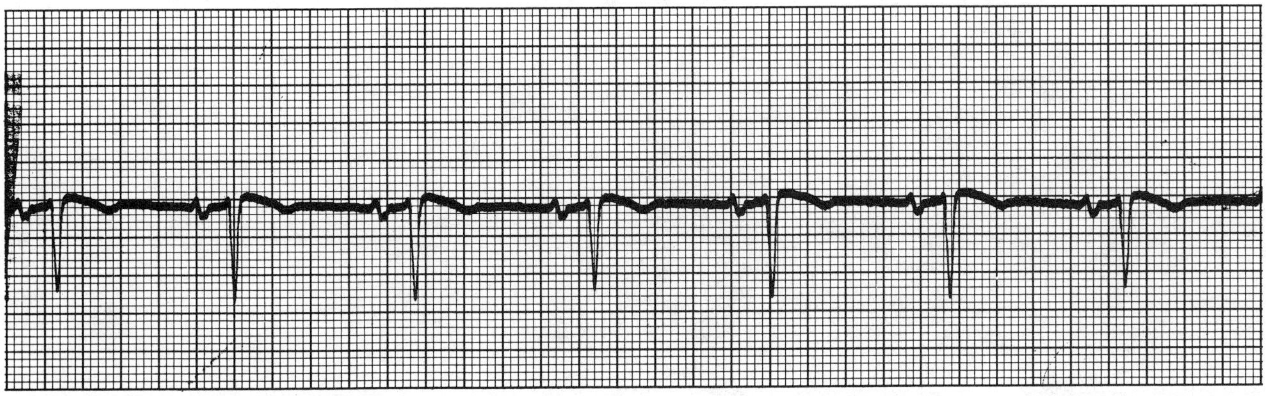

Regular rhythm

If the rhythm is irregular, you must determine how it is irregular. It may be totally irregular, with no pattern to the irregularity.

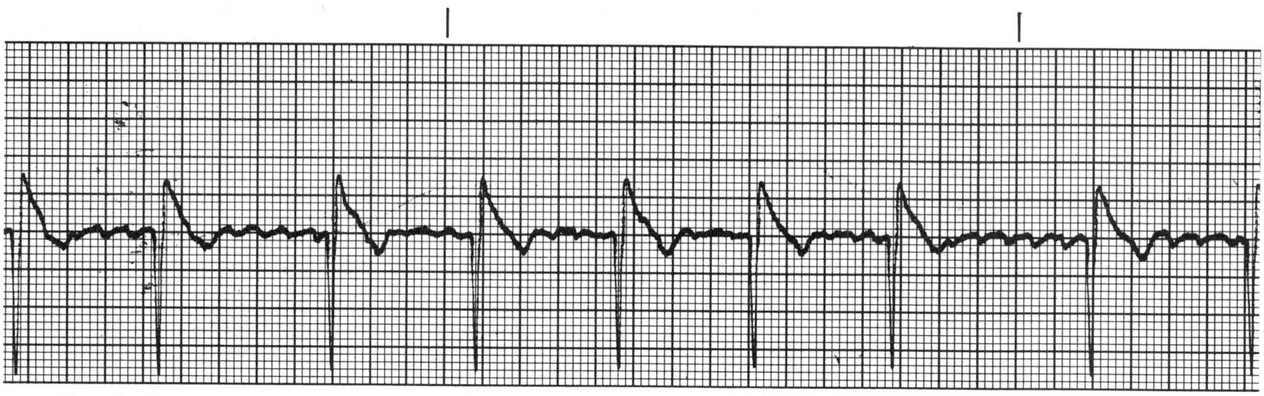

Irregular rhythm

It may be a regular underlying rhythm, but may contain early beats, late beats, or pauses that make the overall pattern irregular.

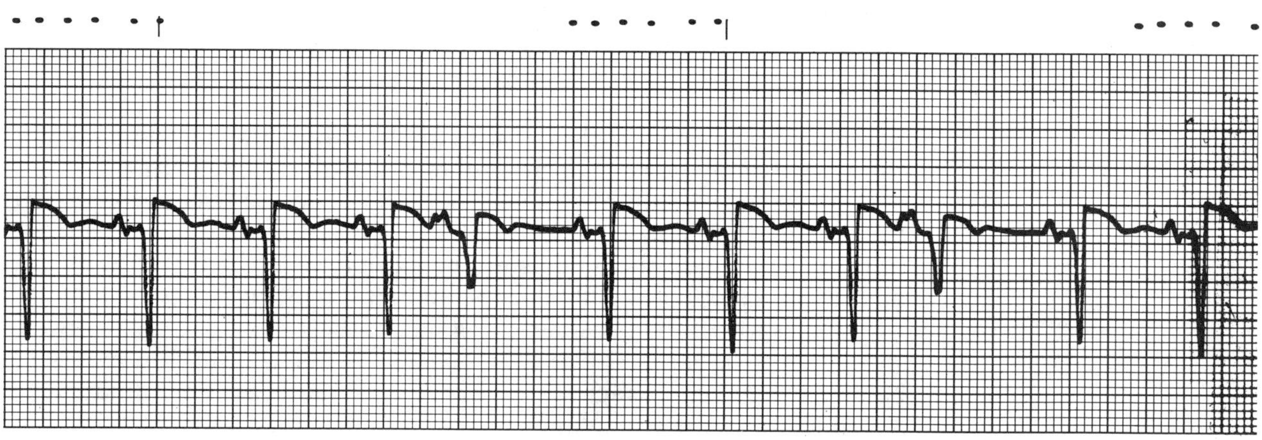

Regular rhythm with early beats

It may be irregular because the rate is changing, either speeding up or slowing down, or both speeding and slowing.

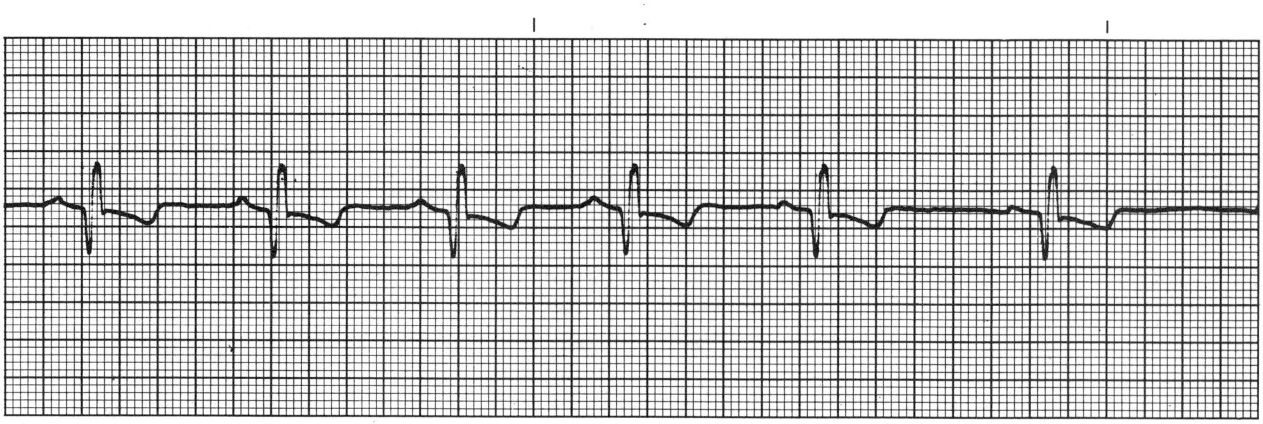

Irregular rhythm/changing rate

The rhythm may be irregular in a repeating pattern that makes it regular in its irregularity.

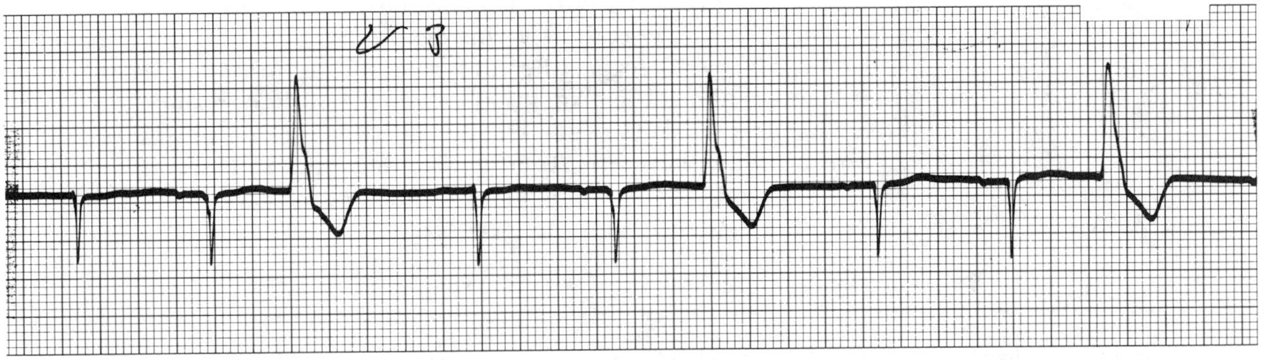

Regular-irregular rhythm

Another thing that must be examined is whether or not the atrial and ventricular rhythms are both regular. There are certain dysrhythmias with a difference in atrial and ventricular rhythms as one of their chief characteristics.

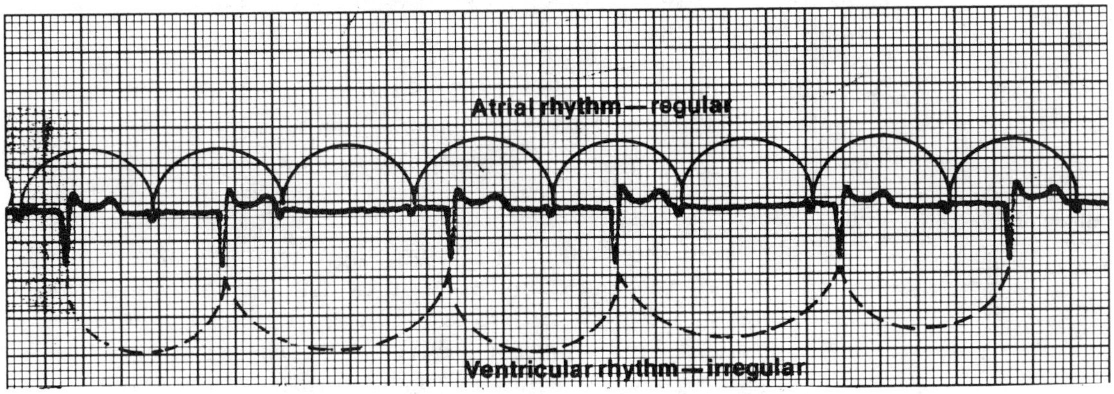

Atrial and ventricular rhythm patterns

When looking at the atrial rhythm, you obviously measure from P wave to P wave—the P-to-P interval. Of course, the ventricular rhythm is determined by clocking between QRS complexes—the R-to-R interval.

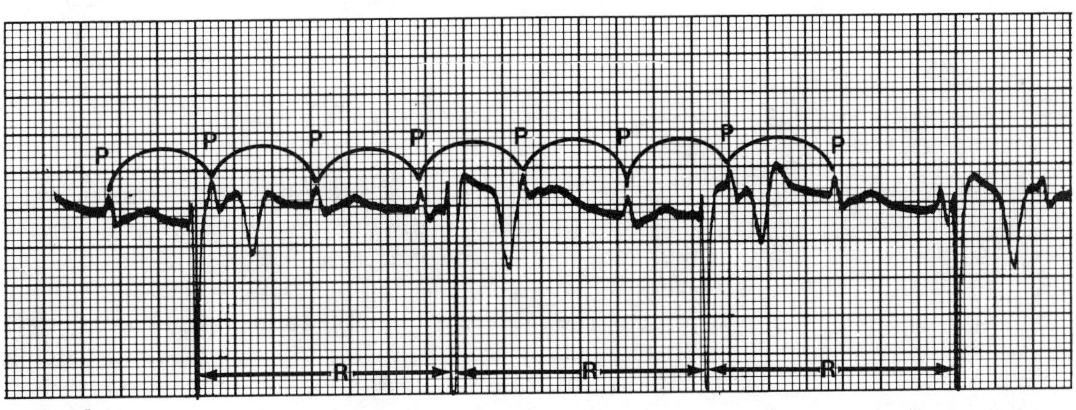

P-to-P and R-to-R intervals

THE RATE

The method of rate measurement is determined by the rhythm. If the rhythm is irregular, the best means of determining the rate is to take a 6-second ECG strip, count the number of complexes in the 6 seconds, and multiply by 10 to get the rate per minute. Most ECG paper has time markers above the grid, every 3 seconds, although some manufacturers put the markers every second. If, for some reason, the markers are not present, there are 30 large, 5-mm blocks in 6 seconds of ECG paper. Remember, the paper moves under the stylus of the ECG machine at the rate of 25 mm per second.

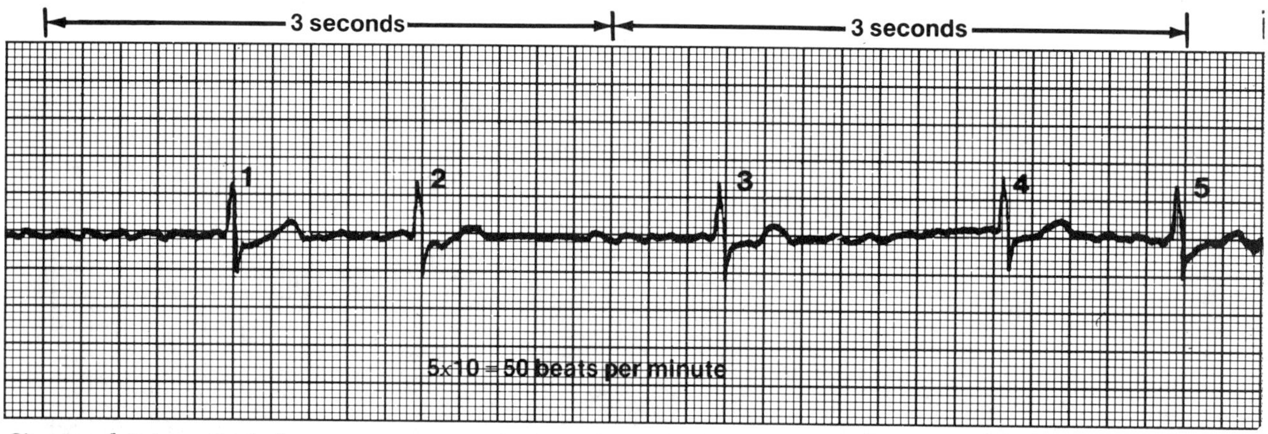

Six-second strip method of rate determination

If the rhythm is regular, there is a way of arriving at a more accurate rate than that obtained by using the 6-second strip method. This more accurate method is based on the fact that there are 1500 1-mm squares in 1 minute of ECG paper. The most accurate way of determining the rate would be to count the number of 1-mm squares between complexes, and divide that number into 1500, which would give you the rate per minute. However, this method is somewhat cumbersome, so a rate table has been devised making use of the fact that there are 1500 1-mm squares in 1 minute.

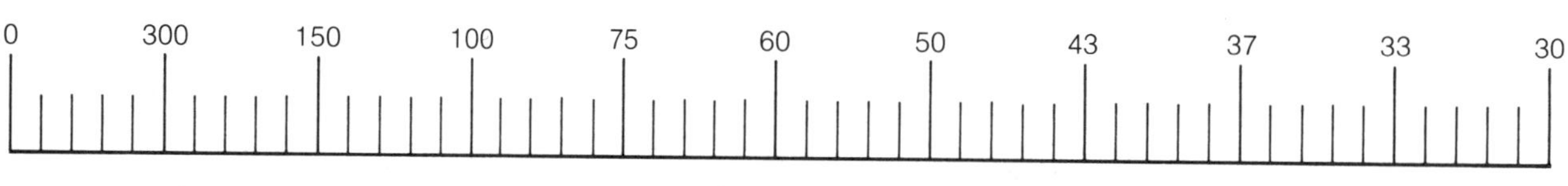

If there are five 1-mm squares or one large 5-mm block between complexes, the rate (by dividing 5 into 1500) would be 300 per minute. If there are ten 1-mm squares or two large 5-mm blocks between complexes, the rate would be 150 per minute (1500 ÷ 10), and so on. If you memorize the rate for each of the large 5-mm blocks, you can determine the rate quickly with no math or tools such as rate calculators involved.

Now, this really sounds simple, but what happens when the number of squares between complexes is not a multiple of the five small 1-mm squares? Perhaps there are 13 1-mm squares between QRS complexes. What can you do then? You could divide the 13 1-mm squares into 1500 and get the rate (115.3846). But this is a lot of trouble, and do you really need a rate that accurate? There is a shortcut that gives a reasonably accurate rate and, better still, doesn't take a lot of time or require a pocket calculator. If we go back to the rate scale, and refine it a little, it becomes useful, no matter how many small squares are between the complexes.

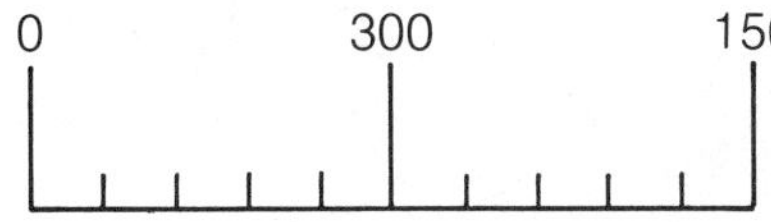

If you look at the rate scale, between the 300 mark and the 150 mark, there are five small squares. The difference in rate between 300 and 150 is 150 beats per minute. If you divide the 150-beat difference by the five small squares, each square would be worth 30 beats per minute. So, if we filled in the rates for each small square, it would look like this:

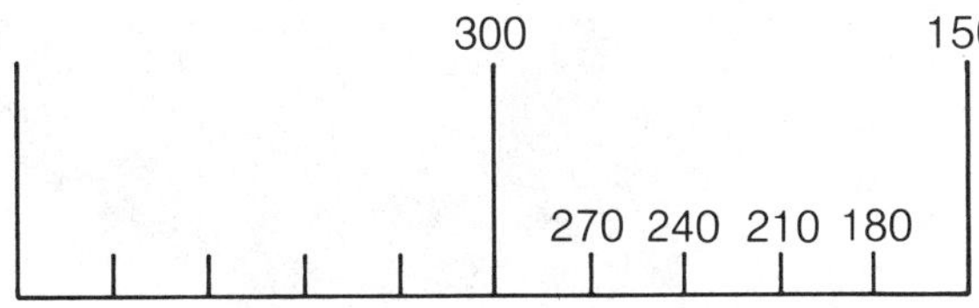

If there were seven small squares between complexes, the rate per minute would be 240.

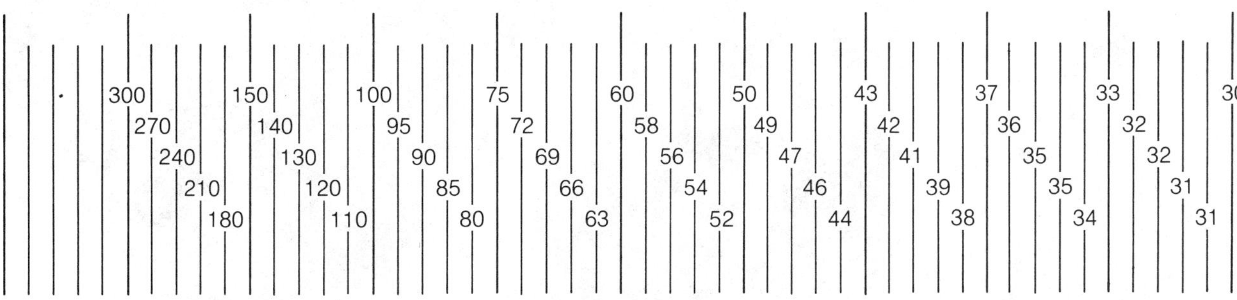

Between 150 and 100, there is a difference of 50 beats per minute. Dividing the 50-beat difference by the five small squares determines that the rate goes by increments of 10 beats per minute between 150 and 100. Between 100 and 75, the rate increments go by 5 beats per minute. Between 75 and 60, the rate changes by increments of 3 beats per minute. Between 60 and 50, it changes by 2 beats per minute; between 50 and 43, by 1.5; below 43, each square equals about 1 beat per minute.

This method does not give exact rates, but is close enough for purposes of dysrhythmia interpretation. The beauty of this method is that one carries everything needed to figure out the rate around in their head, not their pocket. It's necessary to memorize the 300–150–100 and so forth markers, but as this tool is used, it becomes second nature. Eventually, it becomes automatic knowledge that the rate changes in increments of 5 beats per minute between 100 and 75, and so on.

With these two methods of rate determination, one can discover the rate of any dysrhythmia. ECG calipers make the task much easier. Setting the interval between two complexes, and moving the caliper points across the strip determines whether the rhythm is regular or not. By using that one-interval set on the calipers, put the left-hand caliper point on a dark line, and starting with the *next* dark 5-mm line, count 300–150– and so forth, and get the rate. Without calipers, a small strip of paper will suffice. Merely put the edge of the strip of paper under the baseline of the ECG, and mark the interval between two complexes on the paper strip. Then use the two marks on the paper strip as caliper points. I would recommend investing in a pair of calipers for work with monitored patients. It really will make dysrhythmia interpretation a lot easier (Fig. 4-1).

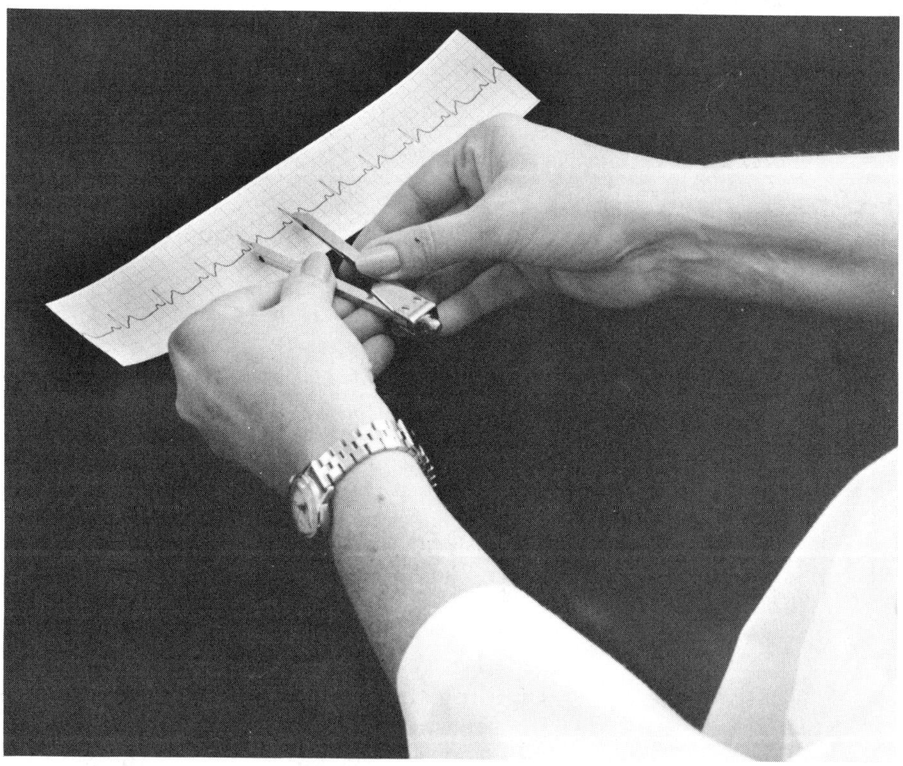

Figure 4-1 Demonstration of the use of calipers to determine rhythm and regularity of heart rate.

Now, knowing the two methods of rate determination, here are some examples of ECG rhythm strips to practice on.

Rate Strip Interpretation

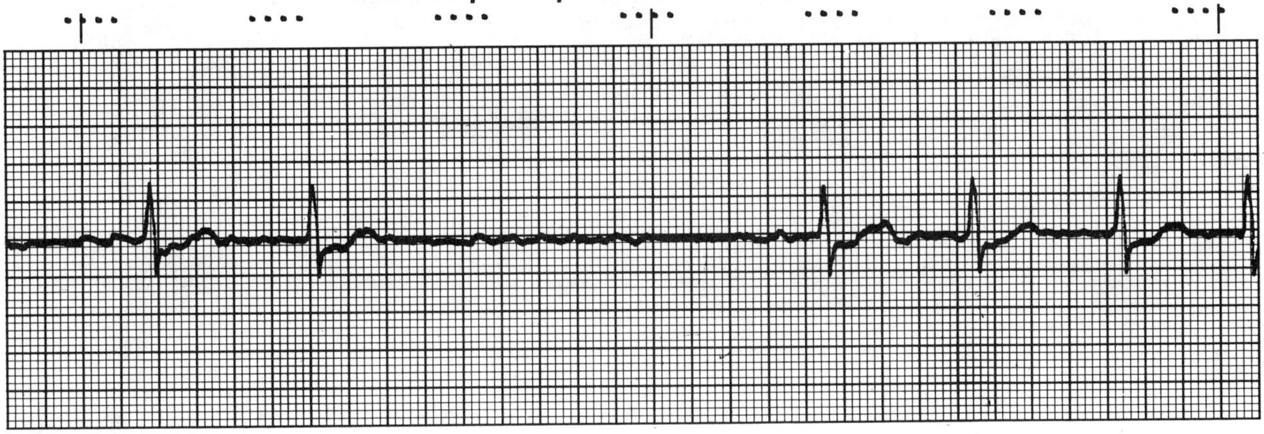

Practice strip 1

Practice Strip 1. This rhythm strip is quite obviously irregular, so the appropriate way to determine the rate is with the 6-second strip method. There are five QRS complexes within the two 3-second markers at the top of the strip. Multiplying the five QRSs by 10, you arrive at the rate, which is 50 beats per minute.

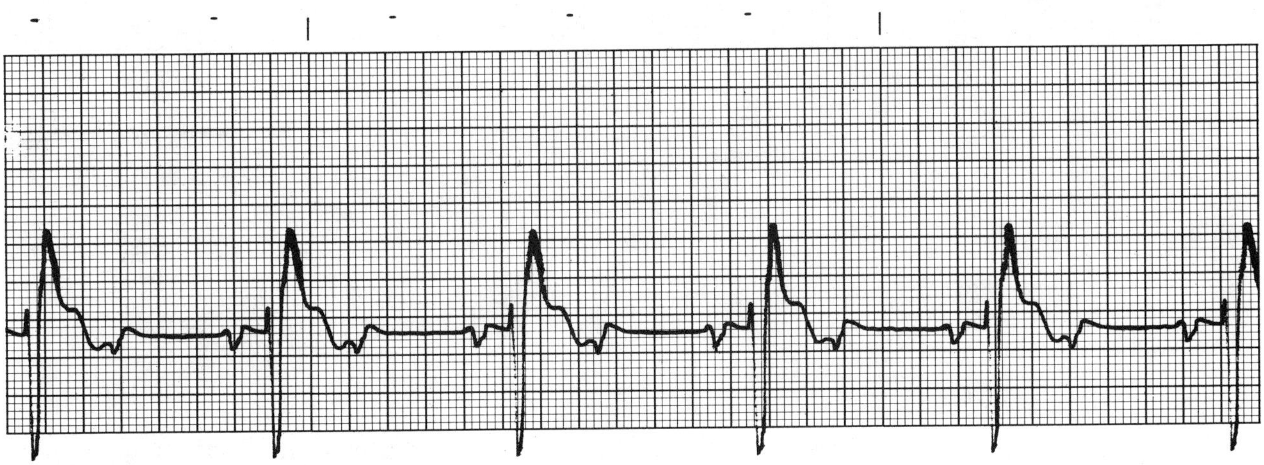

Practice strip 2

Practice Strip 2. In this strip, there are more P waves than QRS complexes, so the atrial rate will be greater than the ventricular rate. Both rhythms are regular, so the 300–150–100 method is the most accurate way to find the rate. There are three large blocks and one small square between P waves, so the atrial rate is 95 beats per minute. There are six large blocks and two small squares between the QRS complexes, so the ventricular rate is 47 beats per minute.

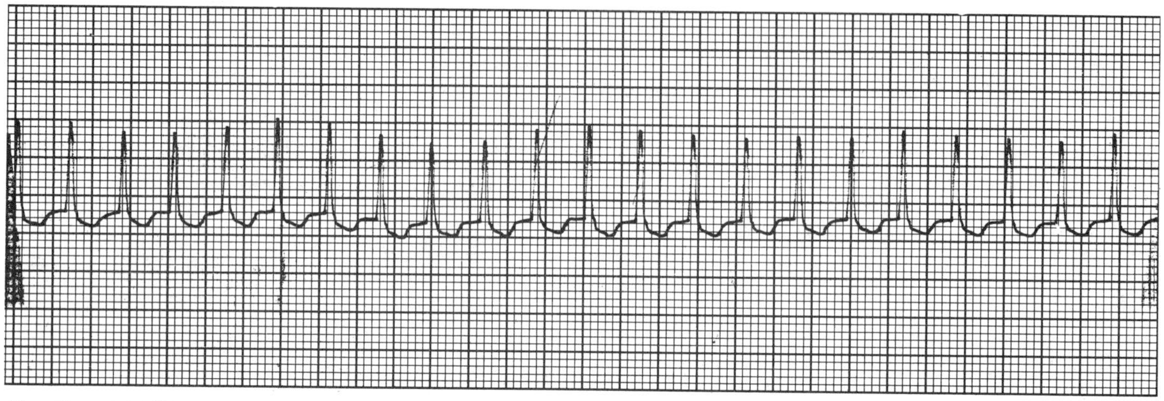

Practice strip 3

Practice Strip 3. This fast rhythm is regular and there are one large and two small squares between QRS complexes. The ventricular rate is 240 beats per minute. There is no obvious atrial activity, so the atrial rate cannot be determined.

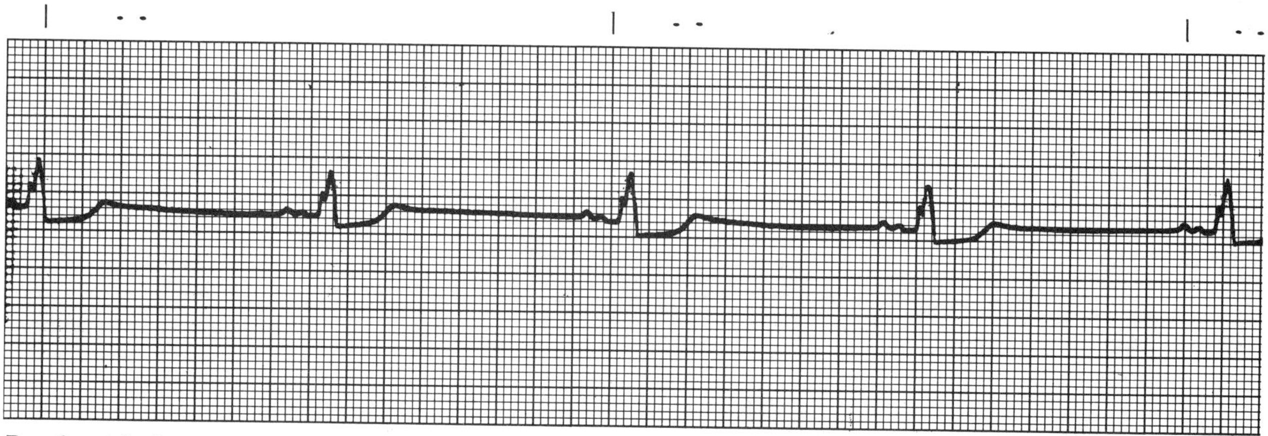

Practice strip 4

Practice Strip 4. This very slow rhythm is slightly irregular, but there is not more than three, small squares difference between complexes. Thus, it is considered regular. There are eight large blocks between complexes, so the rate is 37 beats per minute. All the P waves and QRS complexes are related, so the atrial and ventricular rates are identical.

Knowing the whys and hows of rate determination, let's look at the whats, namely, what to look for. First of all, what is the rate? Is it fast? Or slow? If the rhythm changes abruptly, what is the new rate? In a rhythm that is irregular only because there are early or late beats, but with a regular underlying rhythm, find the rate of the regular beats.

Determine if the atrial and ventricular rates are the same. If all the P waves and QRS complexes are connected, then, of course, the atrial and ventricular rates will be the same. But the two rates will be different if P waves are present without QRS complexes, or QRS complexes without P waves. Of course, the atrial rate is determined by measuring the P-to-P interval, and the ventricular rate by using the R-to-R interval.

THE P WAVES After assessing the rhythm and the rate, the next parameter to examine is the P wave. Determine if there are P waves present in front of all beats. Also, compare the configuration of the P waves; they should all be the same shape. P waves should be no wider than 0.11 second. Again, it is necessary to know what the normal P wave for this patient looks like in the lead being observed. If there is an FLB, look carefully to determine if there is a P wave associated with it. If there are no obvious P waves present, examine the strip for some other form of atrial activity such as flutter or fibrillation waves.

THE PR INTERVAL The first thing to determine is the length of the PR interval. Is it within the normal range of 0.12 to 0.20 second? To find the PR interval, begin measuring where the slope of the P wave first leaves the isoelectric line. Stop measuring at the first deflection of the QRS complex, whether it goes in a negative or positive direction. If the first deflection of the QRS complex is negative or downward in direction, what is really being measured is a PQ interval, not a PR. After measuring the PR interval of what has been determined to be a normal beat, check to see that all the PR intervals have the same duration. If the PR intervals change, see if there is a pattern to the change. Or, are they all different, with no pattern? Also check the PR intervals of any FLBs that are present.

Measure the following PR intervals

1.

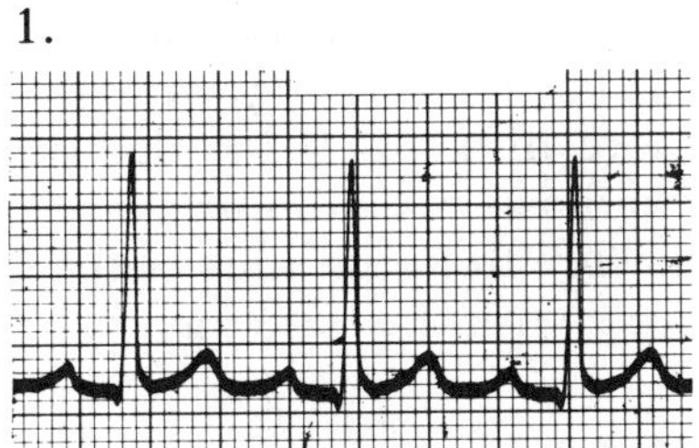

2.

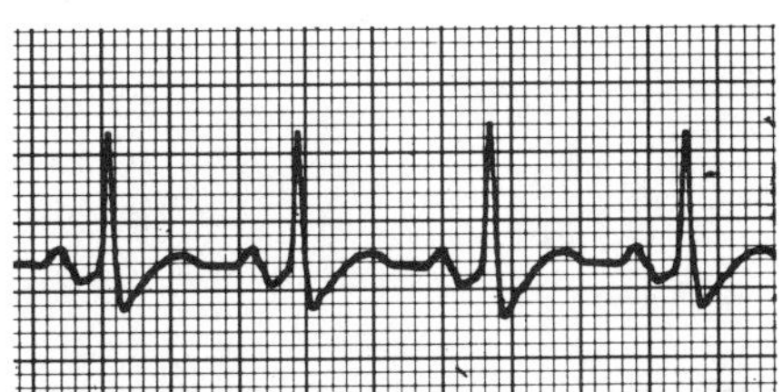

3.

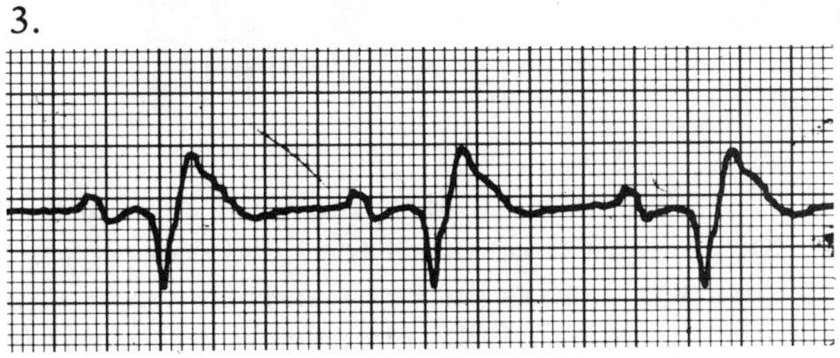

Answers

1. The PR interval in this strip measures 0.20 second.

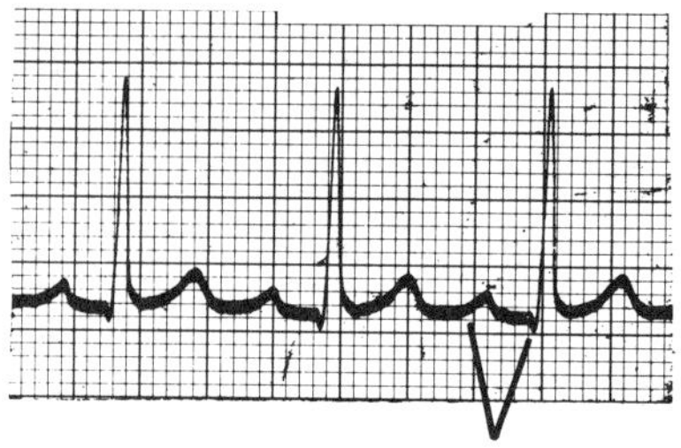

2. The PR interval in this strip measures 0.16 second.

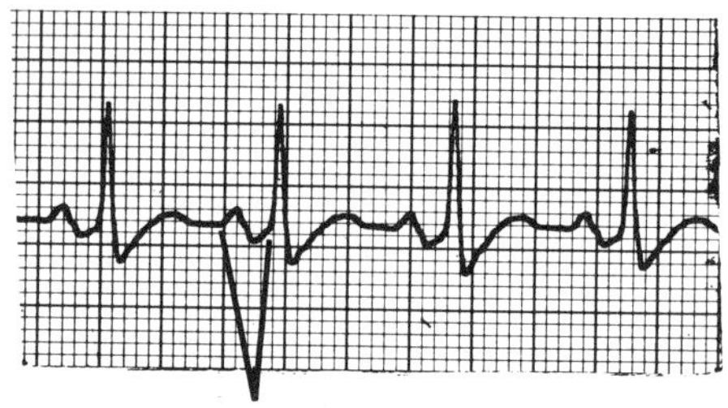

3. The PR interval in this strip measures 0.28 second.

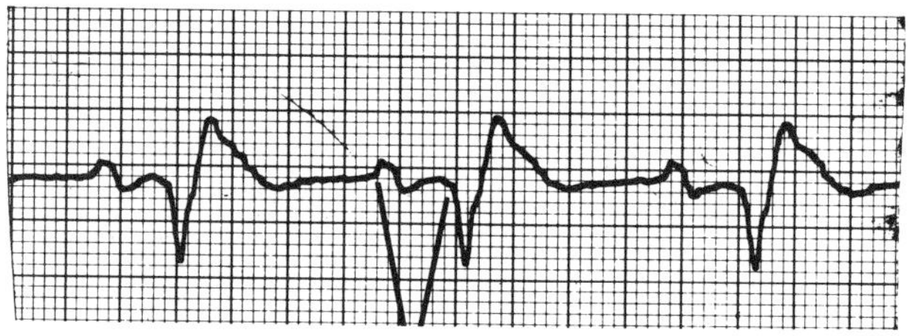

THE QRS DURATION The QRS complex should measure between 0.06 to 0.12 second. Begin measuring the QRS complex from the end of the PR interval measurement. The QRS duration ends at an arbitrary place called the J junction or J point. The J junction is defined as that point where the S wave stops and the ST segment starts. The J junction may be located right on the baseline, making the measurement simple. Unfortunately, when the ST segment becomes displaced by injury or drugs, the J junction gets pulled along with the ST segment, making the measurement more difficult. If the decision is that the J junction is located above the baseline, drop an imaginary line from the J to the baseline and measure from the start of the QRS to the place the imaginary line intersects with the baseline.

Isoelectric

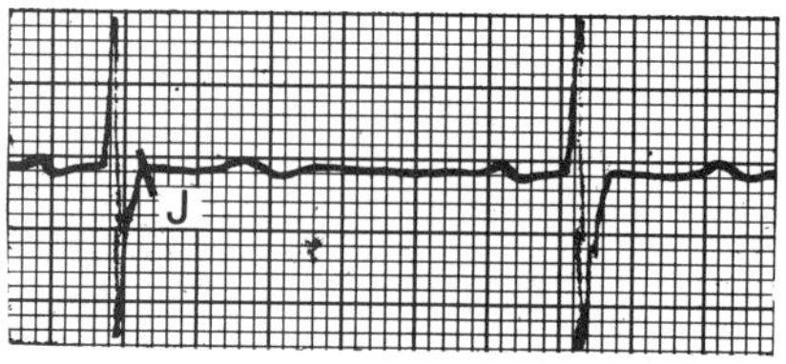

Elevated

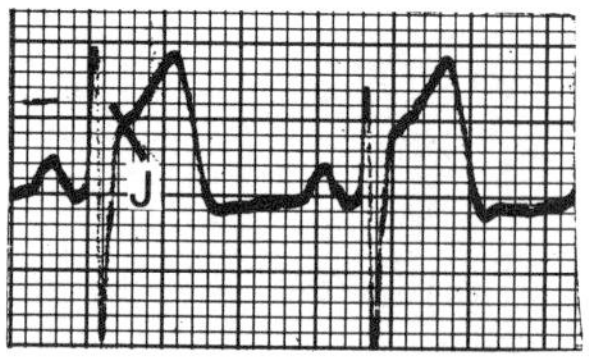

Depressed

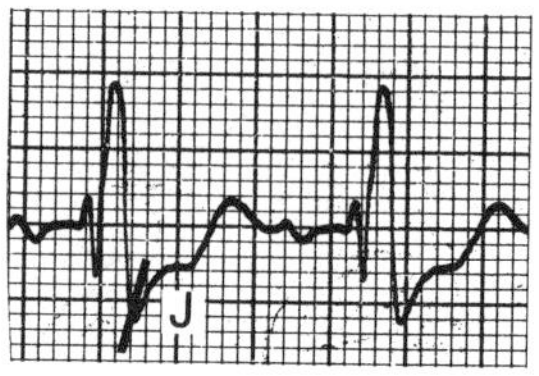

After determining the QRS duration of the normal beats, check the configuration of all the QRS complexes for any change in shape or duration. Also be sure that every P wave is followed by a QRS complex, and that every QRS complex is preceded by a P wave.

Mark the J junction and measure the QRS duration on the following strips.

1.

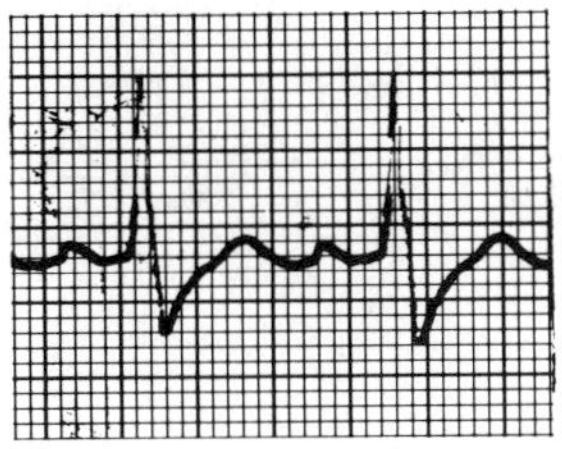

2.

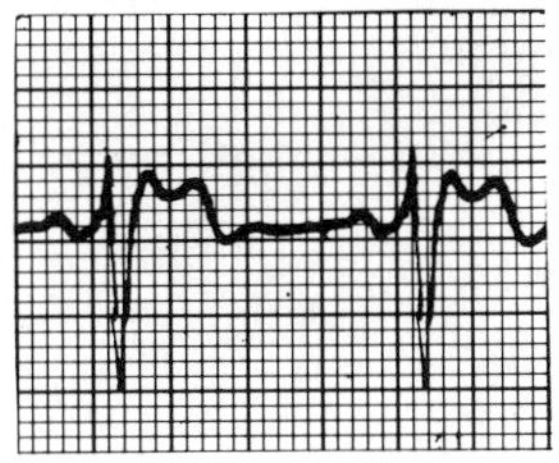

3.

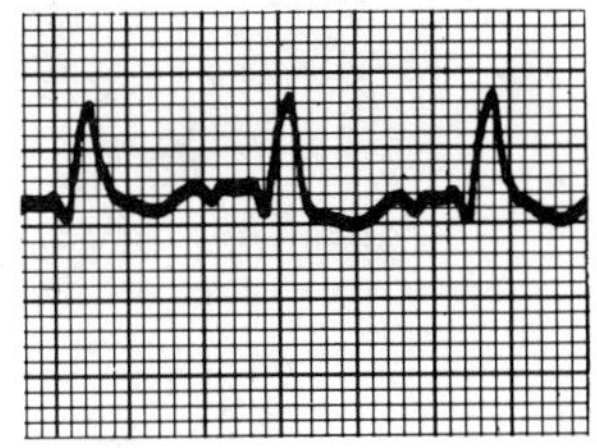

4.

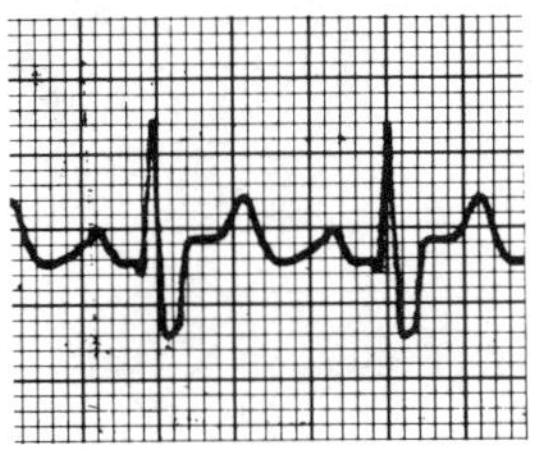

5.

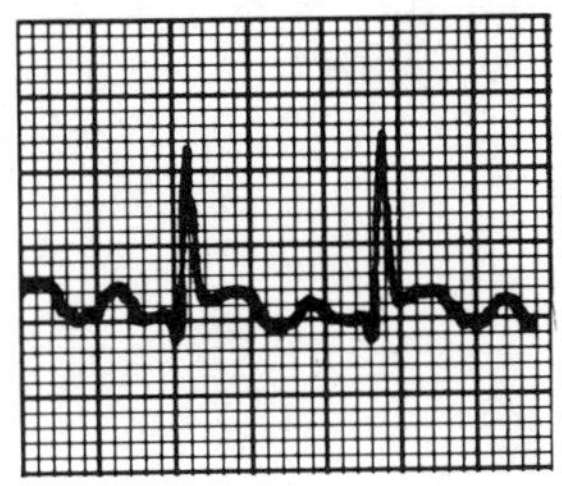

6.

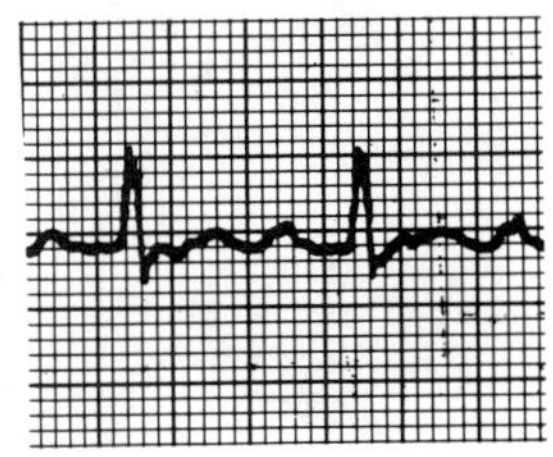

Answers

1.

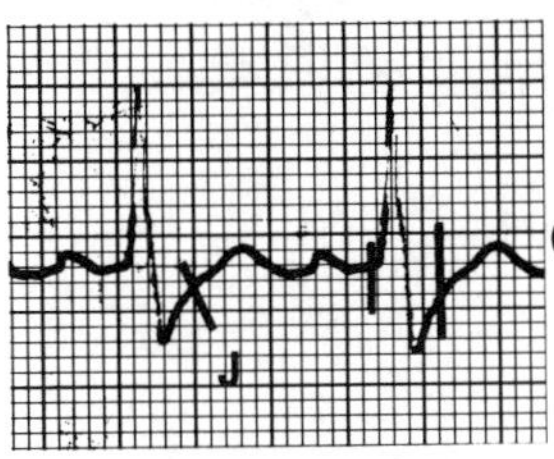

0.16 second

2.

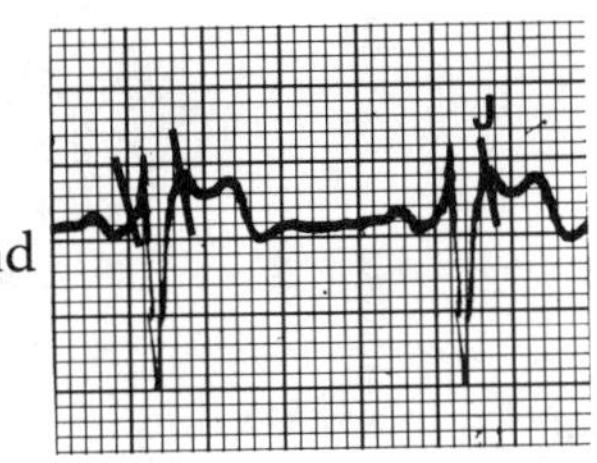

0.12 second

3.

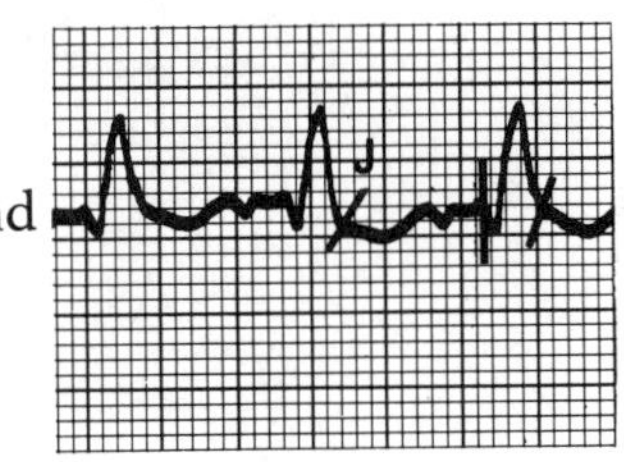

0.20 second

4.

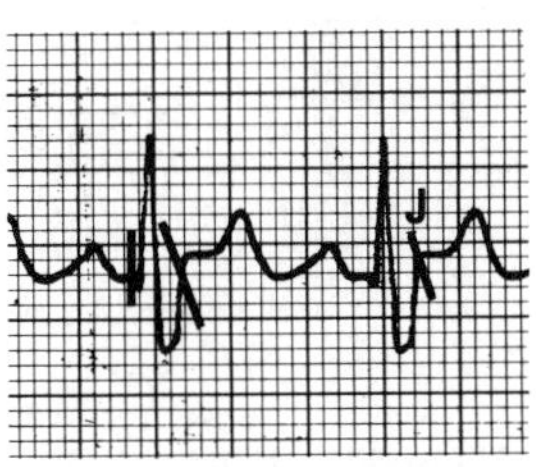

0.14 second

5.

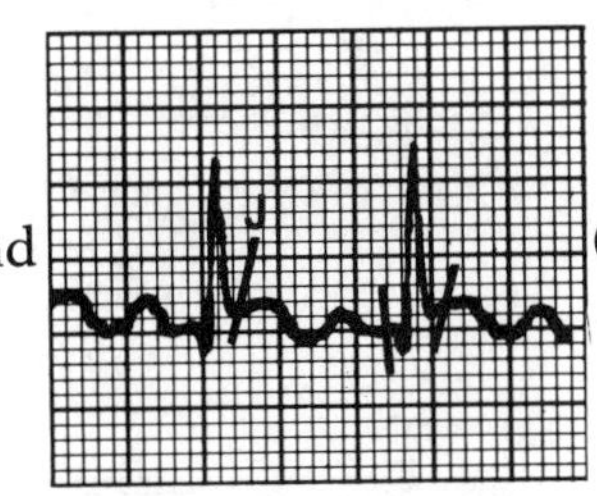

0.10 second

6.

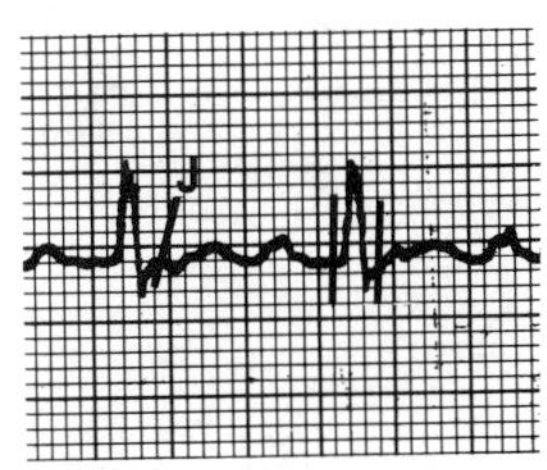

0.12 second

THE INTERPRETATION Once all five parameters have been thoroughly examined, all of the information that is needed to make a complete and correct interpretation of any dysrhythmia is available. When making the interpretation, first mention the underlying rhythm, if present, and then include any other abnormalities or rhythm changes, *e.g.*, NSR with multifocal PVCs or sinus bradycardia with first degree AV block.

Measure the PR interval, QRS duration, and rate on the following tracings.

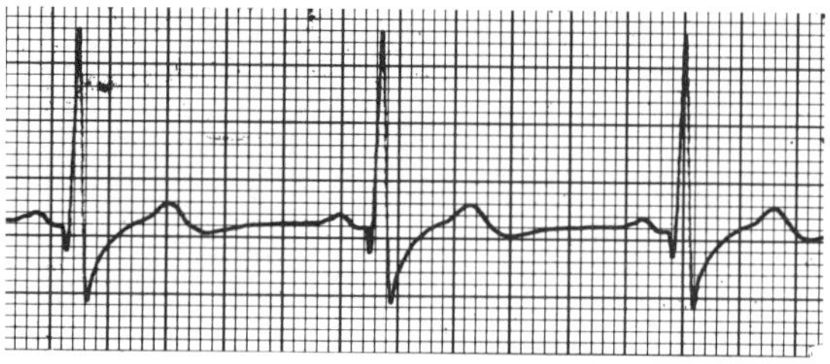

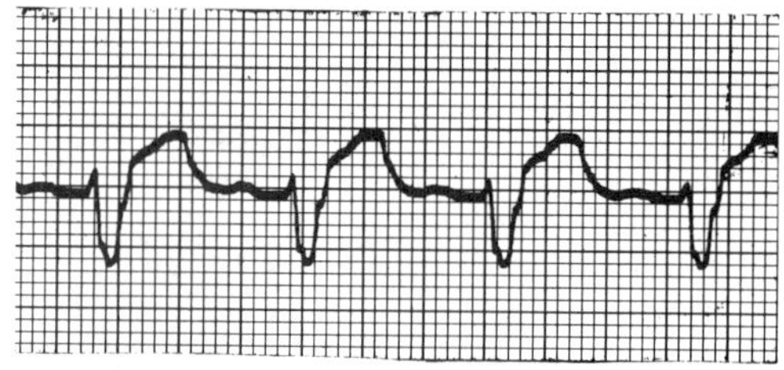

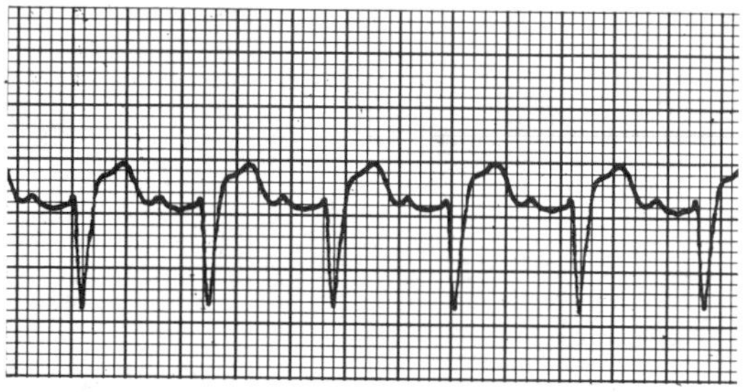

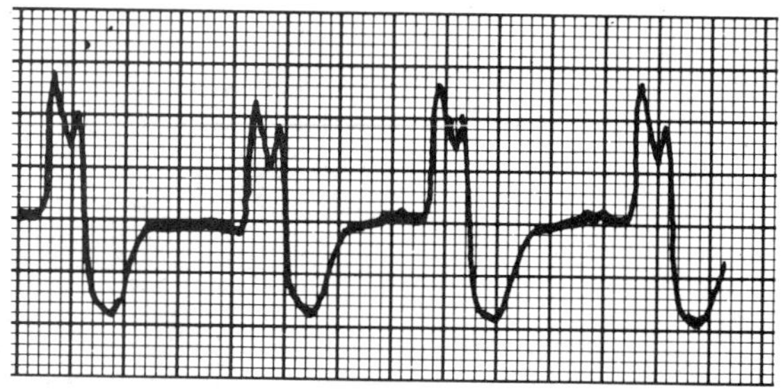

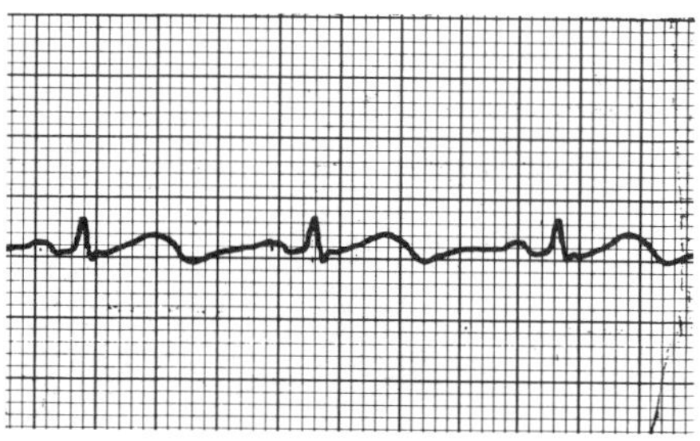

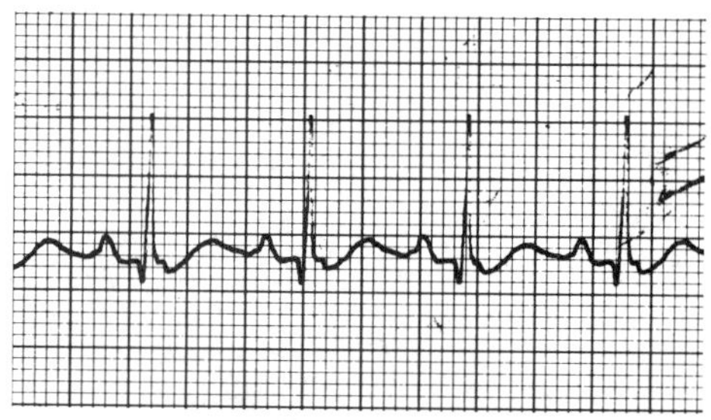

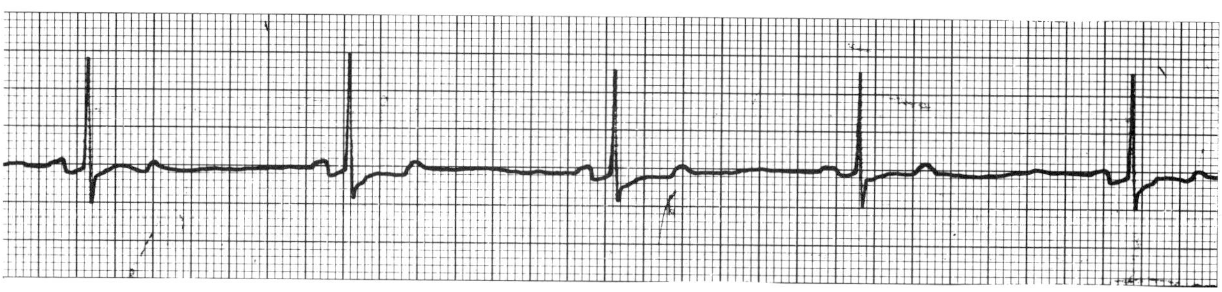

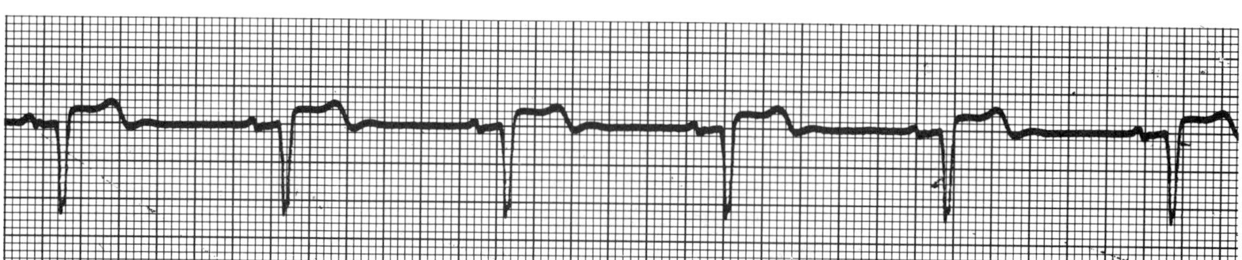

Answers

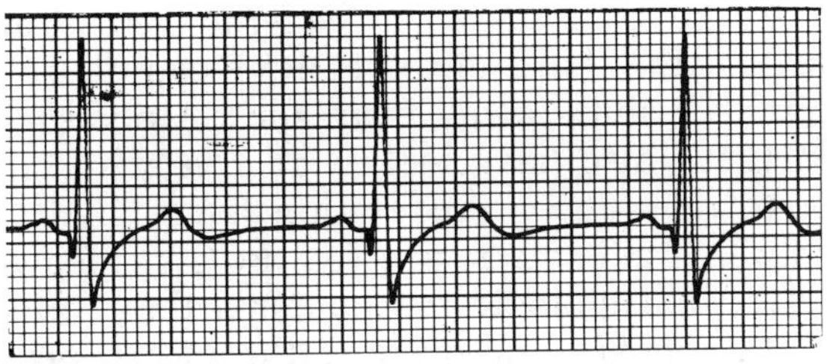

Rate: 58 PR: 0.16 QRS: 0.12

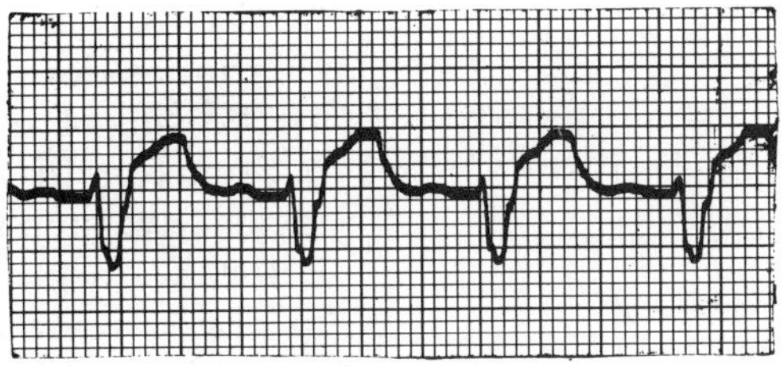

Rate: 95 PR: 0.20 QRS: 0.14

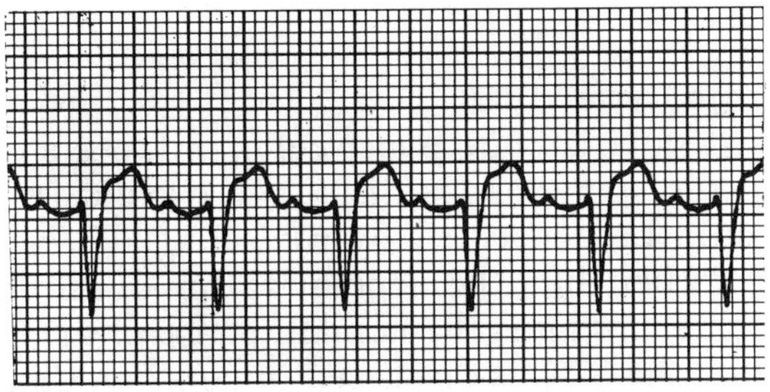

Rate: 135 PR: 0.16 QRS: 0.10

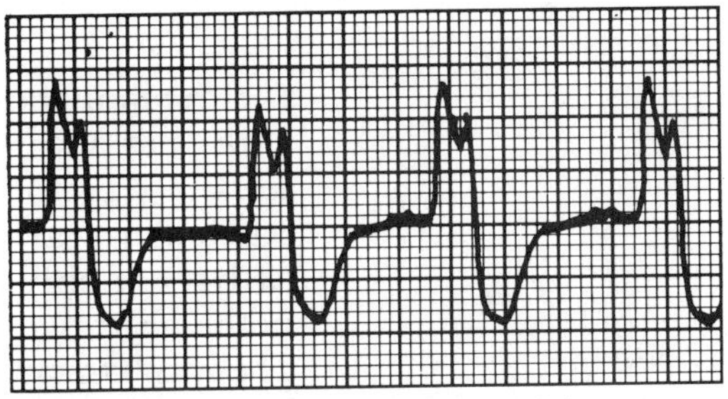

Rate: 85 PR: 0.16 QRS: 0.16

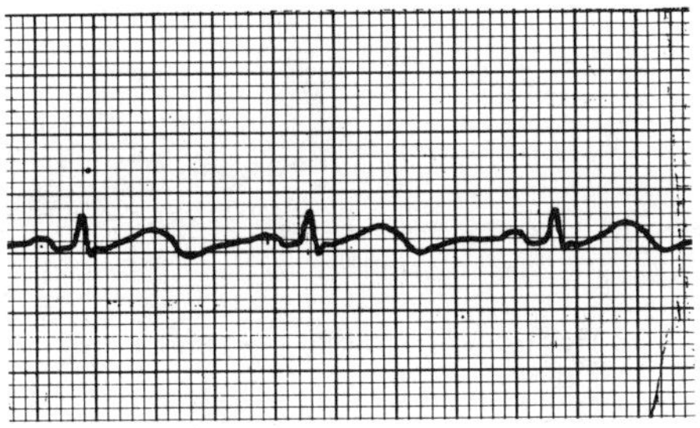

Rate: 80 PR: 0.16 QRS: 0.08

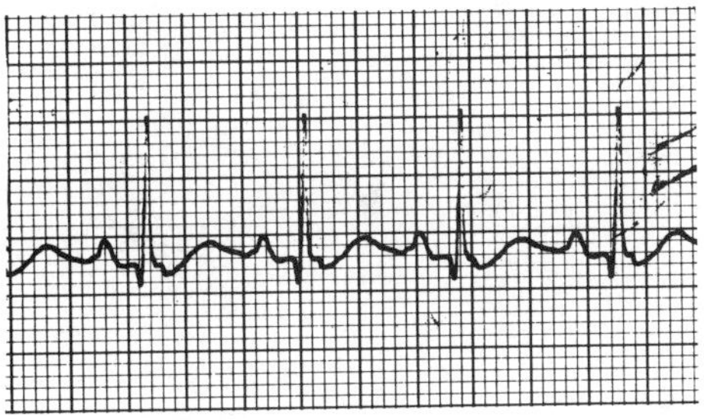

Rate: 110 PR: 0.16 QRS: 0.10

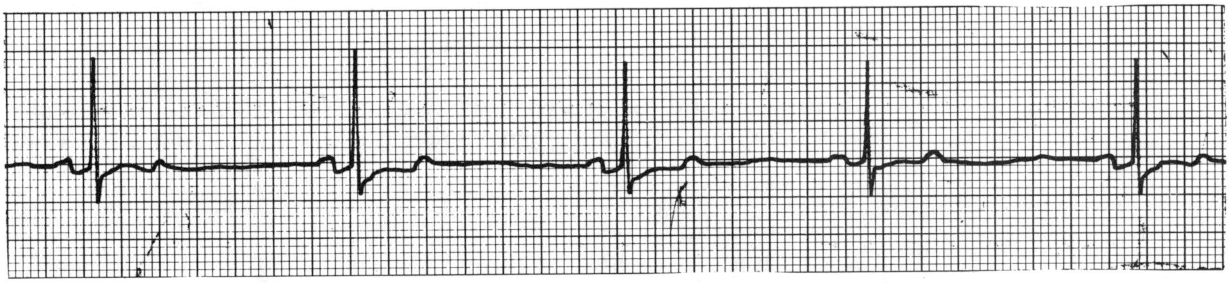

Rate: 50 (6-second strip) PR: 0.20 QRS: 0.06

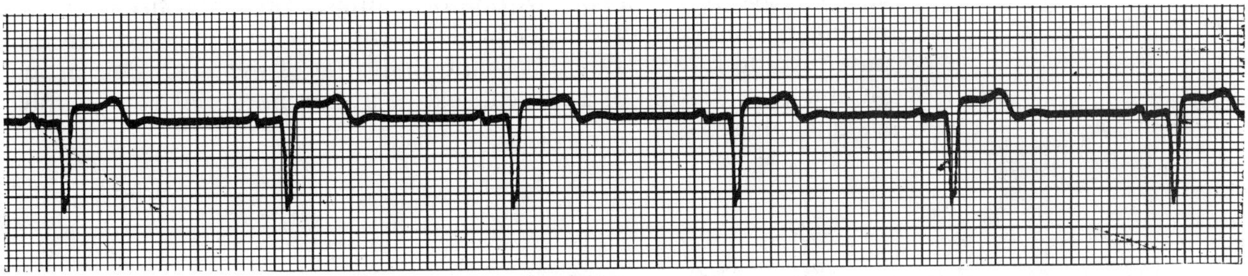

Rate: 52 PR: 0.18 QRS: 0.08

ELECTROPHYSIOLOGY REVIEW

So far in this chapter we have discussed in general terms how dysrhythmias develop and how the shape of the PQRST complex changes as the site of the pacemaker shifts away from the SA node to lower pacemakers in the heart. We also have looked at a very specific and logical five-step method to aid in the interpretation of any rhythm strip. Before we begin to apply this information to real ECG strips, we need to briefly review the electrophysiologic mechanisms that control the normal depolarization of the heart, and produce the special properties inherent in myocardial tissue—automaticity and conductivity.

The Spontaneous Discharge Cycle

Cells that automatically depolarize, the pacer cells, produce a characteristic waveform called the spontaneous discharge cycle (SDC). This particular waveform would be generated by recording the electrical activity of only one cell, rather than the depolarization of all the cells in the heart, which, of course, produces the familiar shape of the PQRST. The mechanism generating the SDC is discussed in detail in Chapter 2, but as a brief review, the SDC has four phases:

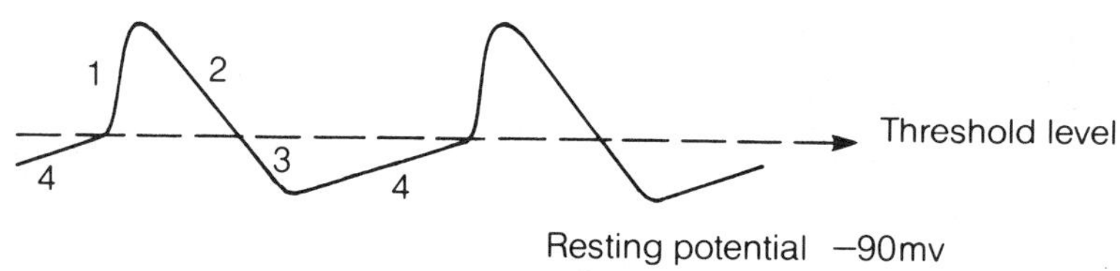

Phase 1—rapid depolarization; *Phase 2*—absolute refractory period; *Phase 3*—repolarization; and *Phase 4*—slow diastolic depolarization.

Every cell in the heart capable of pacemaking activity goes through this process, and the cell with the fastest SDC will be in control of the heart's rhythm. The fastest pacemaker is usually located in the SA node.

Action Potential Curve

Cells with a slower SDC or those with no pacing capabilities are activated by a conducted wave of depolarization from the SA node. If we were to look at the depolarization of a single cell being fired off by a propagated or conducted wave of electrical activity, the waveform generated would have a different shape than that of the SDC. This propagated depolarization of a cell causes the action potential curve, which has four phases.

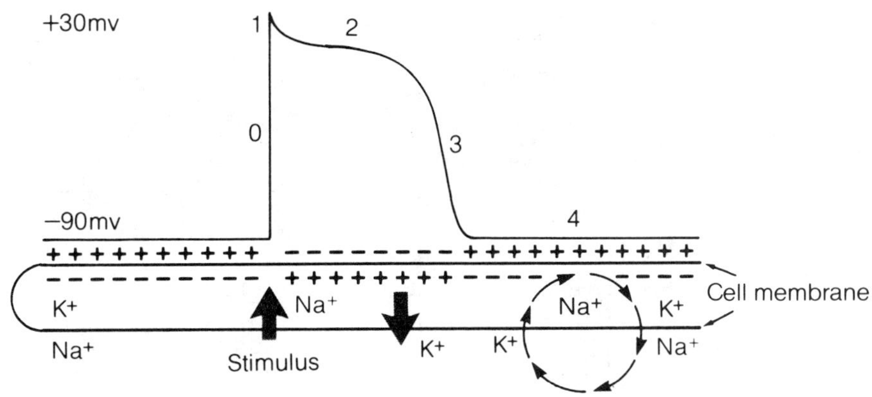

Phases 0 and *1* are produced by depolarization of the cell; *Phase 2* is the absolute refractory period; *Phase 3* is the partial refractory period when repolarization is occurring; and *Phase 4* occurs when the cell has reached its resting potential and is fully repolarized and ready to be stimulated again.

Dysrhythmias will develop because of abnormalities in either automaticity, the SDC, or in conductivity, the action potential. If the SDC of the SA node is altered, different sinus dysrhythmias will result. Greatly slowing the SDC of the SA node permits the development of escape beats on rhythms. If the SDC of an ectopic pacing focus is accelerated, premature beats, tachycardias, flutters, or fibrillation occur. If the conducted wave of depolarization is altered, the AV block or bundle branch block occurs.

Now, to begin our discussion of dysrhythmias, we will look at the SA node, its normal rhythms, and the dysrhythmias that result when its automaticity or conductivity is altered. In each strip, a *normal beat* (if present) is highlighted with a darker tracing.

NORMAL SINUS RHYTHM

Normal sinus rhythm (NSR), the usual rhythm of the heart, results when the SA node is going through its SDC at a rate of 60 to 100 times a minute, and is the fastest pacemaker in the heart. (See strip on following page.)

Criteria

RHYTHM NSR will have a regular rhythm, but the R-to-R interval may vary as much as three small squares and still be considered regular.

RATE The rate will be between 60 to 100 beats a minute.

P WAVES The most important criterion for NSR is the presence of a normal P wave in front of every QRS complex. The term *normal* P wave is a relative one, and means normal for that particular patient in the lead being monitored.

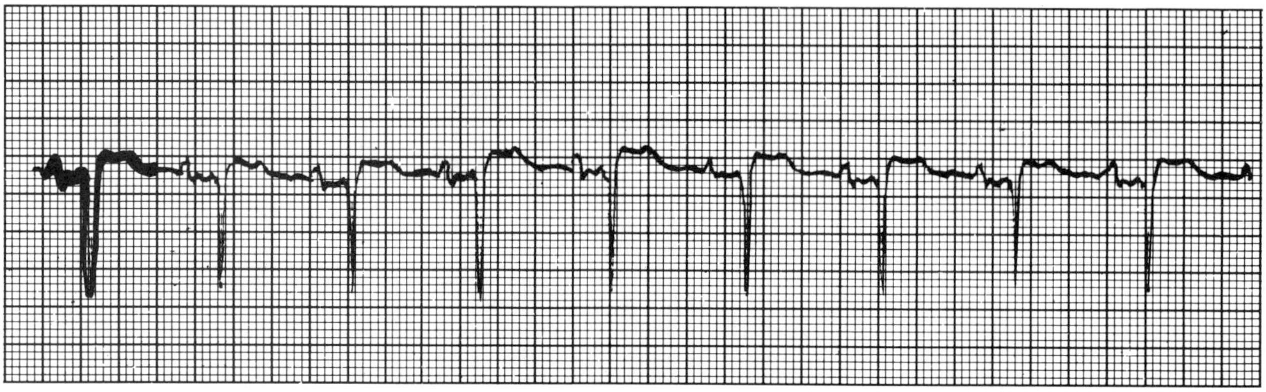

Normal sinus rhythm

PR INTERVAL Assuming there are no conduction defects present in the AV node, the PR interval should be within the normal limits of 0.12 to 0.20 second. The PR interval should be constant in each beat.

QRS DURATION Assuming there are no conduction defects present in the bundle branches, the QRS duration should be within the normal limits of 0.06 to 0.12 second. All the QRS complexes should have the same configuration and be preceded by a P wave.

Actually, all the criteria for NSR are met when there is a regular rhythm, at a rate of 60 to 100 per minute, with normal P waves. If there are no conduction problems lower in the heart, then the PR interval and QRS duration also will be normal. But either or both of these measurements could be prolonged or abnormal when conduction defects are present; however, the underlying rhythm will still be NSR.

Hemodynamic Effects

NSR produces the most effective cardiac contraction and provides a normal cardiac output if the contractility of the myocardium is unaltered. The normal rate of NSR allows adequate time for ventricular filling between beats, thus providing an optimal stroke volume. The presence of a P wave and a normal PR interval ensures that atrial contraction occurs at the optimal time before ventricular stimulation, thus providing the 15% to 30% of atrial kick that produces the most effective contraction of the ventricular myocardium (Starling's law).

Therapy

Obviously, no treatment is needed for NSR.

SINUS ARRHYTHMIA

Sinus arrhythmia is a variation of NSR still considered a normal rhythm in most circumstances. Sinus arrhythmia occurs when changing intrathoracic pressure due to the respiratory cycle causes increases and decreases in vagal stimulation to the SA node, thus accelerating and retarding its SDC. As inhalation occurs, vagal tone decreases, and the rate of SA node depolarization speeds up. Exhalation increases vagal

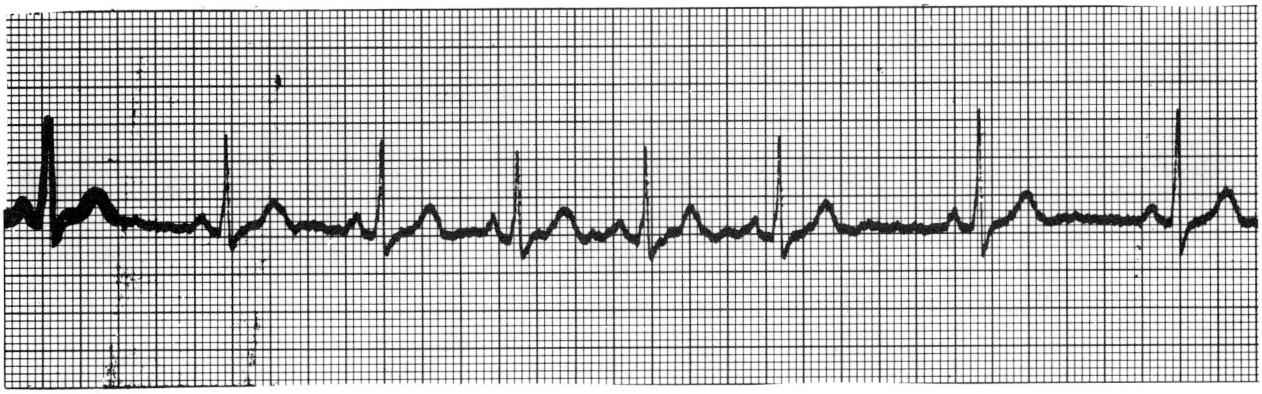

Sinus arrhythmia

tone, which in turn slows the rate of depolarization of the SA node. This phenomenon is frequently seen in children and is also normal in adults. There are also nonrespiratory versions of sinus arrhythmia.

Criteria

RHYTHM The rhythm in sinus arrhythmia will be irregular. It speeds and slows in cycles that may correspond to the patient's respirations.

RATE The rate, which must be determined by the 6-second strip since the rhythm is irregular, will probably be within normal limits. Sometimes there will be a sinus arrhythmia in the presence of a sinus bradycardia.

P WAVES There will be a normal P wave present in front of every QRS complex.

PR INTERVAL The PR interval will be within the normal range of 0.12 to 0.20 second constant throughout the strip if there are no AV conduction defects.

QRS DURATION The QRS complexes will measure between 0.06 and 0.12 second if no conduction defect is present in the bundle branches. Each QRS complex should have the same configuration and should be preceded by a P wave.

Hemodynamic and Clinical Considerations

Sinus arrhythmia will not produce any alteration of the patient's hemodynamic status unless an excess of vagal tone should cause the overall rate to drop into the bradycardic range. Sinus arrhythmia seen with a bradycardic rate is likely to be caused by digitalis toxicity. A nonrespiratory sinus arrhythmia may be caused by cardiac disease, frequently acute MI.

Therapy

Sinus arrhythmia will usually not require any treatment unless the underlying rate is bradycardic and the patient is symptomatic from the slow rate.

5

SUPPRESSION DYSRHYTHMIAS

SUPPRESSION

Now that you are familiar with the common rhythms generated in the sinoatrial (SA) node, let's take a close look at what can happen when suppression of the conduction system alters the automaticity or conductivity of the heart's electrical activity, and the dysrhythmias resulting from this suppression.

CAUSES AND EFFECTS OF SUPPRESSION

The causes of suppression and the resulting effects on the heart are covered in detail in Chapter 4. As a brief review of the more common factors, increased vagal tone or decreased sympathetic stimulation will produce suppression of the electrical activity of the heart, as will hyperkalemia, increased intracranial pressure, cold, or fibrosis of the myocardium.

No matter what the causative factors may be, the effects on the rhythms of the heart are the same. If automaticity is affected, the spontaneous discharge cycle of the predominant pacemaker, usually the SA node, will be slowed, or even stopped. If the sinus rate becomes bradycardic enough, or the pause is long enough, the next fastest pacemaker lower in the heart will be allowed to reach the threshold level, and complete its spontaneous discharge cycle (SDC). This mechanism is called the escape phenomenon. The lower pacemaker is, of course, slower than normal, and depending on the amount of suppression of the SA node, the slower pacing focus may be in control of the heart for only one or two escape beats, or it may become the predominant pacemaker, and an escape rhythm begins.

If conductivity is affected by suppressive influences, the resulting dysrhythmias will exhibit changes that are characteristic of slowed or blocked conduction. Because the rate of impulse conduction through the heart is decreased, the time taken for complete depolarization of the atrial or ventricular myocardium is increased. These changes will slow on the ECG as widened PR and QRS intervals. If conduction of the impulse is blocked completely, the changes on the ECG will be seen as missing parts of the PQRST complex or absent beats.

SUPPRESSED AUTOMATICITY

SINUS BRADYCARDIA

Sinus bradycardia is just a variation of normal sinus rhythm (NSR), but, depending on the circumstances, a patient may be in serious difficulty because of the slow rate. The SDC of the SA node is suppressed, and the resulting slow-rate dysrhythmia will be less than 60 beats per minute.

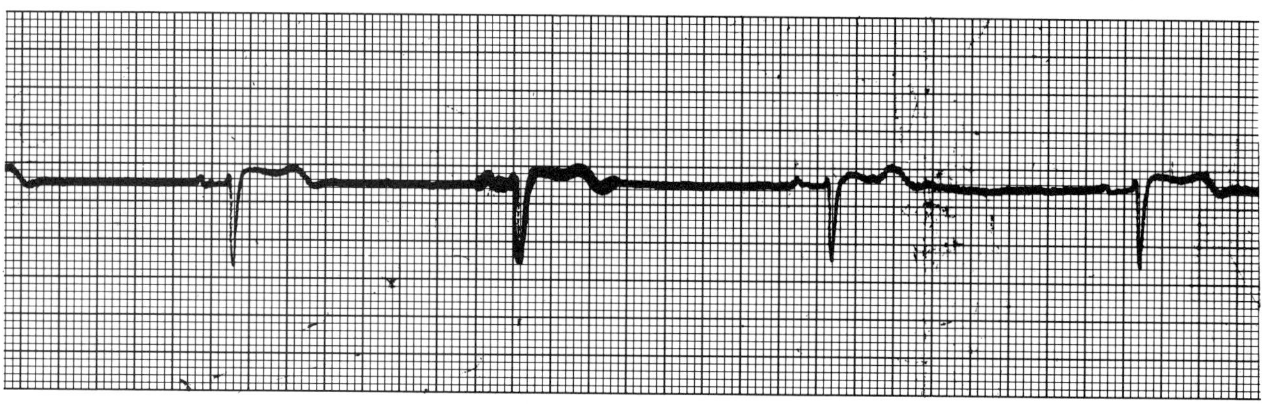

Sinus bradycardia

Criteria

RHYTHM The rhythm in sinus bradycardia will be regular, plus or minus three small squares.

RATE The rate will be less than 60 beats per minute.

P WAVES There will be a normal P wave in front of every QRS complex.

PR INTERVAL The PR interval will be within the normal limits of 0.12 to 0.20 second, and will be constant throughout the strip, if no lower conduction defect is present.

QRS COMPLEX The QRS complex will be within the normal limits of 0.06 to 0.12 second in duration, assuming there are no conduction abnormalities. The QRS configuration will be the same in all beats.

Hemodynamic and Clinical Considerations

Sinus bradycardia may occur as a physiologic response to sleep, and the mere fact that a patient's heart rate is less than 60 is no reason to be alarmed and start the atropine. Well-conditioned athletes may have a resting heart rate of less than 50 beats per-minute. However, a patient with a diseased heart and decreased contractility may be in trouble when his or her rate drops below 50.

If you remember the formula for calculating the cardiac output

$$\text{Heart rate} \times \text{stroke volume} = \text{cardiac output}$$

you know that the rate is directly proportional to the output. However, as the rate begins to slow, the stroke volume will increase because of the prolonged filling time, and the cardiac output will be maintained. But, when the stroke volume reaches its maximum and the rate continues to drop, the cardiac output will decline sharply. The rate where this decrease in output occurs varies from person to person. Once the break-even point is passed, the patient will become symptomatic. The blood pressure will drop and the patient may become short of breath. The patient will experience a change in level of consciousness that may be exhibited as merely restlessness and confusion, or there may even be a loss of consciousness. The patient may become pale, cyanotic, or have cool, clammy skin. The patient also may be thrown into acute left ventricular failure, because the slow rate may cause a back up in volume and pressure behind the left ventricle.

Therapy

The treatment for sinus bradycardia begins with atropine. Atropine blocks vagal stimulation, allowing the beta_1 sympathetic effects on the heart to predominate and thus increase the rate and contractility.

Sinus bradycardia is an instance where you definitely want to be sure you are treating the patient, not the monitor. Although the rate drops, the patient does not necessarily need therapy. If it is needed, then the atropine should be given as the first-line drug, but one must be careful of the amount given. Too much will produce a tachycardia, and too little may worsen the bradycardia.

If atropine is ineffective, isoproterenol may be given as the second-line pharmacologic agent. Unfortunately, isoproterenol has many serious side-effects, including increased ventricular irritability that may precipitate ventricular tachycardia or fibrillation. Because isoproterenol is a pure beta stimulator, it increases both the heart rate and contractility, but it also greatly increases myocardial oxygen consumption. If the oxygen supply to the myocardium is restricted because of coronary artery disease, isoproterenol can cause anginal attacks, or even precipitate myocardial infarction (MI).

If both atropine and isoproterenol are ineffective, or the symptomatic bradycardia becomes chronic, a transvenous pacemaker should be used to prevent the patient's heart rate from dropping below the level that provides normal hemodynamic function.

THE LATE BEATS (ESCAPE BEATS)

Late beats, beats that occur after the next sinus beat is expected, are called escape beats. Escape beats happen only when the SA node defaults as the pacemaker, or when conduction of the sinus impulse is blocked from reaching lower pacing foci to depolarize them. Escape beats occur when the wave of depolarization from a normal sinus impulse does not arrive at the time it should. A slower pacing focus, located lower in the heart, is allowed to reach its threshold level, complete its SDC, and send a wave of depolarization to stimulate the rest of the heart. Since the pacing foci that initiate escape beats have a slower SDC, it takes them longer to reach the threshold and automatically depolarize. The pause before the escape beat is known as the escape interval. The escape interval is usually constant since it represents the SDC length of the slower pacing focus. The longer SDC is the reason that *escape beats are always late*. The lower pacemaker that escapes may be located in the atria, atrioventricular (AV) junction, or the ventricles.

Criteria

RHYTHM The underlying rhythm may be regular, but the overall rhythm of the strip will be irregular because of the pauses produced by the longer SDC of the escape beat.

RATE The rate of the underlying rhythm is likely to be slow because of the suppression, and the overall rate will be even slower because of the pauses before the escape beats.

P WAVES If the underlying rhythm is sinus in origin, there will be normal P waves present in front of the sinus beats. The P wave configuration of the escape beat changes with the location of the lower pacemaker.

Atrial Escape Beats Atrial escape beats will have P waves present, but they will be abnormal and change in configuration from the sinus P wave.

Junctional Escape Beats Junctional escape beats will have the same P wave criteria as any beat arising in the AV junction. There may be no visible P wave, or a retrograde P wave may be positioned in front of or behind the QRS complex.

Ventricular Escape Beats Ventricular escape beats will have no associated P wave.

PR INTERVAL The underlying sinus rhythm will probably have a PR interval that is within normal limits, assuming no conduction defects in the AV node.

Atrial Escape Beats Atrial escape beats will have a PR interval that is likely to be within normal limits, but will probably differ from the PR measurement of the sinus complexes.

Junctional Escape Beats Junctional escape beats will have a PR interval of less than 0.12 second if a retrograde P wave is present in front of the QRS complex.

Ventricular Escape Beats Ventricular escape beats will have no PR interval, since there is no P wave associated with this beat.

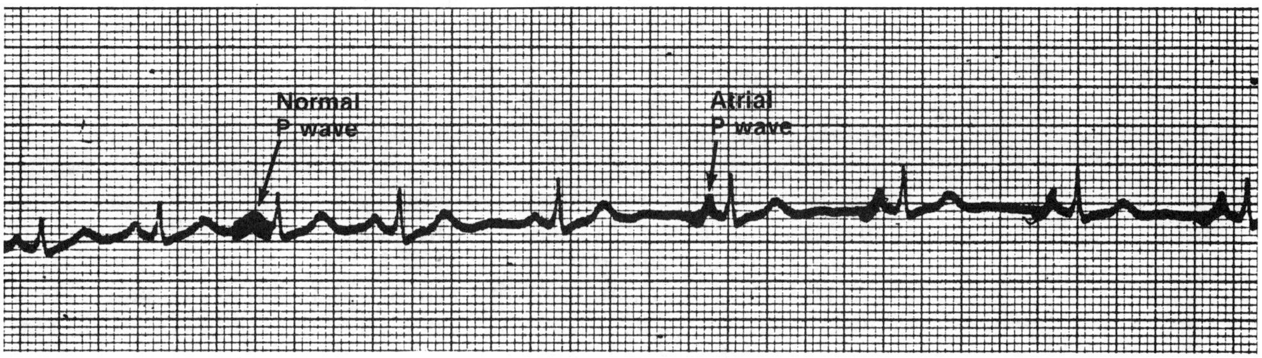

Atrial escape beats

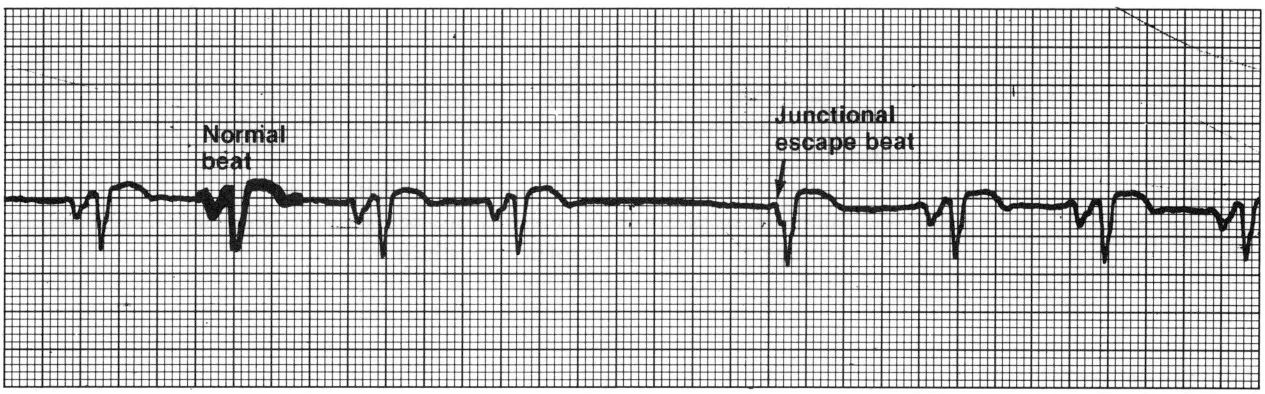

Junctional escape beat

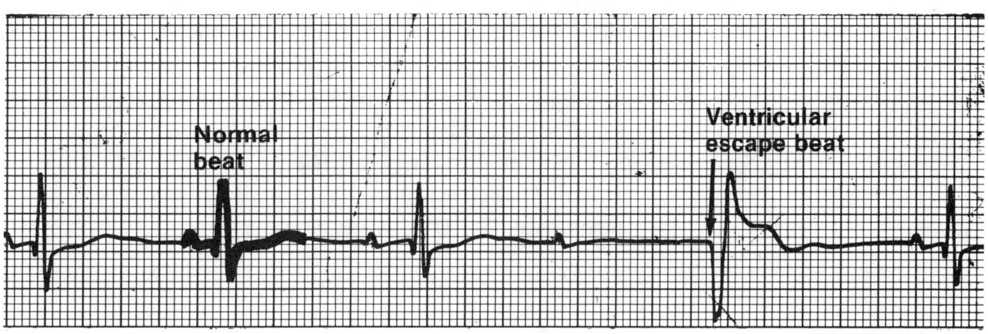

Ventricular escape beat

QRS COMPLEX The underlying sinus rhythm will have normal QRSs if no conduction defect is present in the bundle branches.

Atrial Escape Beats Atrial escape beats should have a normal QRS complex.

Junctional Escape Beats Junctional escape beats *must* have normal QRS complexes.

Ventricular Escape Beats Ventricular escape beats will have a QRS with all of the footprints of any ventricular beat—a wide, bizarre QRS with the ST segment and T wave going in the opposite direction of the main QRS deflection.

Hemodynamic and Clinical Considerations

The hemodynamic effects of escape beats are not caused by the escape beats themselves, but occur because of the underlying slow rates and pauses in the rhythm. The escape mechanism is actually a means of keeping the heart beating when the sinus node slows, stops, or is blocked from supplying a stimulus to the ventricles. If the underlying rate is slow enough, the patient can experience all of the same symptoms that are produced by sinus bradycardia.

Therapy

The cardinal rule in an escape situation is *escape beats are never treated!* They prevent extremely slow rates or even asystole. Ventricular escape beats in particular, because of their configuration, tend to elicit the lidocaine reflex in anyone watching a monitor. But *never* give any suppressive drug when the escape mechanism is present. If lidocaine is given to someone with ventricular escape beats, the lower pacing focus that is trying to keep the heart going is wiped out. When treatment is necessary, treat the suppression, not the escape! Therapy, if needed, is the same as that for sinus bradycardia.

THE SLOW RHYTHMS

The slow rhythms are also caused by the escape mechanism. In fact, six or more escape beats in a row are called an escape rhythm. Again, something either slows, stops, or blocks the sinus impulses, allowing the slower pacing focus to gain control of the heart. However, when escape rhythms are present, the sinus node has defaulted and can't regain the pacing function as it did when a few escape beats occurred. If the sinus node slows enough, the lower pacing focus may be located in the atria, the AV junction, or the ventricles. If the problem is present, not because of sinus suppression but because of AV block, the lower pacemaker can only be located in the AV junction or the ventricles. If complete blockade of the bundle branches is present, the lower pacing focus must be in the ventricles.

WANDERING ATRIAL PACEMAKER

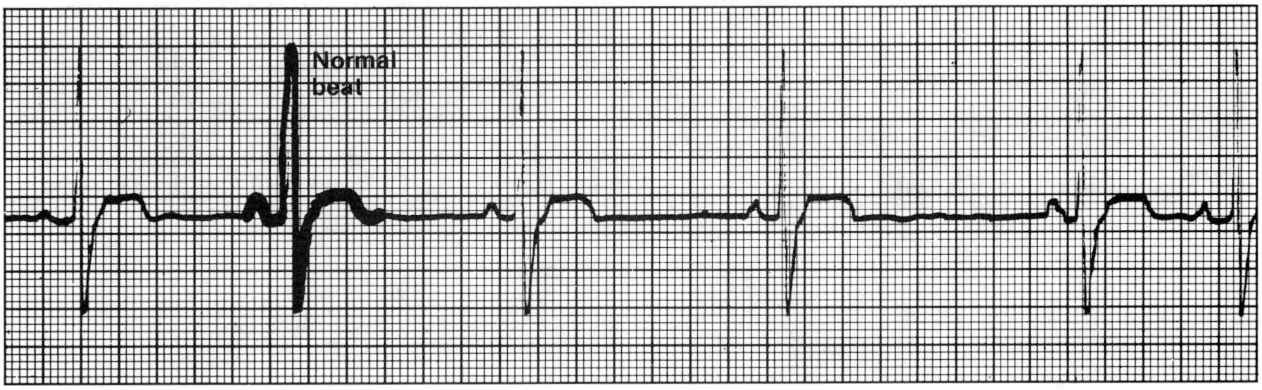

WAP

Wandering atrial pacemaker (WAP) occurs when the SA node is slowed, and its SDC is very close in rate to other pacing foci located in various places in the atrial myocardium. The focus that reaches its threshold and fires itself off first is in control of the heart, either for one beat or perhaps for two or three consecutive beats. The focus that "gets there first with the most" will be the pacemaker.

Criteria

RHYTHM The rhythm in WAP will be irregular because of the slightly different SDC lengths of the various atrial foci and the SA node.

RATE Since there is an escape rhythm, the rate will probably be slow.

P WAVES There will be P waves in front of every beat, but the atrial beats will have a different P wave configuration than the sinus P wave. Actually, each time a different atrial focus fires, the P wave changes shape.

QRS COMPLEX All of the QRS complexes should be normal in duration and identical to the sinus QRSs.

Hemodynamic and Clinical Considerations

WAP is not likely to alter the hemodynamic status of the patient, unless the rate becomes too slow. A similar rhythm will occur because of irritability in the atria, rather than suppression. Irritability speeds the SDCs of the atrial foci, so they usurp the pacing function from the SA node. This produces a WAP at a normal rate. If the irritability increases even more, you may see a WAP at a tachycardic rate known as multifocal atrial tachycardia (MAT) or chaotic atrial mechanism (CAM).

Therapy

WAP usually is not treated, but if the rate is slow enough to make the patient symptomatic, the underlying sinus suppression is treated as in sinus bradycardia. No suppressive drugs should be given.

JUNCTIONAL RHYTHM

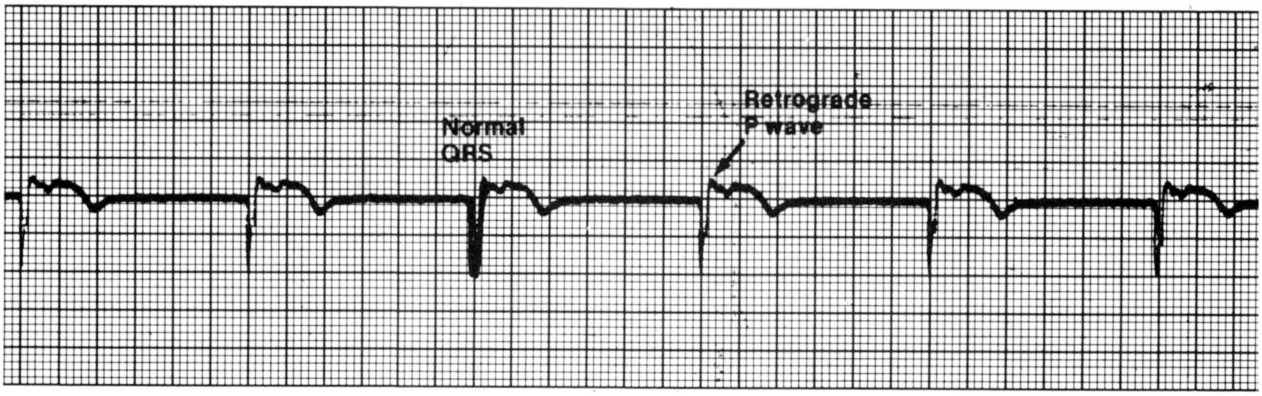

Junctional rhythm

A junctional rhythm will occur when the next fastest pacemaker is located in the AV junction after the SA node defaults or if the AV node is blocking all conduction from the sinus node.

Criteria

RHYTHM The rhythm generated by a junctional focus will be regular, plus or minus three small squares.

RATE The rate will be between 40 to 60 beats per minute, the rate that is inherent in AV junctional tissue.

P WAVES As with any junctional beat, there may be no P waves visible, or a retrograde P wave may be present, located in front of or behind the QRS complex.

PR INTERVAL The PR interval will be less than 0.12 second if a retrograde P wave is positioned in front of the QRS complex.

QRS COMPLEX All of the QRS complexes will be normal and identical to the sinus QRS complexes.

Hemodynamic and Clinical Considerations

Junctional rhythm may not cause any real hemodynamic changes, but the slow rate, coupled with a loss of atrial kick if no P wave is present in front of the QRS complex, may be enough to cause problems in the patient with an injured heart or decreased contractility. If this is the case, the cardiac output may drop, along with the blood pressure, causing all of the symptoms that are produced by any slow-rate dysrhythmia. It may throw the patient into acute left ventricular failure if he or she was only marginally compensated before this dysrhythmia began.

Therapy

If the rate and loss of atrial kick have compromised the patient's cardiac output and therapy is needed, the junctional rhythm itself is not treated, but the suppression causing the rhythm is. The therapy would be the same as that of sinus bradycardia. No suppressive drugs should be given.

VENTRICULAR RHYTHM (IDIOVENTRICULAR RHYTHM)

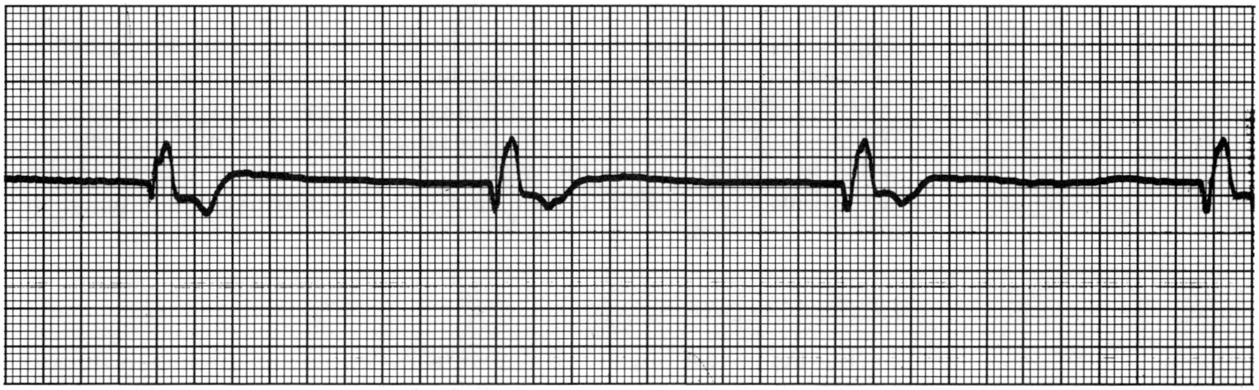

Idioventricular rhythm

Ventricular rhythm is the most dangerous of the escape rhythms. It occurs only when all of the higher pacemakers are either suppressed or blocked from reaching the ventricles, allowing the very slow, ventricular pacing focus to reach its threshold and fire.

Criteria

RHYTHM The rhythm may be regular, plus or minus three small squares. However, ventricular foci are not very dependable, so it may be somewhat irregular.

RATE The rate will be *slow*, 20 to 40 beats a minute, the rate inherent in ventricular conduction tissue.

P WAVES There will be no P waves associated with the QRS complex.

PR INTERVAL There will be no PR interval.

QRS COMPLEX The QRS complex will have all the same footprints as any ventricular beat. The QRS will be wide and bizarre, with the ST segment and T wave going in the opposite direction from the main QRS deflection.

Hemodynamic and Clinical Considerations

Ventricular rhythms are very slow and notoriously undependable. They may stop firing at any time, thus leaving the patient in ventricular standstill. There is no atrial kick since there are no associated P waves.

THERAPY A patient in ventricular rhythm is probably going to need either atropine to try to stimulate a higher pacemaker, or isoproterenol to speed up the SDC of the ventricular focus. If these drugs don't work or the rhythm becomes chronic, the patient may need a pacemaker.

SUPPRESSED CONDUCTIVITY

THE SA BLOCKS

SA blocks occur because suppression in the area of the SA node slows and finally blocks conduction of the sinus impulse at the SA junction where the SA nodal fibers connect with the intra-atrial tracts. There are four types of SA block: first-degree; second-degree, type I; second-degree, type II; and third degree. The SA blocks are commonly caused by acute MI or suppressive drugs such as digitalis, quinidine, or propranolol. They are likely to be transient in nature. If this particular type of dysrhythmia becomes a chronic problem, it may be seen as a sick sinus syndrome, or tachy-brady syndrome, where the underlying slow sinus rates alternate with tachycardias that disappear when the atrial rate is kept at a normal level with an atrial pacemaker.

FIRST-DEGREE SA BLOCK

In first-degree SA blocks, all the sinus impulses are conducted through the SA junction to the atria, but there is a constant delay in the conduction time it takes the impulse to leave the SA node and reach the atria. However, because the electrical activity generated by the SA node itself is much too small to be picked up by the surface ECG, there will be no evidence of this decreased conduction present in a normal rhythm strip. Special electrophysiologic studies that involve cardiac catheterization are needed to unmask this dysrhythmia.

SECOND-DEGREE SA BLOCK, TYPE I (SINUS WENCKEBACH)

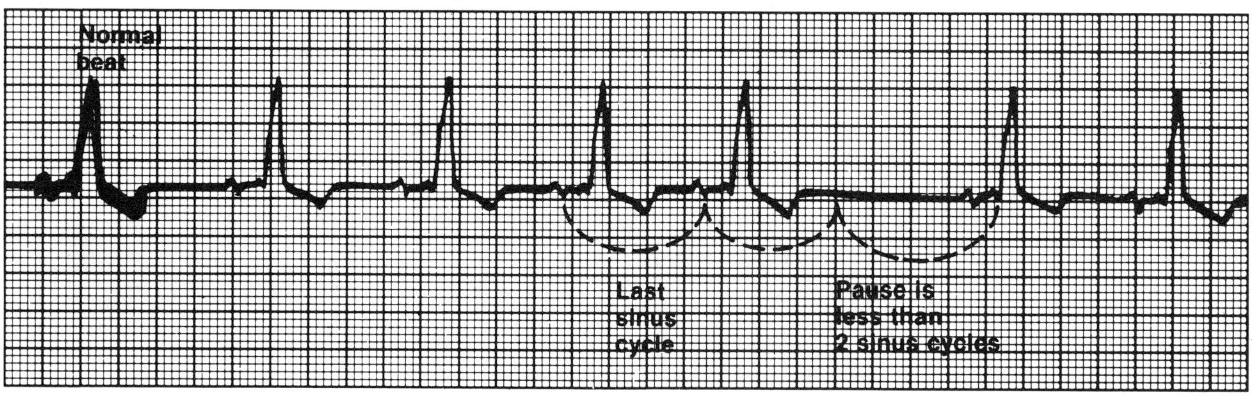

2° SA block type I (Sinus Wenckebach)

Second-degree SA block is a form of incomplete block, since some impulses are conducted from the SA node and some are blocked. Second-degree SA block, type I, is also known as sinus Wenckebach.

Electrophysiologically, the SA node is firing regularly, but there is a progressively increasing delay in the time it takes the impulse to move through the SA junction and into the atria. The delay increases with each succeeding P wave, until one impulse is blocked from leaving the SA node altogether. Conduction of the sinus impulse, once it leaves the SA node, is normal through the rest of the heart. The rhythm strip will appear as groups of beats in an irregular rhythm, with pauses between the groups when the sinus impulse is blocked. Many times, sinus Wenckebach will be interpreted as sinus arrhythmia, which it greatly resembles. But sinus arrhythmia will speed and slow in cycles, whereas sinus Wenckebach will become progressively faster until a less-than-compensatory pause occurs, and the progression begins again.

Criteria

RHYTHM The rhythm will be irregular. The P-to-P interval shortens progressively until a pause occurs. The pause will be shorter in length than two of the sinus cycles that precede the pause. After the pause, the next P-to-P interval lengthens and each succeeding P-to-P interval shortens again as the Wenckebach progression reports itself.

RATE The rate will be the same as the underlying rhythm.

P WAVES Each beat will have a normal sinus P wave in front of it. There will be no P wave present during the pause.

PR INTERVAL The PR interval probably will be within normal limits, unless there is a concurrent AV conduction delay present.

QRS COMPLEX The QRS complexes will be normal if no bundle branch block is present. Each QRS complex will be preceded by a P wave. There will be no QRS complex present during the pause.

Hemodynamic and Clinical Considerations

There may be no real hemodynamic alterations, unless the underlying rate is slow.

Therapy

Usually, no treatment is required, unless the rate is very slow, which causes the cardiac output to be compromised. If treatment is necessary, atropine, isoproterenol, or a pacemaker may be used.

SECOND-DEGREE SA BLOCK, TYPE II

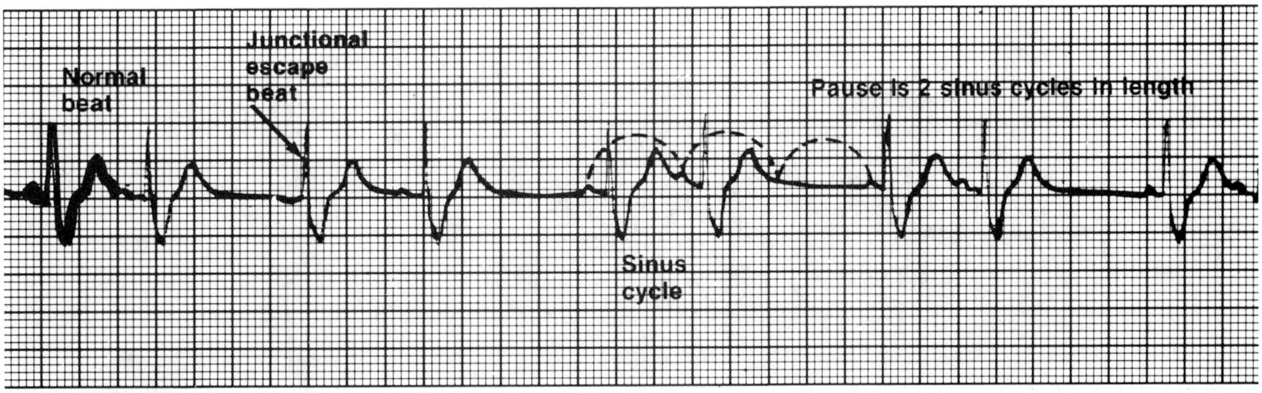

2° SA block type II (exit block with a junctional escape)

Second-degree SA block, type II, is also known as sinus exit block. In this dysrhythmia, the sinus node forms the impulse regularly, but the wave of depolarization is intermittently prevented from exiting the SA junction in a regular pattern.

Criteria

RHYTHM The underlying rhythm will be regular, but there will be pauses that last exactly two, three, or four or more sinus cycle lengths. There may be escape beats present during the pause if it lasts long enough to allow a lower pacing focus to reach its threshold and fire.

RATE The rate will be the same as the rate of the SA node minus the pauses.

P WAVES There will be normal P waves present in front of the sinus beats, but there will be no P waves present during the pause. You will be able to time the P-to-P interval across the pause, and the next sinus P wave will arrive exactly on time.

PR INTERVAL Assuming that the conduction through the AV node is normal, the PR interval of the sinus beats will be within normal limits.

QRS COMPLEX The sinus QRS complexes will be normal if no bundle branch block exists. If any QRS complexes are present during the pause, they will be late beats produced by the escape mechanism. Depending upon the length of the pause, single escape beats or an escape rhythm may be present.

Hemodynamic and Clinical Considerations

There may be no hemodynamic alterations, but if the pauses are frequent or long in duration, or if the underlying sinus rate is slow, the resulting bradycardia may cause a drop in the cardiac output that could produce symptoms in the patient.

Therapy

The treatment, if necessary, will be the same as that of sinus bradycardia.

THIRD-DEGREE SA BLOCK

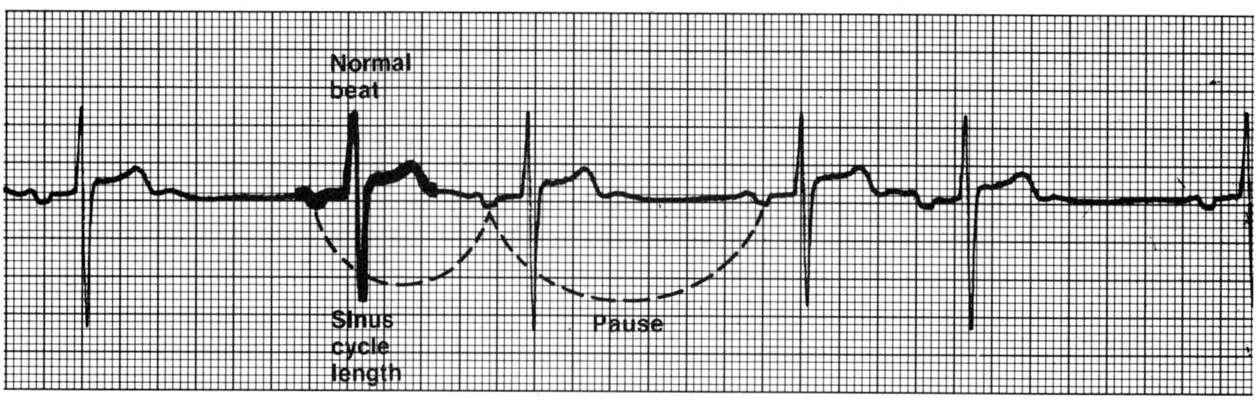

3° SA block (sinus arrest)

In third-degree SA block, the sinus impulse is unable to get out of the SA node entirely, producing pauses in the rhythm. It is nearly impossible to differentiate this rhythm on the surface ECG from a sinus arrest, where the SA node stops firing. Thus, for all intents and purposes, the two terms are considered by some to be interchangeable.

Criteria

RHYTHM There probably will be a regular underlying rhythm, which is made irregular by pauses that are *not* multiples of the sinus cycle length.

RATE The rate may be bradycardic because of suppression of the SA node and because of the pauses.

P WAVES There will be normal P waves present in front of the sinus beats, but there will be no sinus P waves present during the pause. You probably will not be able to clock the sinus P-to-P interval across the pause. If the block is intermittent, the next sinus beat will arrive when the block goes away.

PR INTERVAL The PR interval of the normal beats will be within normal limits if no AV block is present.

QRS COMPLEX The QRS complexes will be normal if no bundle branch block exists. There may be escape beats or rhythms present if the pause is long enough.

Hemodynamic and Clinical Considerations

As with the lower degrees of SA block, hemodynamic alterations will occur as a result of this dysrhythmia if the pauses are long enough to make the overall rate bradycardic.

Therapy

Therapy is the same as sinus bradycardia.

THE AV BLOCKS

If conductivity between the atria and ventricles is suppressed, the AV blocks occur. Just as there are three degrees of SA block, there are also three degrees of AV block. There is a good deal of confusion surrounding the terminology and criteria for the various degrees of AV block. Electrocardiographers and electrophysiologists in separate parts of this country tend to divide the blocks differently and use varying criteria for the identification of these dysrhythmias. There is also a way of dividing the AV blocks according to the site of blocked conduction, for example, the AV node, the His bundle, or the bundle branches. This confusion may seem to be merely an exercise in semantics, but, unfortunately, the degree of severity and the treatment may differ widely as the terminology changes. Our discussion will try to present this material as completely and clearly as possible, but you must be aware that the thinking about these abnormal rhythms and their criteria may be different in your area. In this discussion we will divide the AV blocks into first-degree; second-degree, type I; second-degree, type II; third-degree; and high-grade AV block.

ELECTROPHYSIOLOGY

No matter what you call the block, or where the level of blockade occurs, the results are the same. Conduction of the sinus impulses from the atria to the ventricles is slowed, partially blocked, or completely blocked. This may well slow the rate of the ventricles to the point where the patient will become symptomatic, or there may be a complete cessation of ventricular activity that is lethal if not corrected rapidly.

All of the alterations in conduction that occur from AV block are exaggerations of the normal AV nodal functions. The physiologic delay provided by the AV node to allow time for atrial activation before the ventricles are stimulated is increased and may be prolonged either slightly or significantly. The physiologic filtering of rapid atrial stimuli that protects the ventricle becomes pathologic when the AV node begins filtering sinus impulses at normal rates. Finally, the conduction of impulses may cease altogether and produce total blockade at the AV node. The atria and the ventricles are dissociated completely from each other, and each chamber must be activated by separate pacemakers.

CAUSES

The AV blocks can be produced by many factors, including hyperkalemia; drugs such as digitalis, quinidine, procainamide, beta blockers, and calcium antagonists; and acute MI. In the presence of an inferior wall infarction, AV blocks are seen frequently, since the blood supply of both the inferior wall and the AV node usually is supplied by the right coronary artery. However, when the AV block develops in the face of an anterior-septal infarction, it usually is considered a more serious proposition, and may be treated more aggressively.

FIRST-DEGREE AV BLOCK

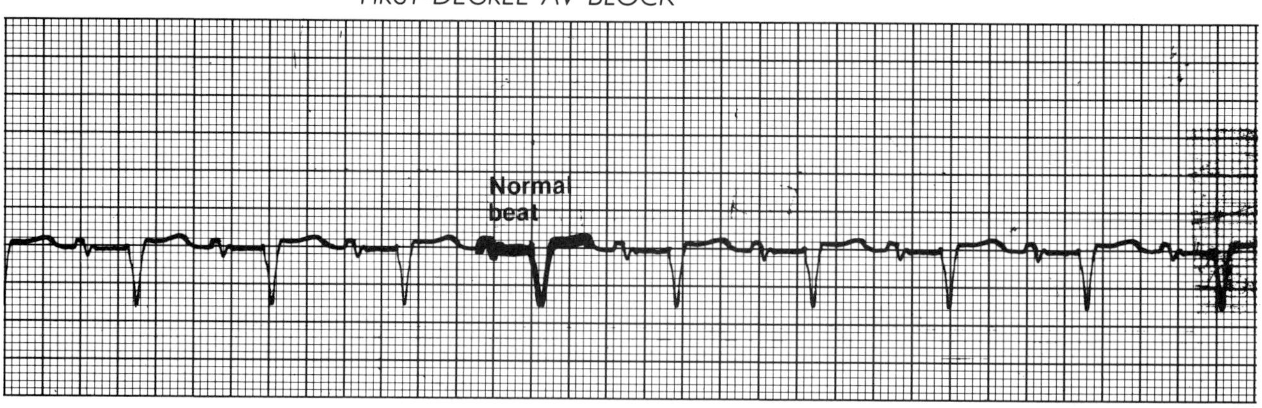

1° AV block

In first-degree AV block, the AV node is delaying conduction for a longer than normal period, but all of the sinus impulses are conducted to the ventricles. The delay in conduction is constant with each sinus beat. This has the effect of consistently increasing the PR interval so it measures more than 0.20 second, the upper limit of normal AV conduction.

Criteria

RHYTHM The rhythm will be regular if the underlying sinus mechanism is regular.

RATE The rate will be the rate of the underlying sinus rhythm.

P WAVES There are normal sinus P waves present before each beat, and all are conducted to the ventricles.

PR INTERVAL The PR interval will be greater than 0.20 second, and it will be constant throughout the strip.

QRS COMPLEX The QRS will be within normal limits if no bundle branch block is present. There will be a QRS after each P wave since conduction is only delayed and not blocked.

Hemodynamic and Clinical Considerations

First-degree AV block will not affect the patient's hemodynamic status. It may be seen in individuals with normal healthy hearts, and is considered a benign situation in this instance. But, in the presence of heart disease, such as acute MI, it must be considered a warning of impending, and possibly dangerous, decreasing AV conduction.

Therapy

The patient with a first-degree AV block probably will not require any therapy. However, the patient should be observed very closely for increasing block.

SECOND-DEGREE AV BLOCK, TYPE I (WENCKEBACH)

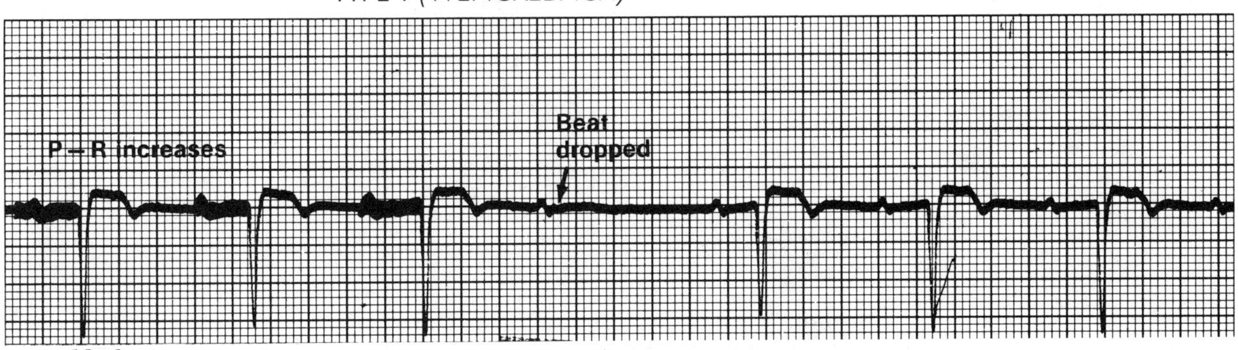

2° AV block, type I

Second-degree AV block is called a form of incomplete block, since only some of the sinus impulses are prevented from reaching the ventricles. Type I, or Wenckebach conduction, occurs when the AV node progressively delays and finally blocks conduction of the sinus impulses from atria to ventricles. On ECG, you will see regular P waves as the sinus node goes through its SDC. However, the AV node will slow conduction more and more, as each successive sinus impulse passes through. This will progressively prolong the PR interval until the AV node remains refractory too long to conduct an impulse, and one P wave is prevented from reaching the ventricular conduction system. A QRS complex is dropped, producing a pause in the rhythm. The next P wave after the pause will be conducted with a PR interval shorter than the last one, since the AV node has had a longer interval after the dropped beat to recover. Then the Wenckebach progression begins again. You will notice that there are groups of beats separated by pauses.

Criteria

RHYTHM Because the SA node is not the problem, the P waves will be regular. The ventricular rhythm will be irregular because of the changing PR intervals and the pauses produced by the dropped QRS complex.

RATE The atrial rate will be the same as the rate in the sinus node. The ventricular rate will be less than the atrial rate, since some QRS complexes are missing.

P WAVES The normal sinus P waves are present, but there will be an occasional P wave that is not followed by a QRS complex.

PR INTERVAL The first PR interval in each Wenckebach progression or group will be shortened. Then, as each successive P wave comes along, the PR increases until one P wave is blocked and one QRS complex is dropped.

QRS COMPLEX The QRS duration will be within normal limits if no bundle branch block is present. Every so often a QRS is dropped, producing the pause in the ventricular rhythm. The dropped QRS and the resulting pause causes the appearance of group beating. There will always be one more P wave than QRS complex in each Wenckebach group. Sometimes there will be a regular pattern in the occurrence of the dropped beats where, for example, every fourth QRS is missing. This conduction pattern, if regular, should be mentioned in the interpretation. The above-mentioned situation would be interpreted as 4:3 conduction (four P waves to three QRS complexes). At other times, the conduction pattern varies from group to group, and should then be interpreted as Wenckebach with varying conduction.

Hemodynamic and Clinical Considerations

Unless the underlying sinus rate is slow, Wenckebach is unlikely to cause any real hemodynamic alterations for the patient. It is viewed as a benign rhythm, particularly when seen with an inferior wall infarction. It should be viewed with more caution when the patient has an anterior-septal infarction, and should always be considered as a warning that a higher degree of block may occur at any time.

Therapy

Usually, therapy is not indicated unless the ventricular rate is particularly slow. However, the patient must be closely observed for signs of increasing block.

SECOND-DEGREE AV BLOCK, TYPE II

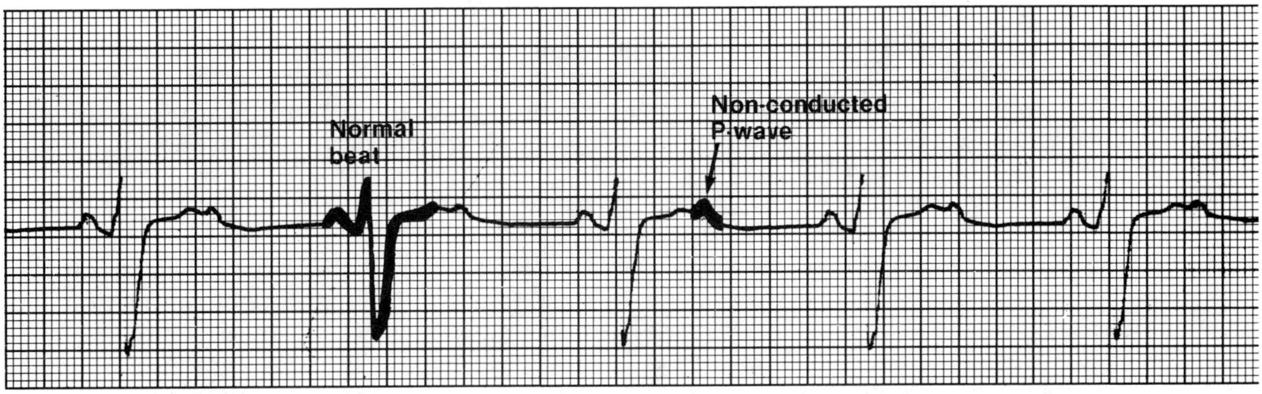

2° AV block, type II

Second-degree AV block, type II, another form of incomplete block, is considered by some to occur at the level of the bundle branches rather than at the AV node or His bundle. Type II block is also called a fixed-ratio block because it usually has a regular pattern of conduction and blockade. In this variety of block, the sinus impulses are prevented from reaching the ventricles more frequently than in Wenckebach conduction. Only one out of every two, three, four, or more P waves makes it through to the ventricles.

Criteria

RHYTHM Because the conduction pattern usually is fixed, both the atrial and ventricular rhythms are regular.

RATE The atrial rate will be greater than the ventricular rate. Because of the fixed conduction pattern, there will be a numerical ratio between the two rates. The atrial rate should be exactly two, three, four, or more times the ventricular rate.

P WAVES The P waves will be present, but not all of them are conducted to the ventricles. Thus, many P waves will not be followed by QRS complexes.

PR INTERVAL The PR interval may be within normal limits or prolonged, but the PR will be constant with each beat.*

QRS COMPLEX The QRS complex may be normal or widened,* and many QRS complexes are missing in a regular pattern of two, three, or more P waves to each QRS. This regular pattern should be mentioned in the interpretation as 2:1, 3:1, 4:1, and so forth, block.

Hemodynamic and Clinical Considerations

This form of second-degree AV block is much more likely to be a danger to the patient, since the ventricular rate probably is very slow because,

**Note*: Since this form of second-degree AV block is considered by some to be at the level of the bundle branches, they list the criteria for this type-II block as having a normal PR interval and a wide QRS duration. Thus, any 2:1 block with a prolonged PR or normal QRS complex would be considered a 2:1 Wenckebach progression rather than a type-II block.

at the very best, it will only be half the atrial rate, and could be as much as a third to a quarter of the atrial rate. As with any slow rate, the cardiac output and blood pressure may drop drastically, causing the patient to become short of breath, restless, and to experience chest pain. If allowed to continue untreated, the patient may lose consciousness, suffer an infarction, or extend the area of infarction he or she already has.

Therapy

Atropine, as an IV bolus, may be the first-line drug when therapy is needed. Atropine blocks vagal tone and often increases conduction and the ventricular rate. If atropine doesn't work, an isoproterenol drip may be used. Isoproterenol causes an increase in $beta_1$ stimulation, which can increase AV conduction. However, extreme caution must be taken when using this drug because it can easily produce ventricular irritability that can result in ventricular tachycardia or fibrillation. The patient in second-degree AV block, type II, may well need a pacemaker. The drug therapy would be used in an attempt to stabilize the patient's condition until the pacer wire can be inserted.

HIGH-GRADE AV BLOCK

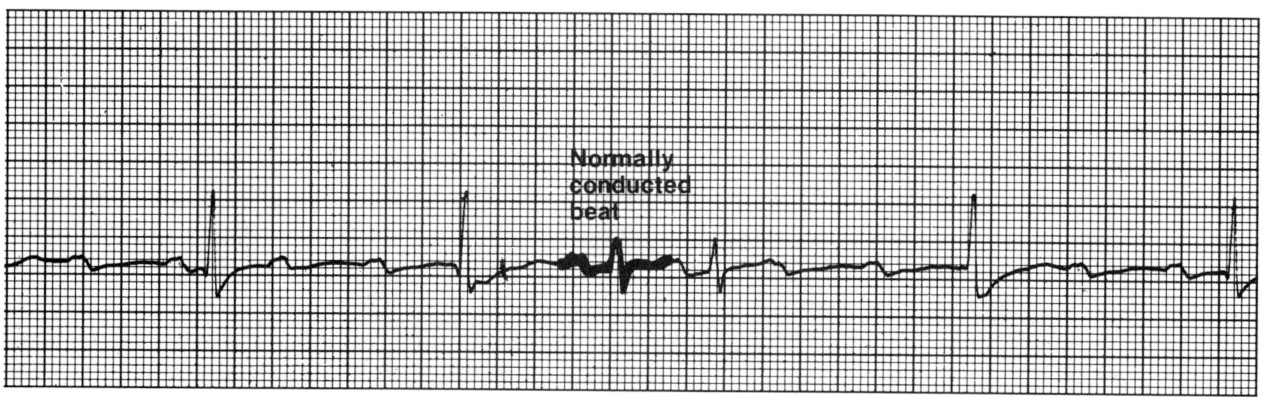

High-grade AV block

High-grade AV block is considered to be an intermediate step between second-degree AV block, type II, and third-degree AV block. In this rhythm, there will be three or more consecutive P waves blocked. This can produce long pauses in the ventricular rhythm, which may allow escape rhythms or beats to occur. It will be impossible to differentiate these escape rhythms during the long pauses from third-degree AV block until a sinus P wave is conducted again.

Criteria

RHYTHM The atrial rhythm will be regular sinus P waves. The ventricular rhythm will be irregular because of the pauses when conduction stops, the possible presence of escape rhythms, and the seemingly early

QRS complex that occurs when conduction of the sinus impulse resumes.

RATE The atrial rate will be the rate of the SA node. The atrial rate will be greater than the ventricular because of the pauses and the slower pacing rate of the lower pacemaker that might escape.

P WAVES The P waves present are normal sinus P waves, but some will not be conducted.

PR INTERVAL The PR may be normal or prolonged, but it will be constant when conduction is present.

QRS COMPLEX The QRS duration will be within normal limits in the conducted beats, assuming no bundle branch block is present. Some QRS complexes will be missing when conduction of the sinus impulse ceases. If an escape rhythm occurs, the QRS complexes may be normal, or wide and bizarre if the lower pacemaker is located in the ventricles.

Hemodynamic and Clinical Considerations

The hemodynamic and clinical considerations are the same as these for third-degree AV block.

Therapy

Therapy is the same as for third-degree AV block.

THIRD-DEGREE AV BLOCK (COMPLETE AV BLOCK)

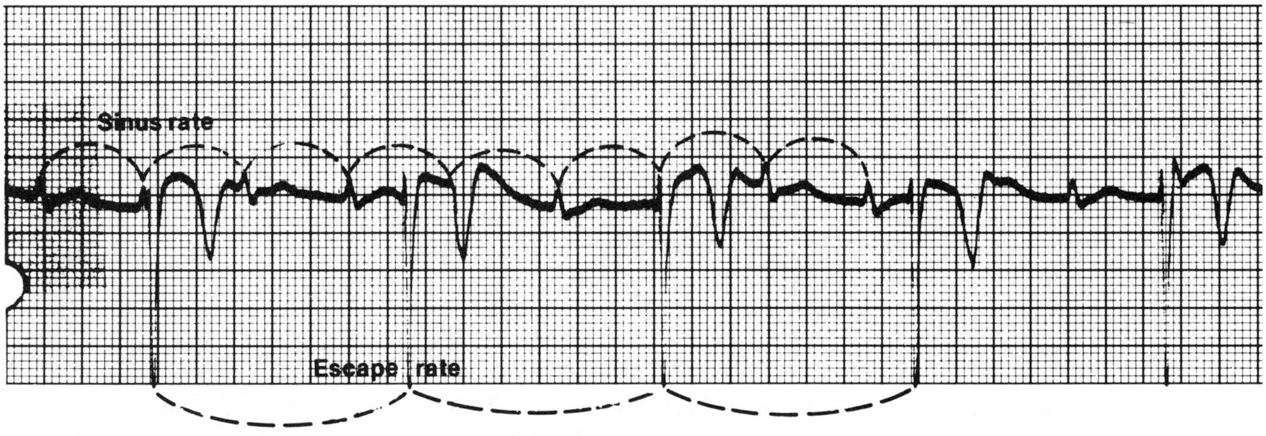

3° AV block with junctional rhythm

In third-degree AV block, the AV node blocks down completely, allowing no sinus impulses to be conducted to the ventricles. The SA node still is depolarizing the atria, but ventricular activation is maintained by the escape of a lower pacing focus. One hopes that the lower focus will arise in the AV junction, producing a junctional rhythm. But, if the entire junction is suppressed, or if the location of the block is at the level of the bundle branches, the lower focus that escapes must be in the ventricles, producing an idioventricular rhythm.

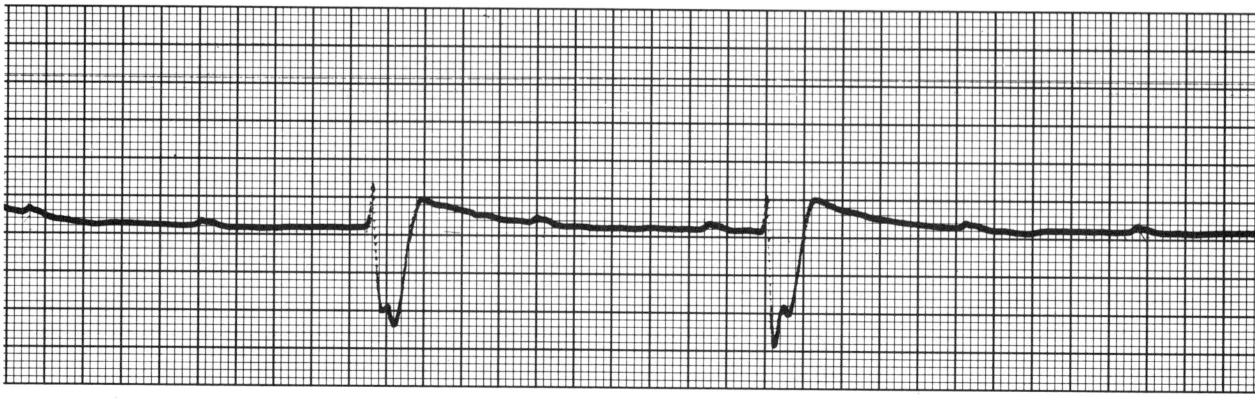

3° AV block with idioventricular rhythm

Criteria

RHYTHM Both the atrial and ventricular rhythms probably will be regular, but they are dissociated from each other.

RATE The atrial rate most likely will be greater than the ventricular rate. The atrial rate may well be tachycardic, particularly if the ventricular rate is slow enough to cause a drop in the cardiac output. The resulting drop in the blood pressure is sensed by the baroreceptors in the carotid sinus and the aortic arch, producing an increase in beta sympathetic tone to the heart in a futile attempt to increase the ventricular rate. Unfortunately, this compensatory mechanism won't work since the AV node can't conduct the sinus impulses, no matter how fast they are.

P WAVES There are sinus P waves present, but none are being conducted to the ventricles.

PR INTERVAL The PR interval appears to vary with each beat. In reality, this is not a PR interval at all because no conduction exists. There are two separate pacemakers running the heart, one in the atria and one in the ventricles. Since these two rhythms are coexisting but dissociated, the atrial and ventricular rhythms are superimposed on each other. There will be some P waves that by chance are sitting in front of QRS complexes; but, since they are not related, what appears to be a PR interval, which, if constant proves conduction, will vary with each beat.

QRS COMPLEX The configuration of the QRS complexes is determined by the location of the lower pacing focus that escapes. If the escape rhythm is coming from the AV junction, the QRS complexes will be normal and probably running at a rate of 40 to 60 beats per minute, which is a junctional rhythm. There probably will be no retrograde atrial stimulation since the AV node is blocked. If the lower pacing focus is located in the ventricles, the QRS complexes will be wide and bizarre, with the ST segment and T waves going in the opposite direction of the main QRS deflection. The rate will be between 20 to 40 beats per minute, which is an idioventricular rhythm.

Hemodynamic and Clinical Considerations

The hemodynamic status of the patient is mostly dependent upon the ventricular rate. If the pacing focus running the ventricles is firing at a nearly normal rate, the patient probably will be in no immediate danger. However, if the lower pacing focus is running at a very slow rate, the patient may be exhibiting all the symptoms produced by a drop in cardiac output.

The other real problem with third-degree AV block is the fact that the lower pacers are not only slow but also very undependable, particularly a ventricular focus, and may stop firing at any time, thus leaving the patient in ventricular standstill.

Therapy

The treatment for third-degree AV block again depends upon the ventricular rate. If the rate is nearly normal, and the patient not too symptomatic, a temporary transvenous pacemaker may be inserted as a safeguard in case the rate drops or standstill occurs. If the rate is slow and the patient is symptomatic, atropine and/or isoproterenol may be used in an attempt to increase the ventricular rate, until the pacing wire can be inserted. Atropine may decrease the amount of block at the AV node by removing vagal tone. Isoproterenol can do the same thing by increasing the beta sympathetic tone. It also may help increase the ventricular rate by increasing the automaticity of the lower pacing focus.

BUNDLE BRANCH BLOCK

When suppression of conductivity is affecting the ventricular conducting system, a bundle branch block (BBB) occurs. One of the bundle branches is unable to pass on the sinus impulse coming from the atria in the normal fashion. BBB can develop as a result of acute MI, rheumatic heart disease, ventricular hypertrophy, congenital deformities, hypertension, or coronary artery disease. It also may develop as an expression of critical rate. The phenomenon of rate-dependent BBB can be a precursor to complete bundle branch block, and is a warning that a serious problem may be impending. Right bundle branch block (RBBB) is usually a transient occurrence, caused by infarction, and disappears as the infarction heals. Left bundle branch block (LBBB) tends to be a stable condition that is more likely caused by preexisting disease rather than an acute infarction.

Before we look at the changes in QRS configuration produced by abnormal depolarization of the ventricles to BBB, a brief review of normal ventricular activation may prove helpful.

NORMAL ACTIVATION OF THE VENTRICLES

The right and left bundle branches (RBB and LBB, respectively) are located in the intraventricular septum. The RBB sends a branch to the papillary muscles, and one to the free right ventricular wall. The LBB divides into two branches: the left anterior fascicle that proceeds down the intraventricular septum to the anterior papillary muscle of the anterior leaflet of the mitral valve, and the posterior fascicle that runs along the inferior wall of the left ventricle to the posterior papillary muscle of the posterior leaflet of the mitral valve.

The normal depolarization of the ventricles begins in the upper part of the septum, which is activated by the LBB. The wave of depolarization through the septum proceeds from left to right. A positive electrode in the V_1 position sees the initial depolarization forces coming toward it, and records a small positive R wave.

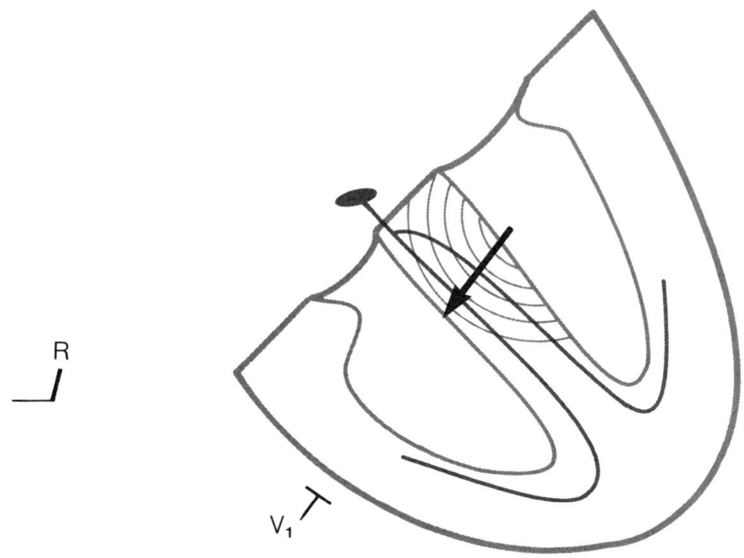

The wave of depolarization then spreads simultaneously to the right and left ventricular walls, from the endocardial to the epicardial surface. The right ventricular forces are cancelled by the much greater activity in the left ventricle, so a positive electrode at V_1 sees only the large wave of electrical activity in the left ventricle moving away from it, which produces a deep negative S wave.

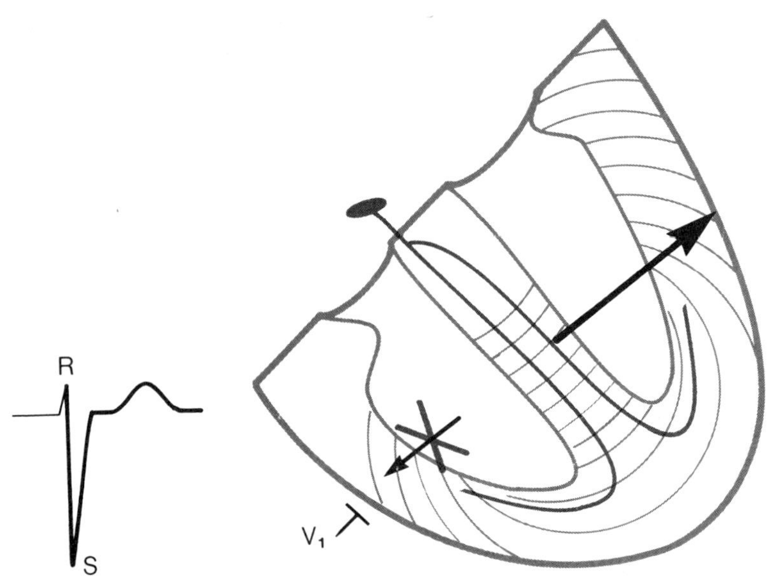

Repolarization through the ventricles proceeds normally so the T wave will be normal.

ACTIVATION OF THE VENTRICLES IN BUNDLE BRANCH BLOCK

When BBB occurs, the ventricle on the unaffected side is depolarized first in the normal fashion, and the impulse then spreads slowly from fiber to fiber through the septum to the ventricle on the blocked side. In BBB, the ventricles are activated one after the other rather than simultaneously.

When BBB is present, the initial QRS deflection will be of normal duration, since the impulse is traveling normally through the unaffected ventricle. The terminal portion of the complex will be widened since the impulse is traveling slowly from fiber to fiber. The QRS complex will be more than 0.12 second in duration. The T wave deflection also is altered because repolarization is abnormal too. The ST segment and T wave will go in the opposite direction from the *terminal* QRS deflection. These ST and T wave changes are called secondary changes resulting from BBB.

RIGHT BUNDLE BRANCH BLOCK

The RBB runs under the endocardium, down the right side of the intraventricular septum. It is a long, thin fiber that has two branches: one that supplies the anterior papillary muscle of the tricuspid valve and one that activates the free right ventricular wall. The blood supply for the RBB comes almost exclusively from the left anterior descending coronary artery. The RBB is blocked easily because the single blood supply and the length and narrowness of the bundle make it very vulnerable to damage.

When the RBB is blocked, the initial activation of the septum is not altered, since septal depolarization normally is initiated by the LBB. A positive electrode in the V_1 position sees the normal wave of septal depolarization from left to right coming toward it, and records the normal R wave usually seen in V_1.

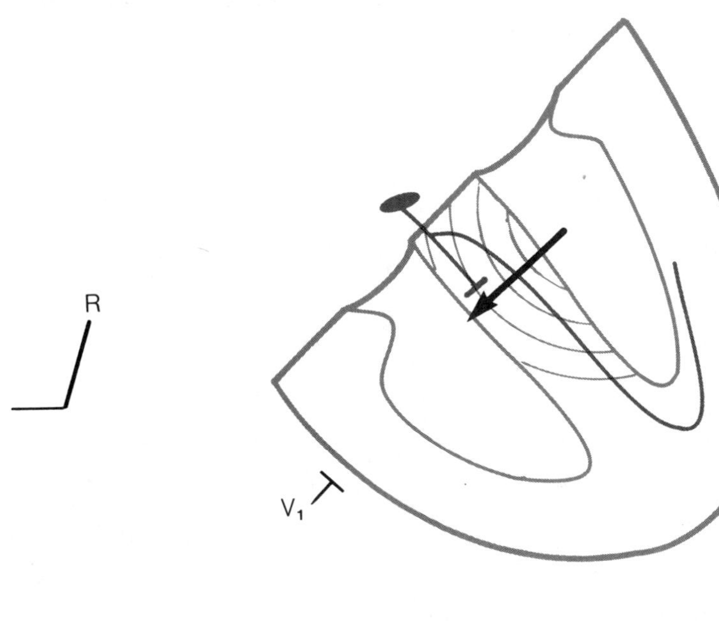

The stimulus continues down the unaffected LBB, and the left ventricle is depolarized in the normal manner. V_1 will see the wave of depolarization in the left ventricle going away from it, and will record a negative S wave. The QRS duration at this point is normal, since the conduction pattern has not yet been altered.

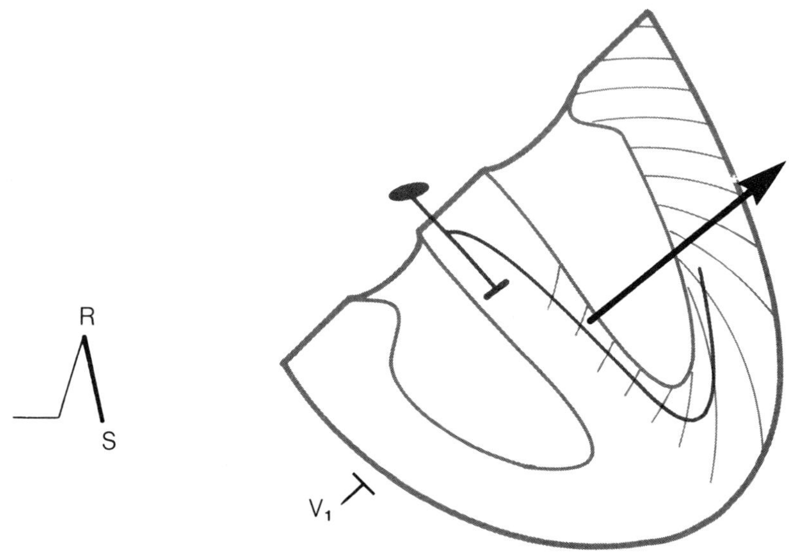

It is after this first deflection that the QRS complex widens, because depolarization of the right ventricle occurs from fiber to fiber rather than through the normal pathway of the RBB and the Purkinje network. Because the left ventricle already has depolarized, the right ventricular forces are unopposed, and are readily seen on the ECG. V_1 sees the wave of depolarization coming through the right ventricle toward it, and records another R wave, called an R′ wave. The ST segment and T wave will be in the opposite direction from the terminal QRS deflection. Since RBBB produces a positive terminal deflection in V_1, the ST segment and T wave will go in the negative direction.

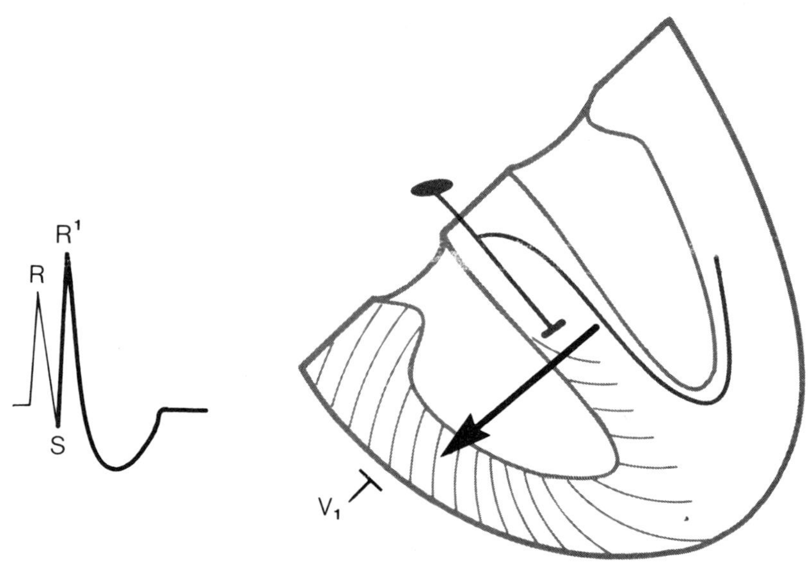

RBBB tends to be considered a less serious disturbance then LBBB. When no acute process is present this may be the case, because LBBB is more indicative of the existence of cardiac disease. However, in the presence of an acute infarction, the development of either RBBB or LBBB is a warning that serious conduction disturbances could develop.

LEFT BUNDLE BRANCH BLOCK

The LBB is located below the endocardium of the left ventricular septum. It begins with the left common bundle and divides into the left anterior fascicle and the left posterior fascicle. The two divisions of the left BB are short, thick fibers that have dual blood supply to portions of them. The blood supply comes from both the right and left coronary arteries.

When the LBB is blocked, the initial activation of the septum is altered. The septum is now activated from right to left by the RBB. The initial wave is receding away from V_1, which produces a Q wave.

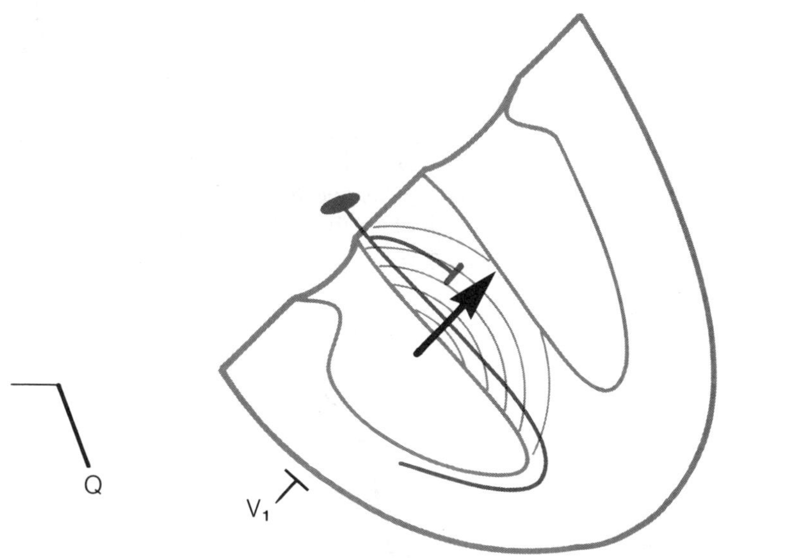

The next part of the ventricles to be activated is the free right ventricular wall. Because there is only a small amount of electrical force generated by the thin right ventricle, it has little effect on the ECG. V_1 may see the small wave of depolarization coming toward it and record a positive notch or R wave on the downstroke of the Q wave, or there may be no evidence of this current showing in the QRS complex at all.

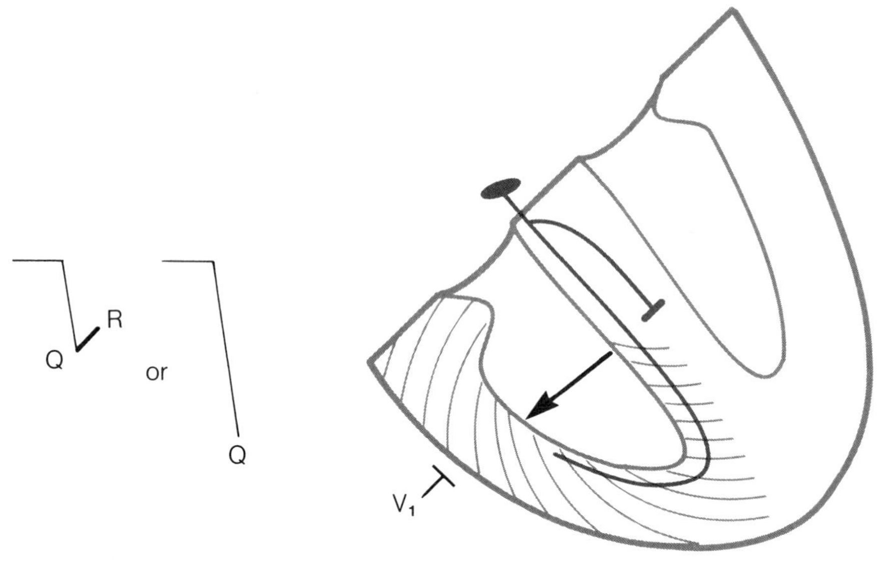

The left ventricle is the last part of the myocardium to be depolarized. This part of the QRS complex will be widened since the left ventricle is being depolarized by fiber-to-fiber transmission of the wave, which takes much longer than normal conduction. V_1 will see the activity in the left ventricle receding away from it, and record a further negative deflection. The T wave and ST segment will show the characteristic secondary changes produced by BBB. In V_1, the terminal QRS deflection in LBBB is negative, so the ST segment and T wave will go in a positive direction.

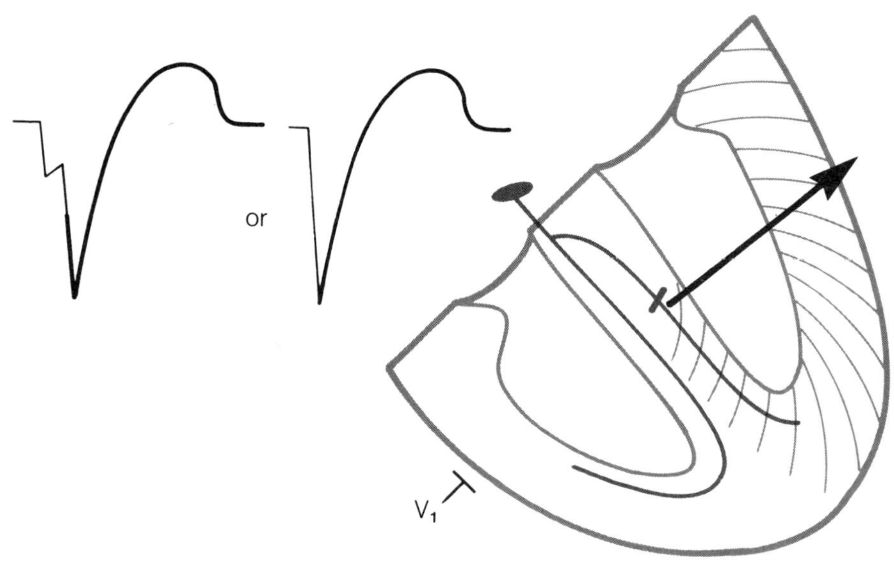

LBBB is considered to be a more serious condition than RBBB because the LBB is a short, thick fiber with a dual blood supply, which requires a more extensive lesion to block conduction. It tends to be a stable condition, rather than a transient occurrence that disappears as the infarction heals. When only one of the two fascicles of the LBB is blocked, it is called a hemiblock.

TERMINAL SUPPRESSION DYSRHYTHMIAS

The following dysrhythmias are the lethal rhythms that are the end result of suppression of automaticity or conductivity in the heart.

PRIMARY VENTRICULAR STANDSTILL

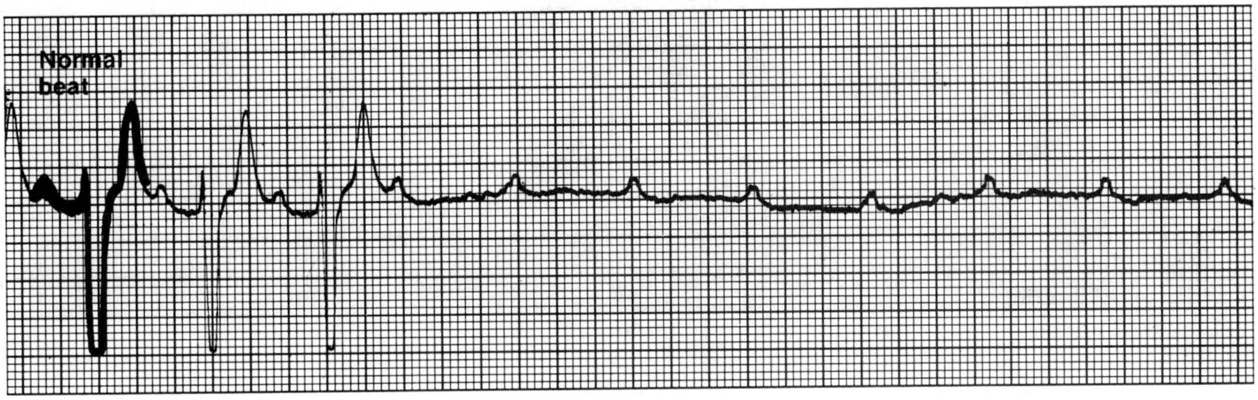

Primary ventricular standstill

Primary ventricular standstill is the end stage of the AV blocks. It occurs when the AV node completely blocks down, but no lower pacemaker escapes. The atria are still being stimulated but the ventricles are not.

Criteria

RHYTHM The atrial rhythm will be regular. There is no ventricular rhythm.

RATE The atrial rate will be whatever the SA node is supplying. The ventricular rate is 0.

P WAVES There will be P waves present, but none of them are being conducted to the ventricles.

PR INTERVAL There are no PR intervals since there is no conduction.

QRS COMPLEXES There are no QRS complexes. There is no conduction from above, and no escape rhythms below the AV node.

Hemodynamic and Clinical Considerations

Since this rhythm is composed entirely of P waves with no QRS complexes, there will be no ventricular contractions, and obviously, no cardiac output. The patient is pulseless, and will be clinically dead shortly if therapy is not instituted rapidly.

Therapy

This is, of course, "Code Blue" time. Cardiopulmonary resuscitation (CPR) must be initiated immediately. The patient needs a pacemaker, but drugs, such as isoproterenol or epinephrine, may be given to try to initiate some ventricular activity. A patient can actually be paced by repeated precordial thumps, but this obviously is not very practical.

SECONDARY VENTRICULAR STANDSTILL

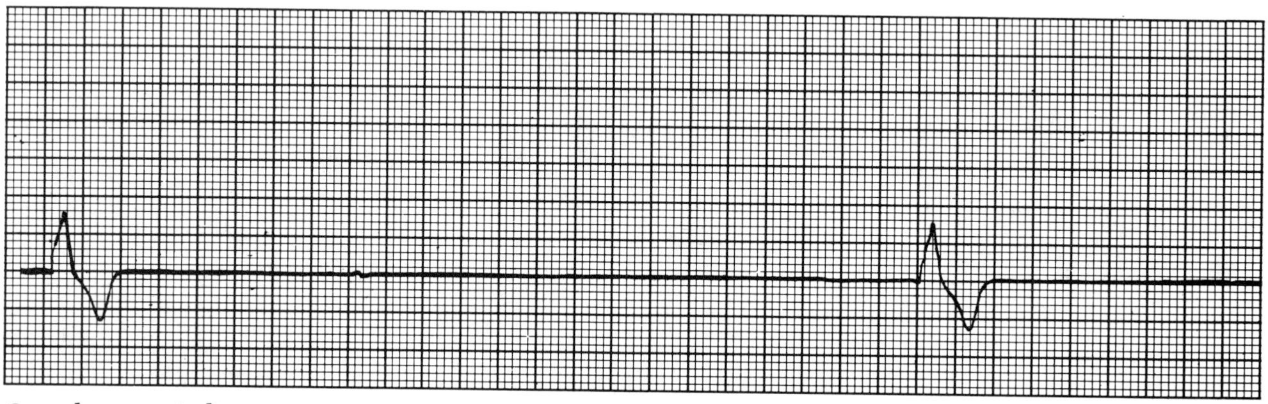

Secondary ventricular standstill

Secondary ventricular standstill may follow primary standstill, or it can occur as the first lethal event. In this rhythm, the atrial activity is missing, but there is evidence of ventricular *electrical* activity. However, this ventricular activity is purely electrical with no resulting mechanical contraction of the muscle. This condition is known as electromechanical dissociation (EMD).

Criteria

RHYTHM There will be no atrial rhythm. The ventricular rhythm may be regular.

RATE The ventricular activity will be slow, but the actual pulse rate is 0.

P WAVES There will be no P waves.

PR INTERVAL There will be no PR intervals.

QRS COMPLEX Wide, bizarre, ventricular complexes usually occur.

Hemodynamic and Clinical Considerations

This rhythm may resemble idioventricular rhythm, and with an ECG alone, it is impossible to differentiate between the two. However, a patient with idioventricular rhythm will have pulses, and the patient in secondary standstill will not. This rhythm is also death-producing unless treated promptly. This rhythm often is seen at the end of the "Code Blue," and usually little can be done to rectify the situation at that point, because the muscle is too far gone to respond to therapy.

Therapy

Therapy is the same as that for primary standstill. The patient needs perfusion and oxygenation. Calcium chloride may be given to try to dissipate the EMD and to resume mechanical contraction. Pacing will not help if the muscle is unable to respond mechanically to electrical stimulation.

ASYSTOLE

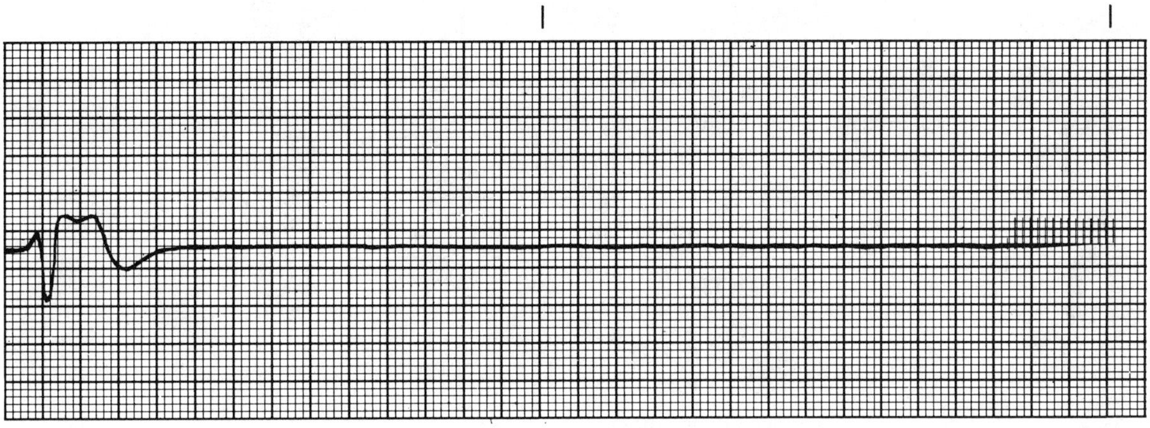

Asystole

In asystole there is no electrical activity at all, and the patient is dead. The ECG shows a flat baseline. Unless some electrical activity can be stimulated with epinephrine, isoproterenol, calcium chloride, or a pacemaker, the patient will not survive. Unfortunately, this rhythm is usually the end of the line, and drug or electrical therapy has little or no success.

PRACTICE STRIPS

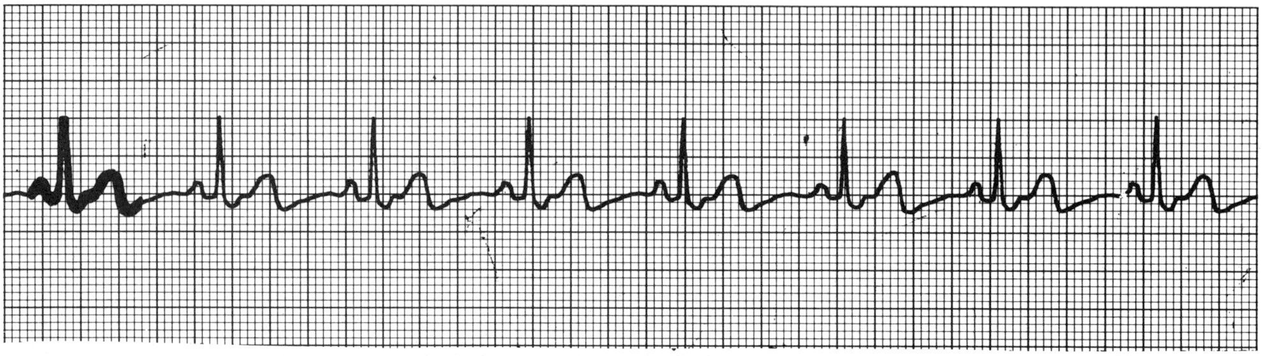

Practice strip 5-1

RHYTHM:

RATE:

P WAVES:

PR INTERVAL:

QRS COMPLEX:

INTERPRETATION:

THERAPY:

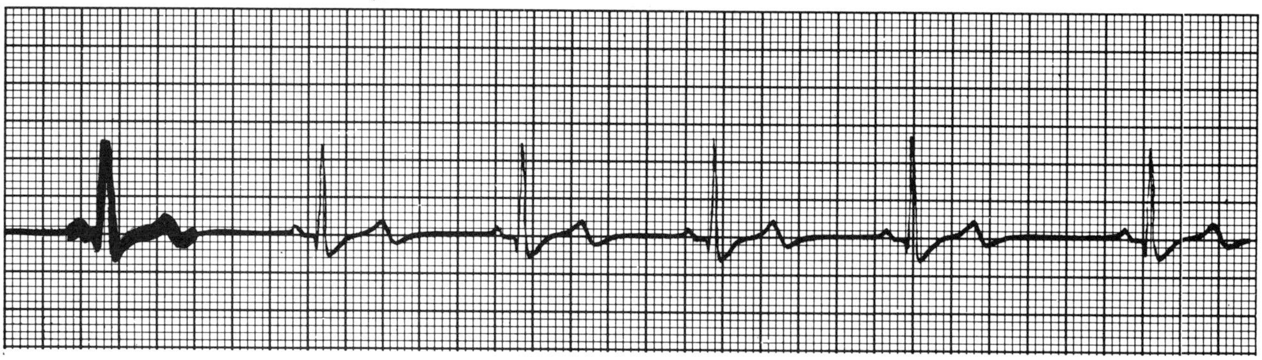

Practice strip 5-2

RHYTHM:

RATE:

P WAVES:

PR INTERVAL:

QRS COMPLEX:

INTERPRETATION:

THERAPY:

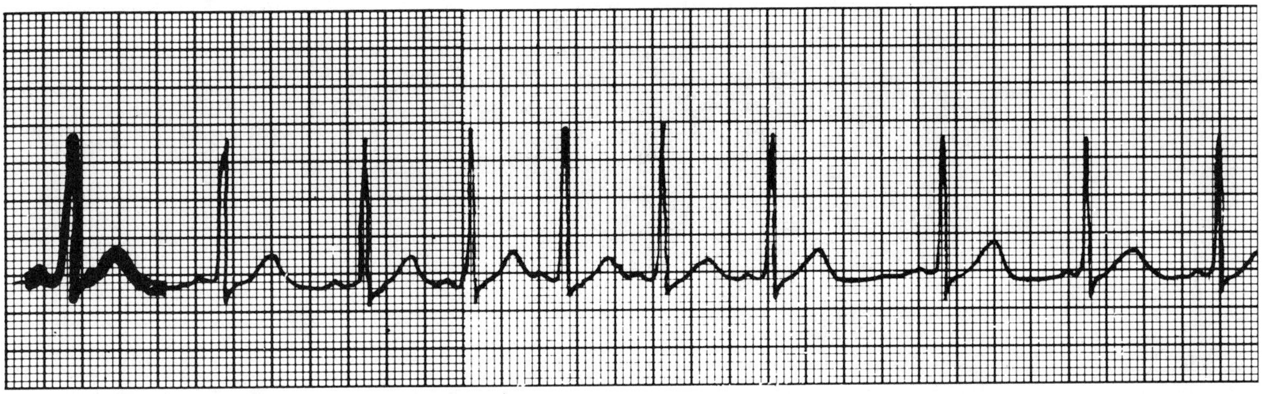

Practice strip 5-3

RHYTHM:
RATE:
P WAVES:
PR INTERVAL:
QRS COMPLEX:
INTERPRETATION:
THERAPY:

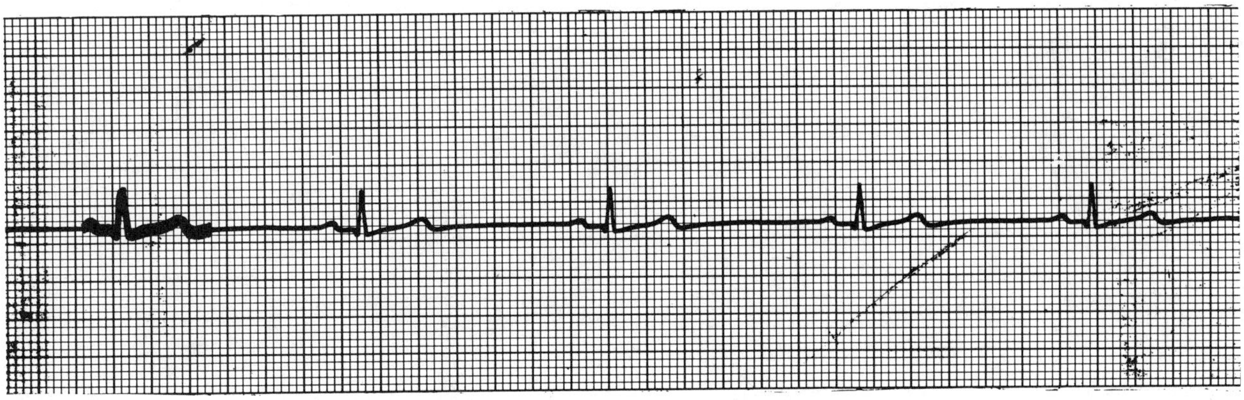

Practice strip 5-4

RHYTHM:
RATE:
P WAVES:
PR INTERVAL:
QRS COMPLEX:
INTERPRETATION:
THERAPY:

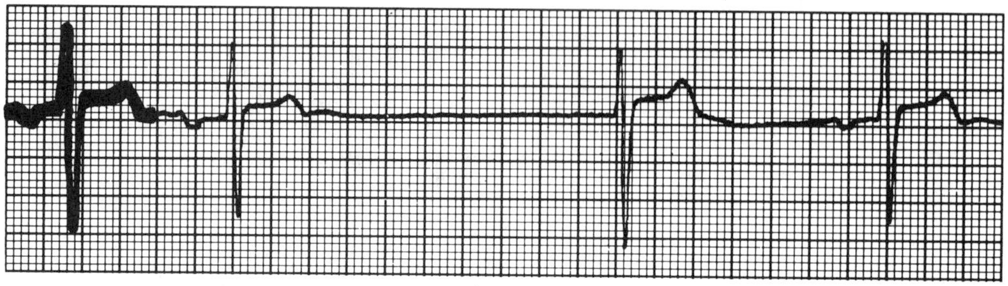

Practice strip 5-5

RHYTHM:
RATE:
P WAVES:
PR INTERVAL:
QRS COMPLEX:
INTERPRETATION:
THERAPY:

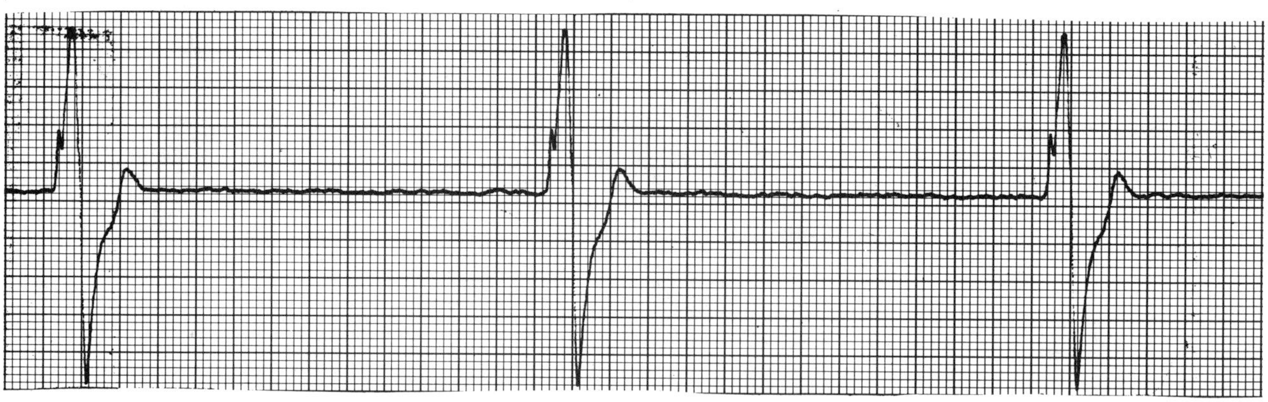

Practice strip 5-6

RHYTHM:
RATE:
P WAVES:
PR INTERVAL:
QRS COMPLEX:
INTERPRETATION:
THERAPY:

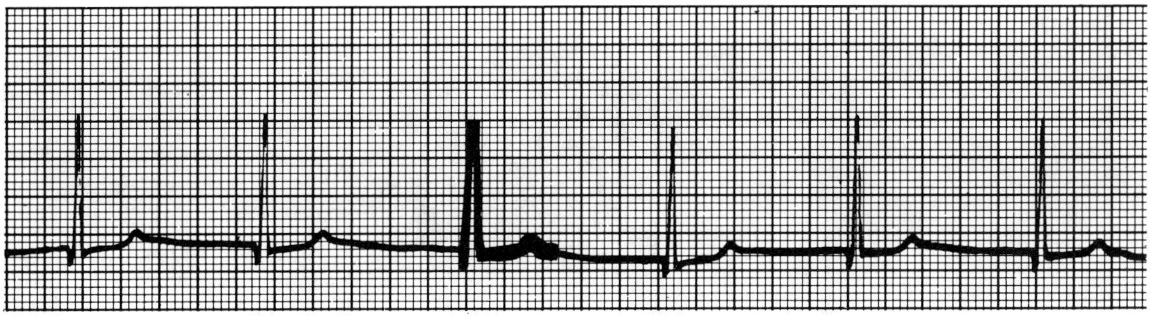

Practice strip 5-7

RHYTHM:

RATE:

P WAVES:

PR INTERVAL:

QRS COMPLEX:

INTERPRETATION:

THERAPY:

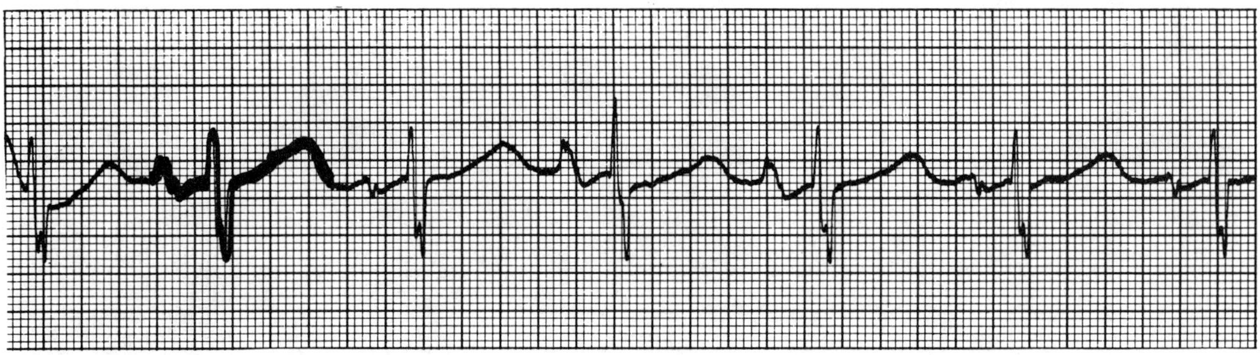

Practice strip 5-8

RHYTHM:

RATE:

P WAVES:

PR INTERVAL:

QRS COMPLEX:

INTERPRETATION:

THERAPY:

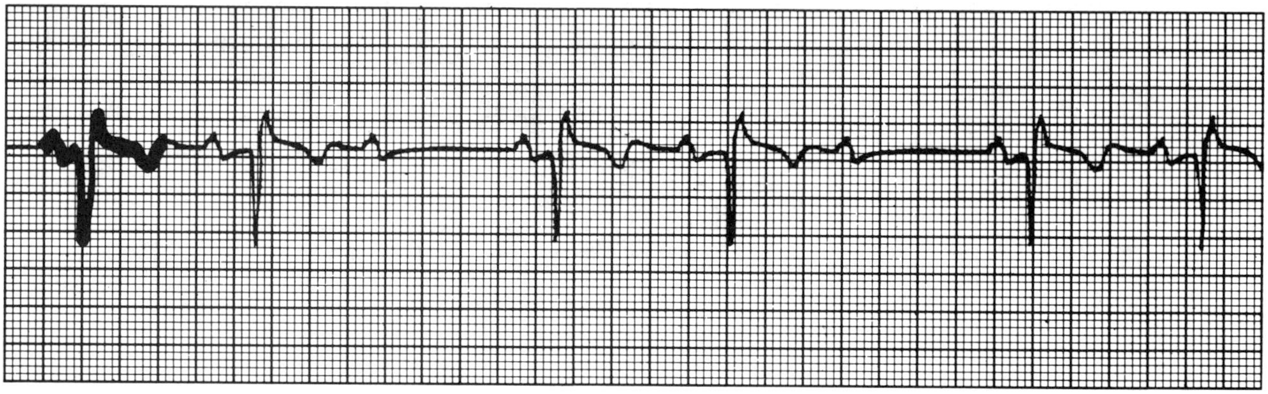

Practice strip 5-9

RHYTHM:
RATE:
P WAVES:
PR INTERVAL:
QRS COMPLEX:
INTERPRETATION:
THERAPY:

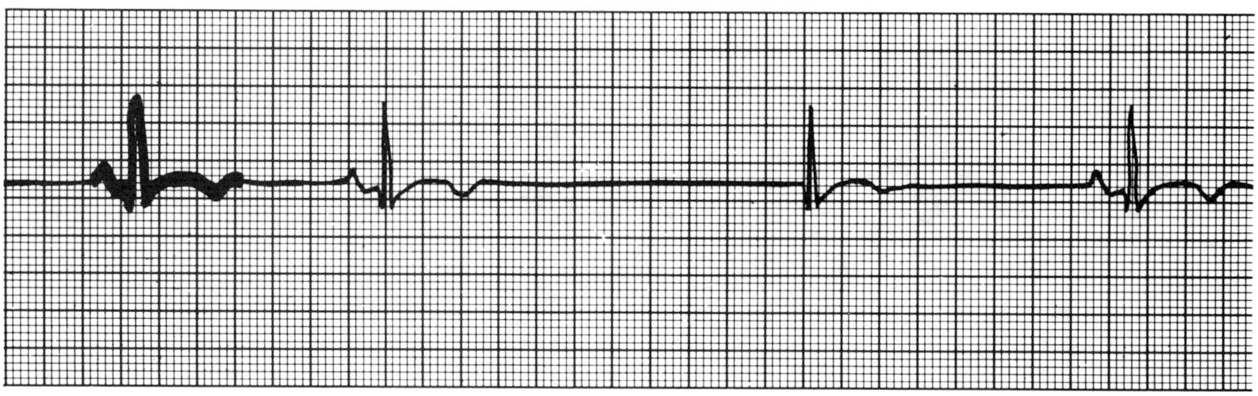

Practice strip 5-10

RHYTHM:
RATE:
P WAVES:
PR INTERVAL:
QRS COMPLEX:
INTERPRETATION:
THERAPY:

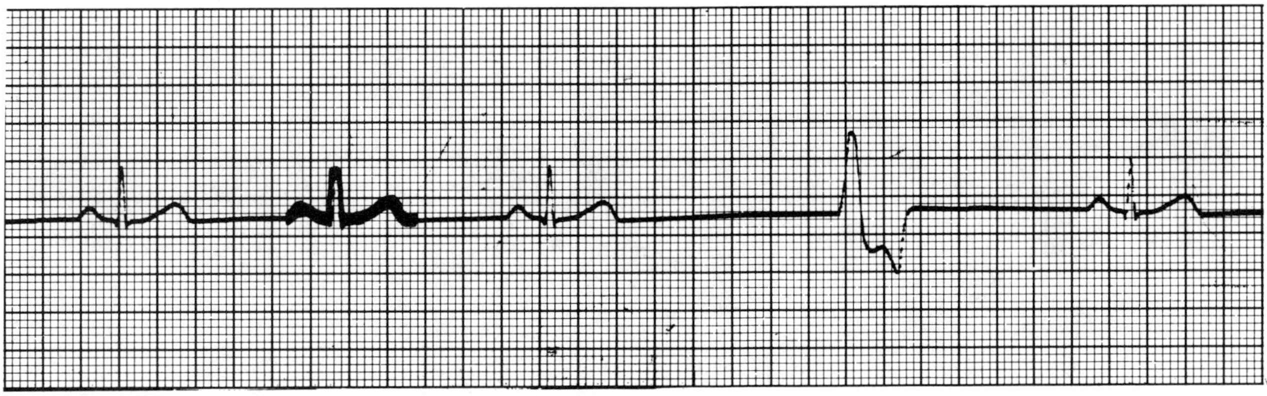

Practice strip 5-11

RHYTHM:

RATE:

P WAVES:

PR INTERVAL:

QRS COMPLEX:

INTERPRETATION:

THERAPY:

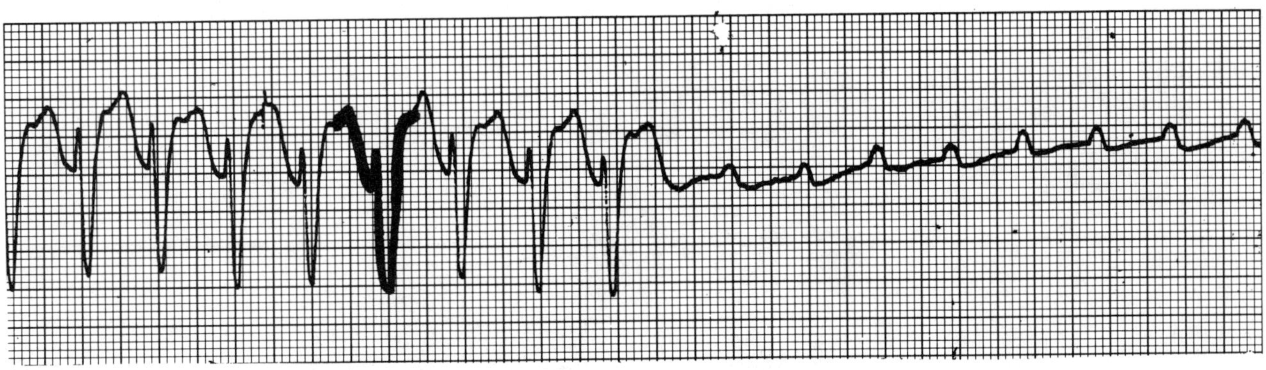

Practice strip 5-12

RHYTHM:

RATE:

P WAVES:

PR INTERVAL:

QRS COMPLEX:

INTERPRETATION:

THERAPY:

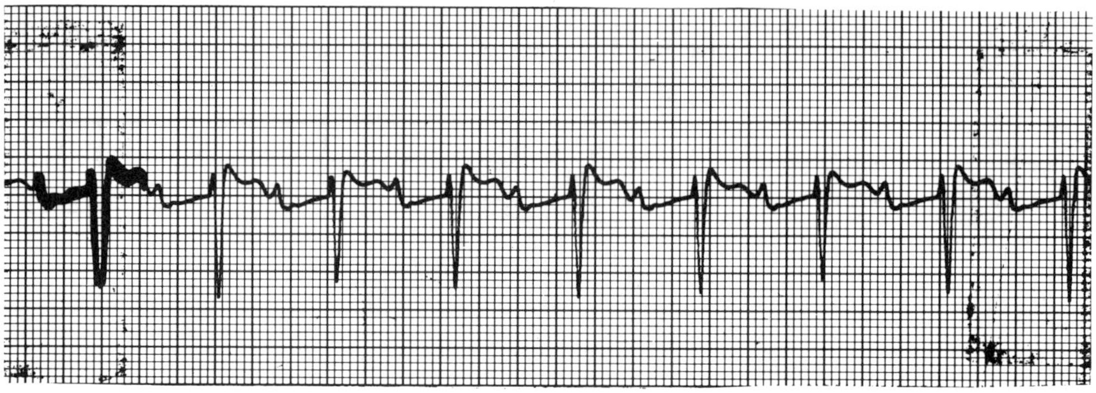

Practice strip 5-13

RHYTHM:

RATE:

P WAVES:

PR INTERVAL:

QRS COMPLEX:

INTERPRETATION:

THERAPY:

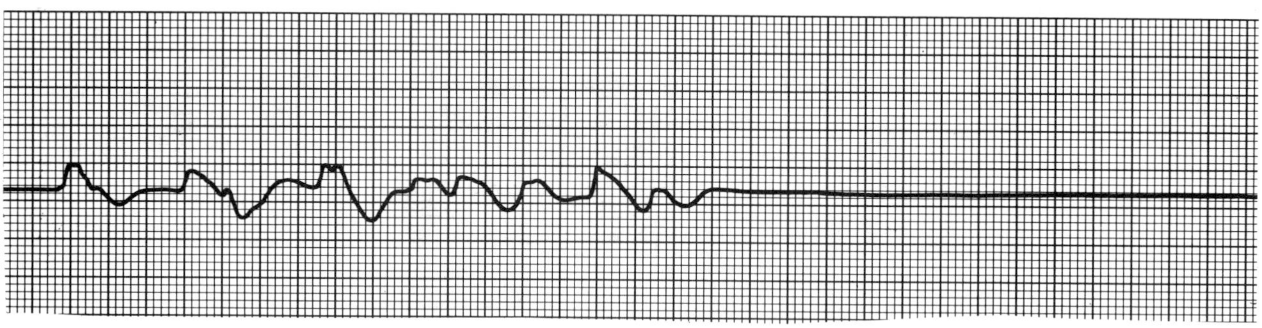

Practice strip 5-14

RHYTHM:

RATE:

P WAVES:

PR INTERVAL:

QRS COMPLEX:

INTERPRETATION:

THERAPY:

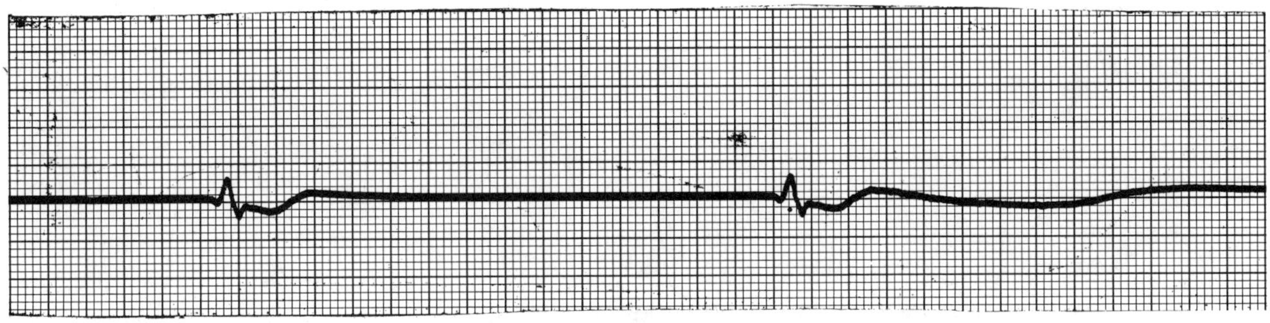

Practice strip 5-15

RHYTHM:
RATE:
P WAVES:
PR INTERVAL:
QRS COMPLEX:
INTERPRETATION:
THERAPY:

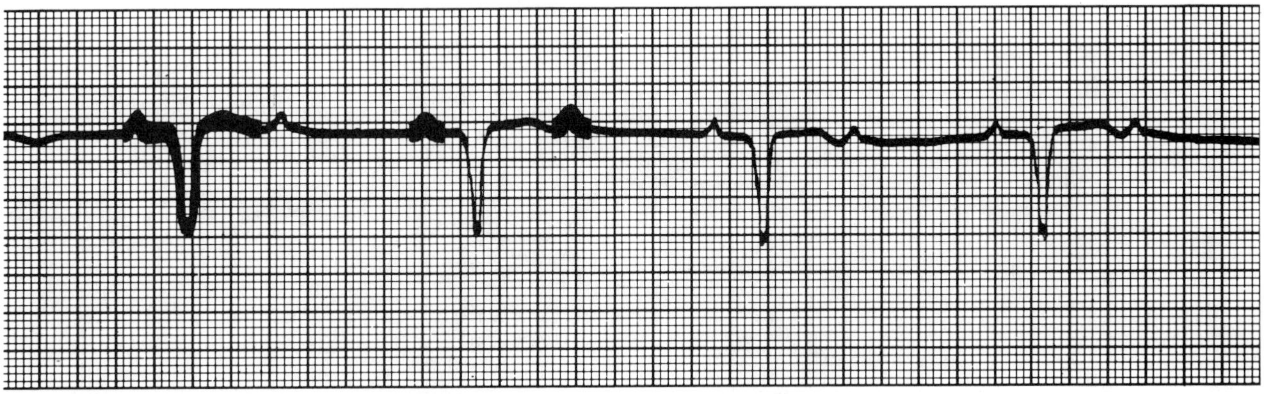

Practice strip 5-16

RHYTHM:
RATE:
P WAVES:
PR INTERVAL:
QRS COMPLEX:
INTERPRETATION:
THERAPY:

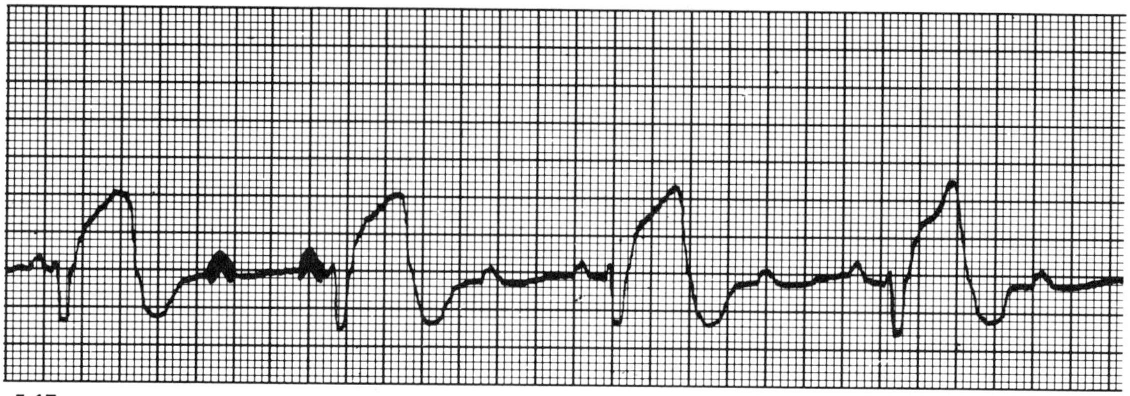

Practice strip 5-17

RHYTHM:

RATE:

P WAVES:

PR INTERVAL:

QRS COMPLEX:

INTERPRETATION:

THERAPY:

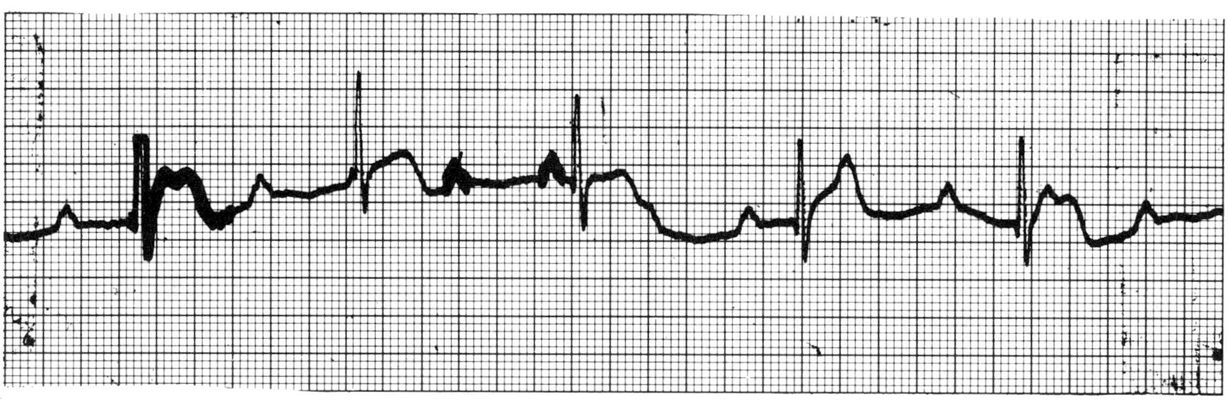

Practice strip 5-18

RHYTHM:

RATE:

P WAVES:

PR INTERVAL:

QRS COMPLEX:

INTERPRETATION:

THERAPY:

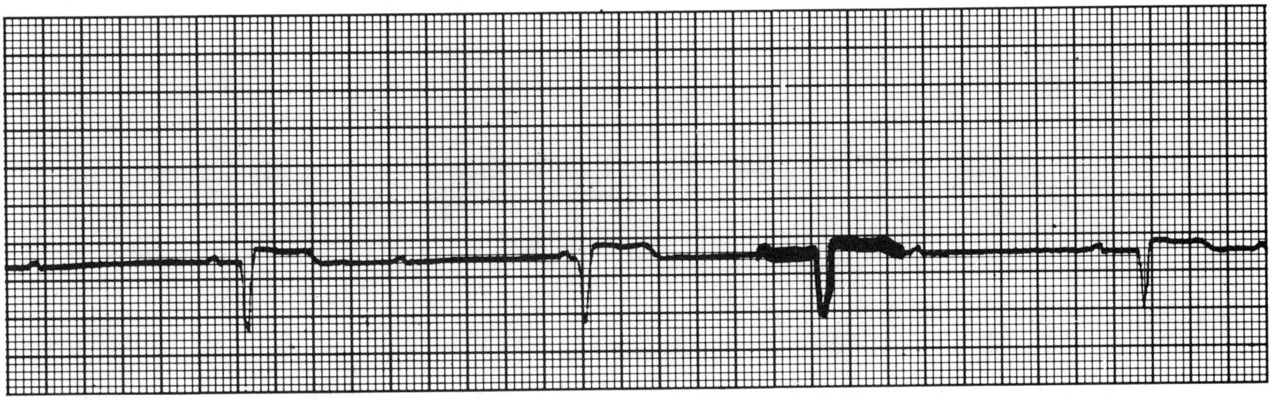

Practice strip 5-19

RHYTHM:

RATE:

P WAVES:

PR INTERVAL:

QRS COMPLEX:

INTERPRETATION:

THERAPY:

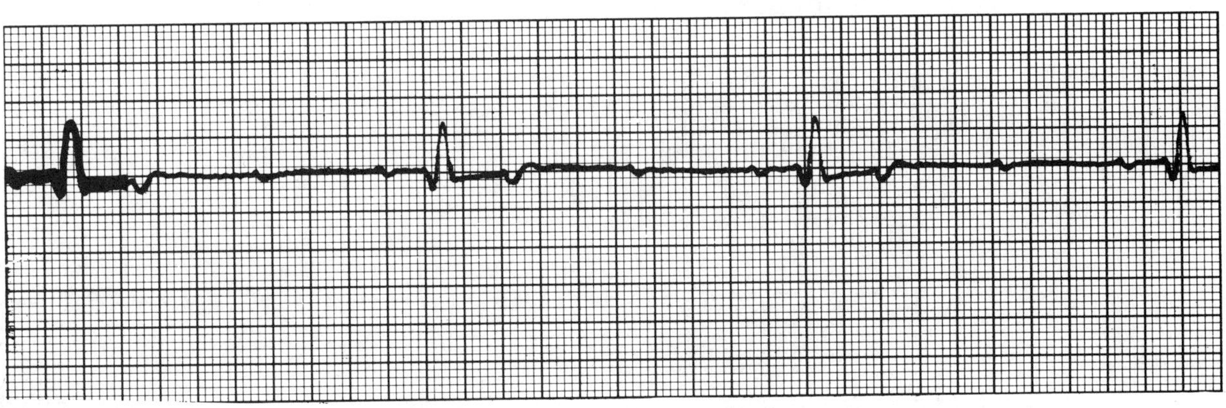

Practice strip 5-20

RHYTHM:

RATE:

P WAVES:

PR INTERVAL:

QRS COMPLEX:

INTERPRETATION:

THERAPY:

ANSWER STRIPS

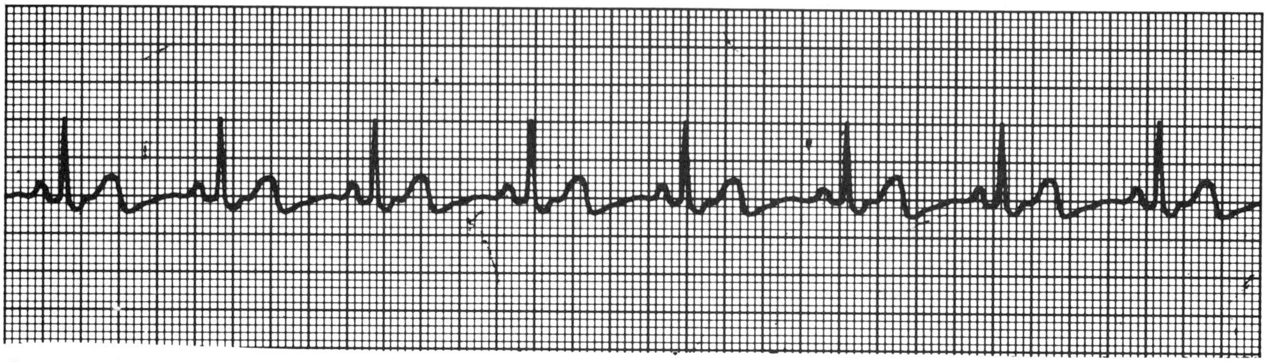

Answer strip 5-1

RHYTHM: *Regular*

RATE: *72*

P WAVES: *Normal*

PR INTERVAL: *0.16*

QRS COMPLEX: *0.12*

INTERPRETATION: *NSR*

THERAPY: *None*

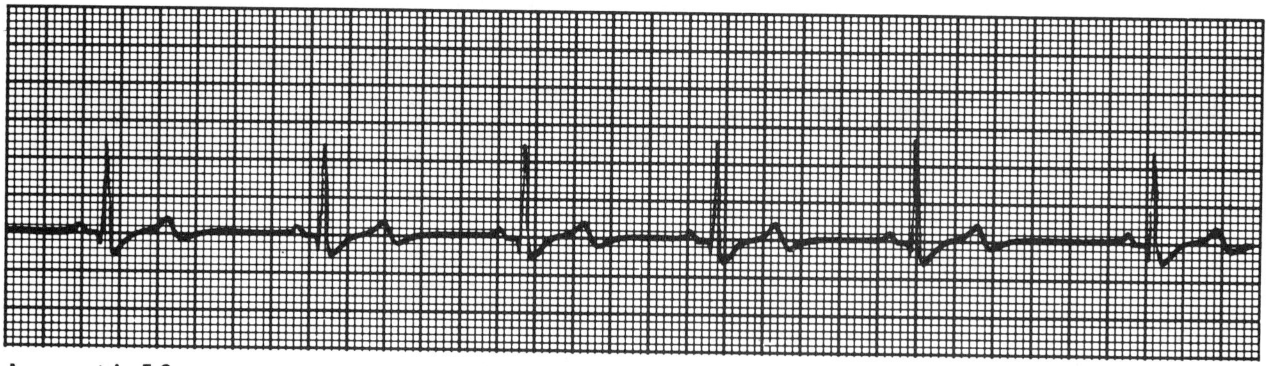

Answer strip 5-2

RHYTHM: *Irregular—speeds and slows*

RATE: *50*

P WAVES: *Normal*

PR INTERVAL: *0.13*

QRS COMPLEX: *0.12*

INTERPRETATION: *Sinus arrhythmia*

THERAPY: *None*

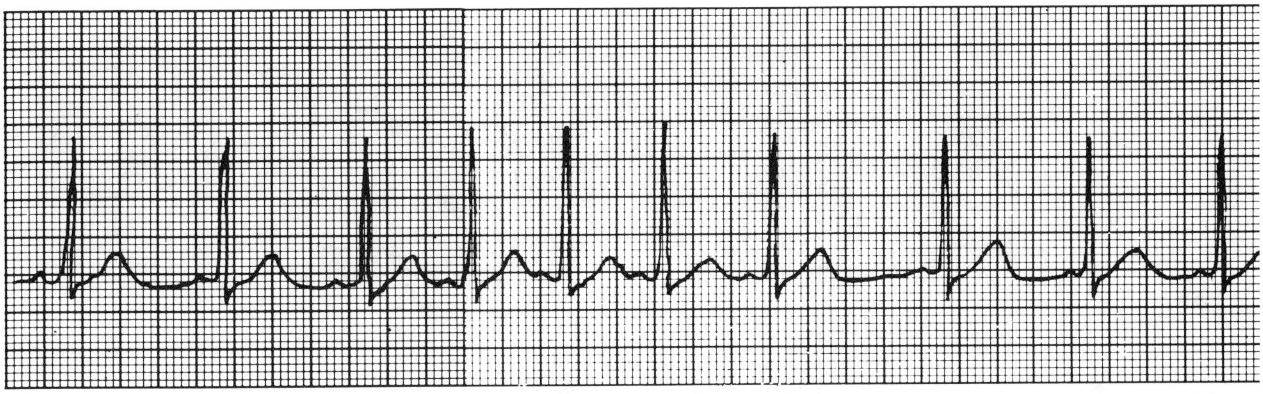

Answer strip 5-3

RHYTHM: *Irregular—speeds and slows*

RATE: *90*

P WAVES: *Normal*

PR INTERVAL: *0.16*

QRS COMPLEX: *0.08*

INTERPRETATION: *Sinus arrhythmia*

THERAPY: *None*

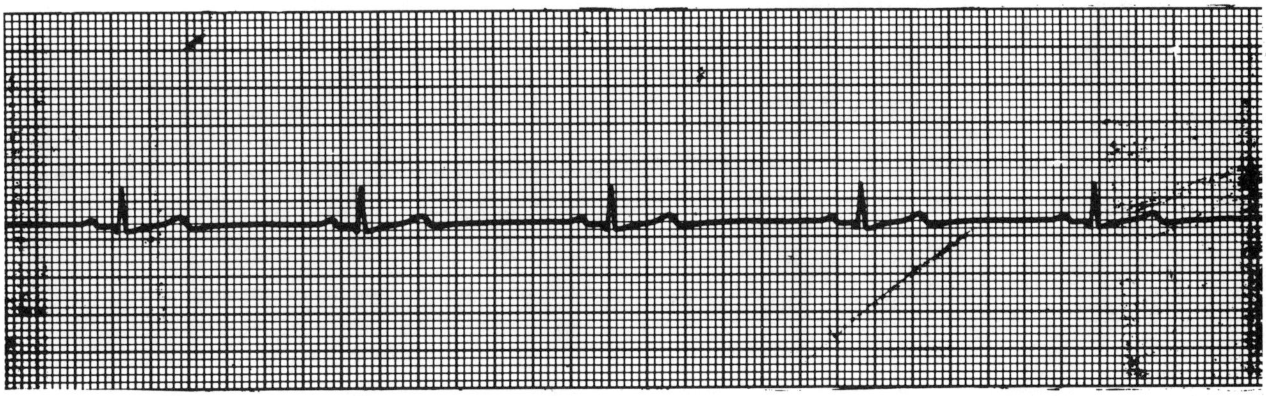

Answer strip 5-4

RHYTHM: *Regular (within three small squares)*

RATE: *45*

P WAVES: *Normal*

PR INTERVAL: *0.16*

QRS COMPLEX: *0.08*

INTERPRETATION: *Sinus bradycardia*

THERAPY: *Check patient; if symptomatic, administer atropine*

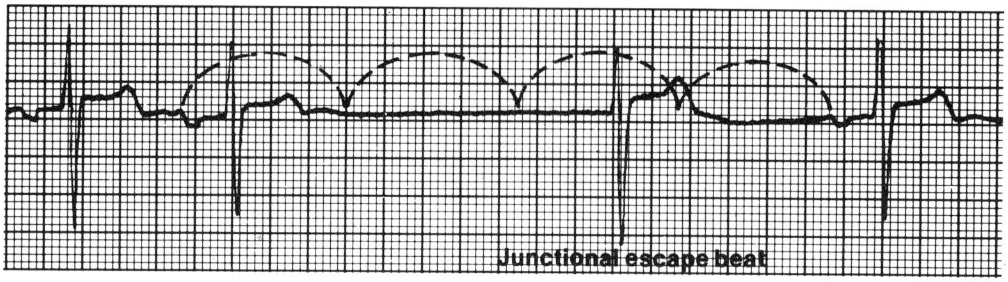

Answer strip 5-5

RHYTHM: *Irregular—pause and late beat, pause is 4 sinus cycles long*

RATE: *Sinus, 70; overall, 40*

P WAVES: *Normal—missing in pause—none in late beat*

PR INTERVAL: *0.26*

QRS COMPLEX: *0.12*

INTERPRETATION: *NSR (with AV block) with 2° SA block (exit block) type II with junctional escape beat*

THERAPY: *Observe patient; if symptomatic administer atropine or isoproterenol, and insert a pacemaker*

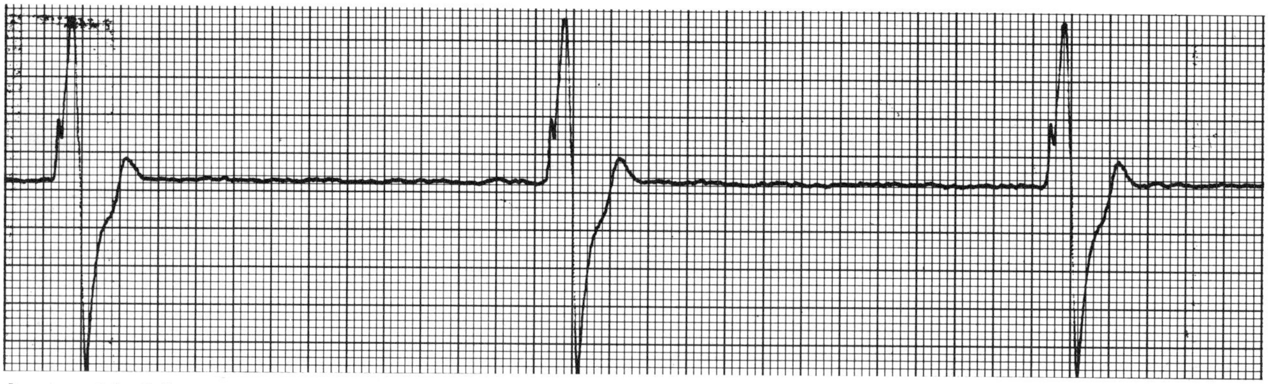

Answer strip 5-6

RHYTHM: *Regular*

RATE: *Less than 30*

P WAVES: *None*

PR INTERVAL: *None*

QRS COMPLEX: *0.24*

INTERPRETATION: *Ventricular rhythm*

THERAPY: *CPR; isoproterenol; pacemaker*

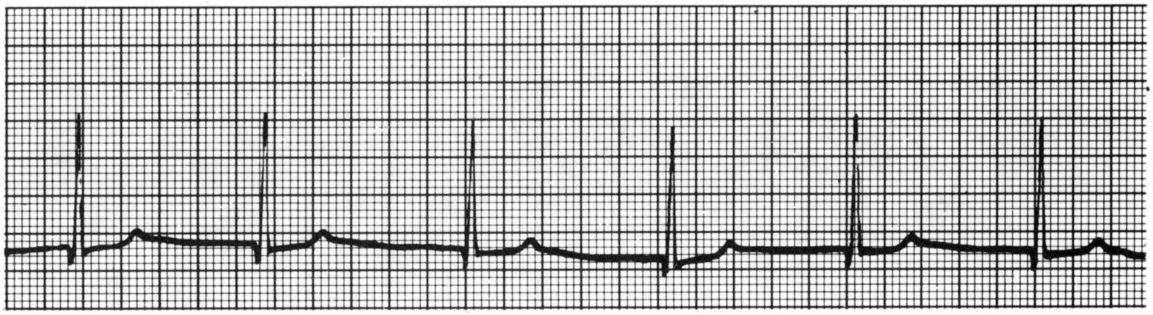

Answer strip 5-7

RHYTHM: *Regular*

RATE: *60*

P WAVES: *None*

PR INTERVAL: *None*

QRS COMPLEX: *0.10*

INTERPRETATION: *Junctional rhythm*

THERAPY: *Watch patient; administer atropine if needed*

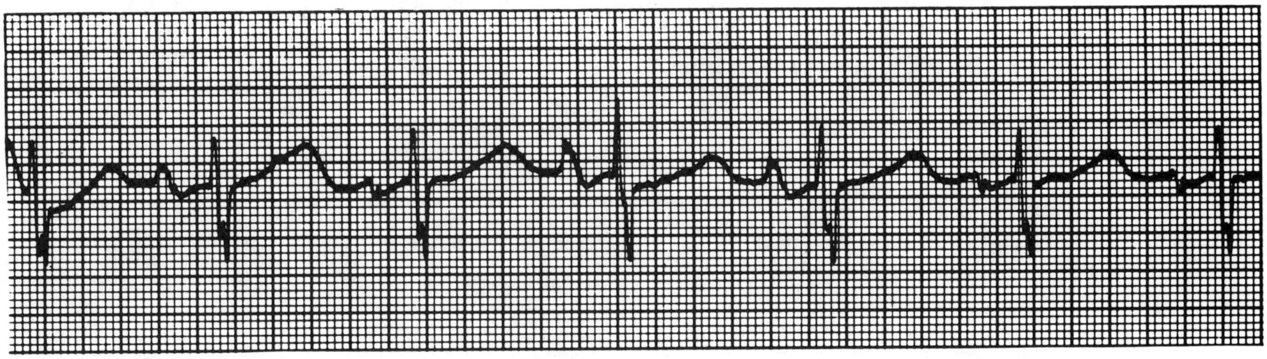

Answer strip 5-8

RHYTHM: *Slightly irregular*

RATE: *60*

P WAVES: *Present—differ in configuration*

PR INTERVAL: *Varies as P wave changes—0.24–0.20*

QRS COMPLEX: *0.10*

INTERPRETATION: *Wandering atrial pacemaker*

THERAPY: *Observe patient; administer atropine if needed*

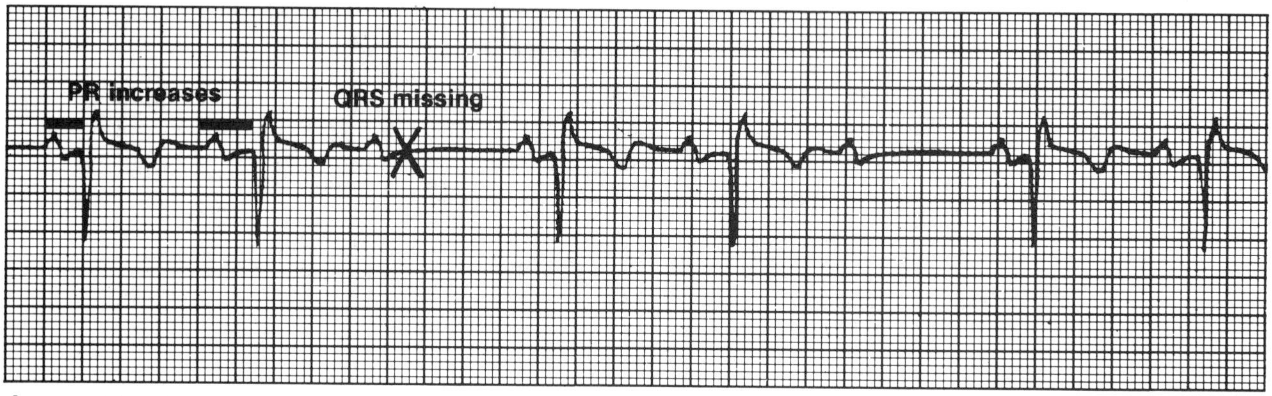

Answer strip 5-9

RHYTHM: *Atrial—regular; ventricular—irregular*

RATE: *Sinus, 72; ventricular, 50*

P WAVES: *Present—not all conducted*

PR INTERVAL: *Increases—0.18 → 0.26*

QRS COMPLEX: *0.10; occasional QRS missing*

INTERPRETATION: *NSR with 2° AV block type I (3:2 Wenckebach)*

THERAPY: *Observe for increasing block*

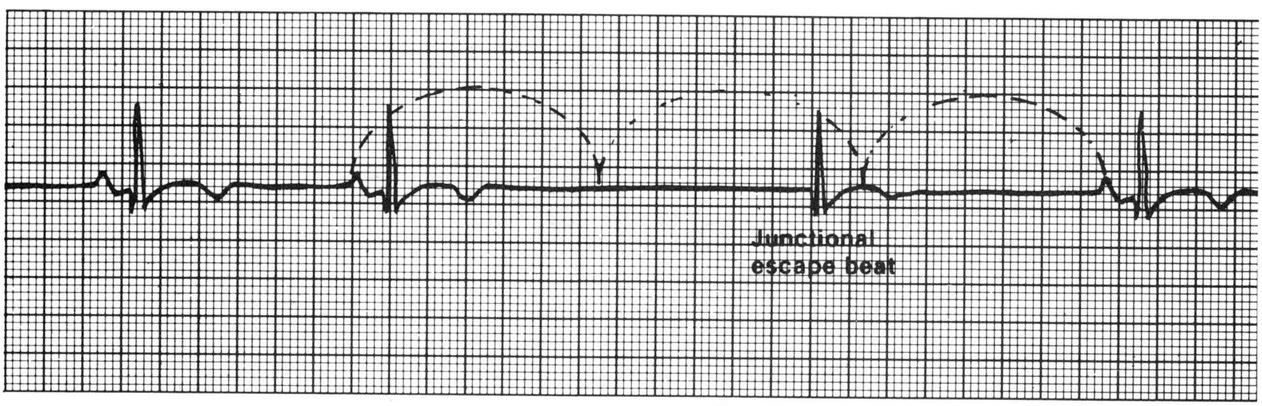

Answer strip 5-10

RHYTHM: *Irregular—pause and late beat—pause is three sinus cycles in length*

RATE: *Sinus, 45; overall, 40*

P WAVES: *Present—none in front of late beat*

PR INTERVAL: *0.18*

QRS COMPLEX: *0.08*

INTERPRETATION: *Sinus bradycardia with 2° SA block (exit block) type II and junctional escape beat*

THERAPY: *Atropine if needed*

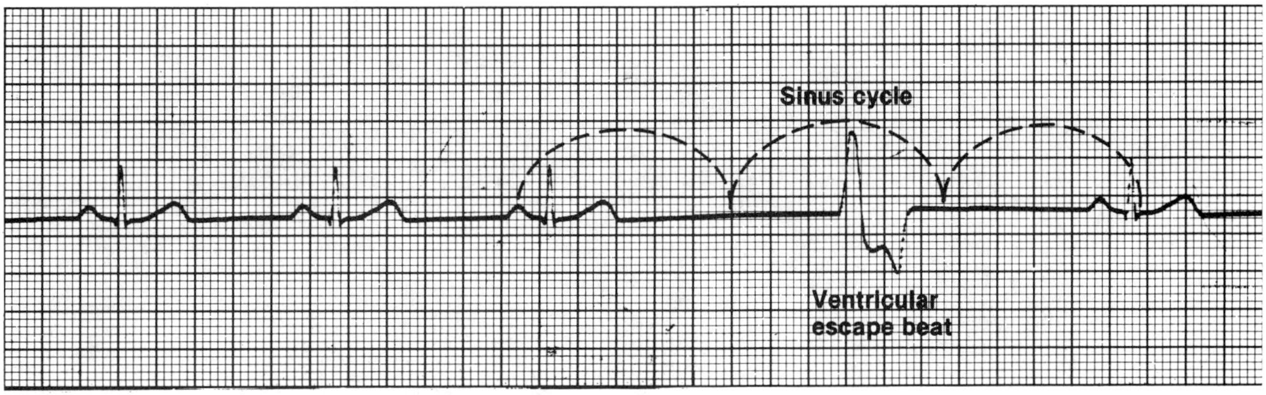

Answer strip 5-11

RHYTHM: *Irregular—pause and late beat; pause is* not *a multiple of sinus cycle*

RATE: *Sinus, 54; overall, 50*

P WAVES: *Present except during pause; none with late beat*

PR INTERVAL: *0.20*

QRS COMPLEX: *0.06—Late beat is wide and bizarre*

INTERPRETATION: *Sinus bradycardia with 3° SA block (sinus arrest) with ventricular escape beat*

THERAPY: *Atropine if needed*

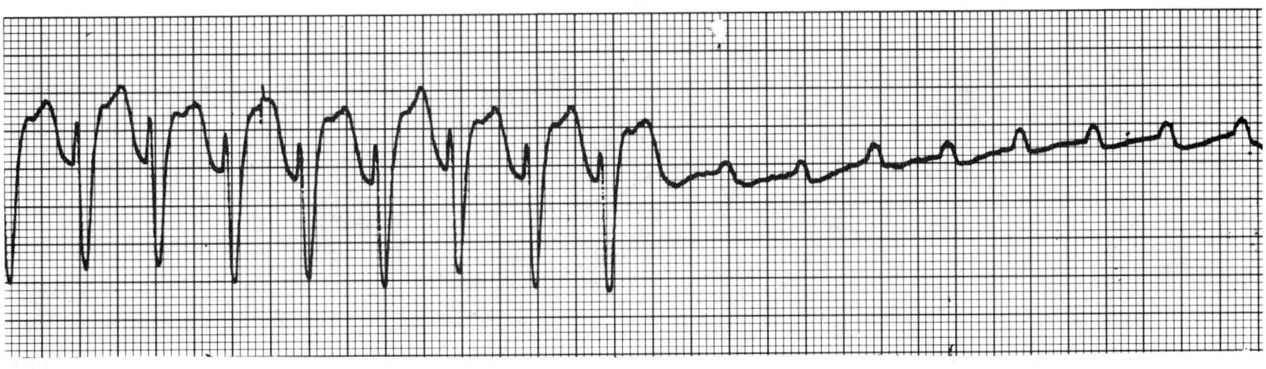

Answer strip 5-12

RHYTHM: *Regular*

RATE: *Sinus, 150; Ventricular, 150 → 0*

P WAVES: *Present—stop conducting to ventricles*

PR INTERVAL: *0.20*

QRS COMPLEX: *0.16*

INTERPRETATION: *Sinus tachycardia with BBB → primary ventricular standstill*

THERAPY: *CPR; pacemaker*

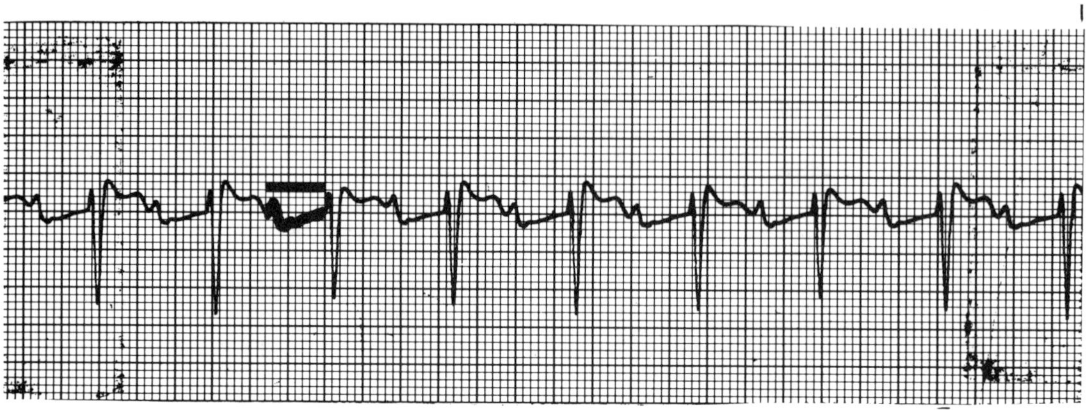

Answer strip 5-13

RHYTHM: *Regular*

RATE: *95*

P WAVES: *Normal*

PR INTERVAL: *0.32*

QRS COMPLEX: *0.10*

INTERPRETATION: *NSR with 1° AV block*

THERAPY: *Observe patient*

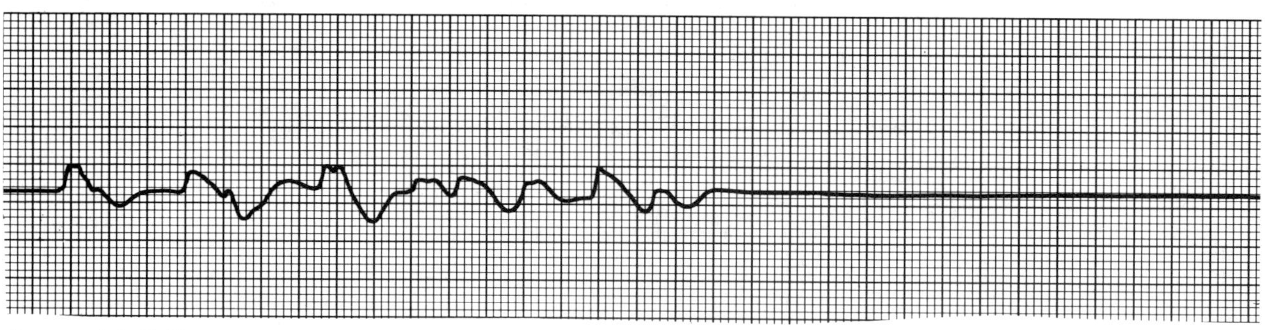

Answer strip 5-14

RHYTHM: *Irregular*

RATE: *?*

P WAVES: *None*

PR INTERVAL: *None*

QRS COMPLEX: *None*

INTERPRETATION: *Agonal rhythm → asystole*

THERAPY: *Code blue; CPR; pacemaker*

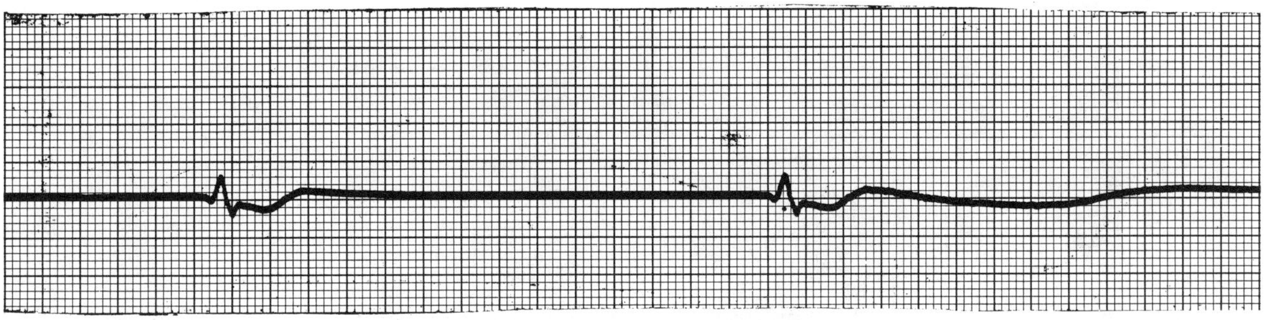

Answer strip 5-15

RHYTHM: *Regular*

RATE: ↓ *20*

P WAVES: *None*

PR INTERVAL: *None*

QRS COMPLEX: *0.16*

INTERPRETATION: *Secondary ventricular standstill*

THERAPY: *Code Blue; CPR; pacemaker*

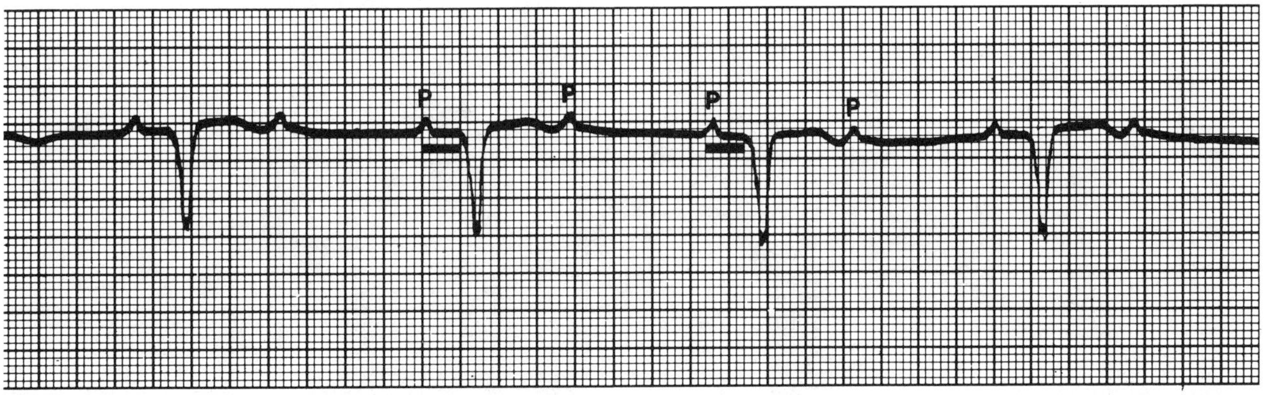

Answer strip 5-16

RHYTHM: *Atrial, regular; ventricular, regular*

RATE: *Sinus, 80; ventricular, 40*

P WAVES: *Present—every other P wave not conducted*

PR INTERVAL: *0.24—constant*

QRS COMPLEX: *0.14*

INTERPRETATION: *NSR with 2° AV block type II 2:1 and Bundle branch block*

THERAPY: *Atropine; isoproterenol; pacemaker*

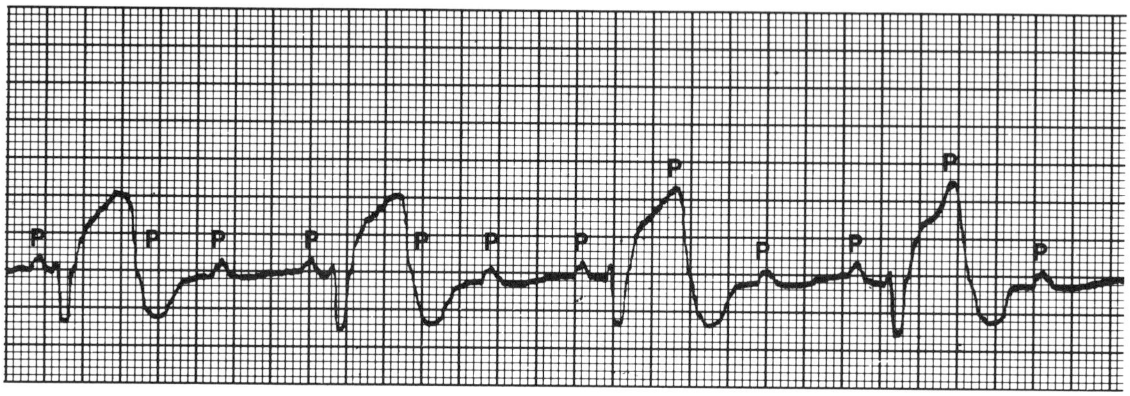

Answer strip 5-17

RHYTHM: *Atrial, regular; ventricular, regular*

RATE: *Sinus, 130; ventricular, 40*

P WAVES: *Present—none are conducted*

PR INTERVAL: *Varies with each QRS*

QRS COMPLEX: *0.14*

INTERPRETATION: *Sinus tachycardia with 3° AV block (lower pacer is in ventricles)*

THERAPY: *Atropine; isoproterenol; pacemaker*

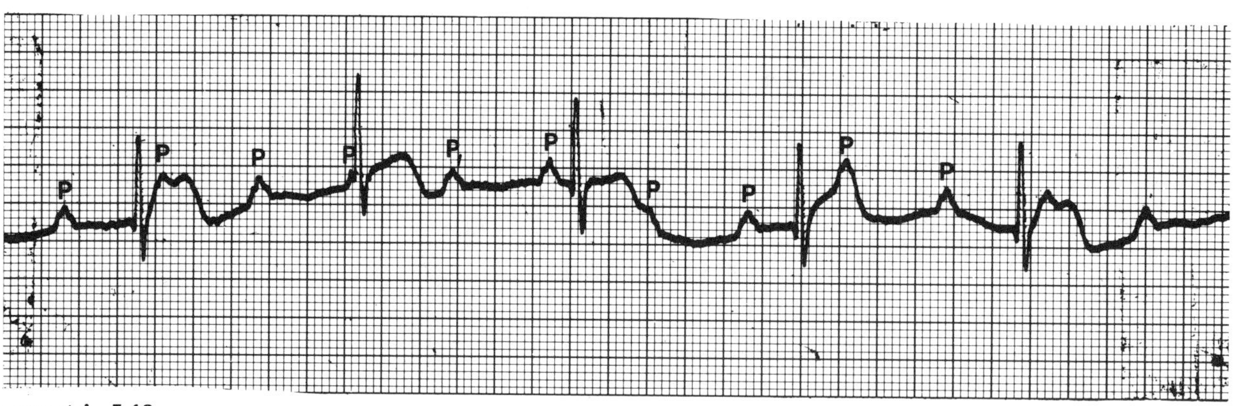

Answer strip 5-18

RHYTHM: *Atrial, regular; ventricular, regular*

RATE: *Sinus, 120; ventricular, 52*

P WAVES: *Present—none are conducted*

PR INTERVAL: *None—varies with each QRS*

QRS COMPLEX: *0.08*

INTERPRETATION: *Sinus tachycardia with 3° AV block (lower pacemaker is junctional)*

THERAPY: *Atropine; isoproterenol; pacemaker*

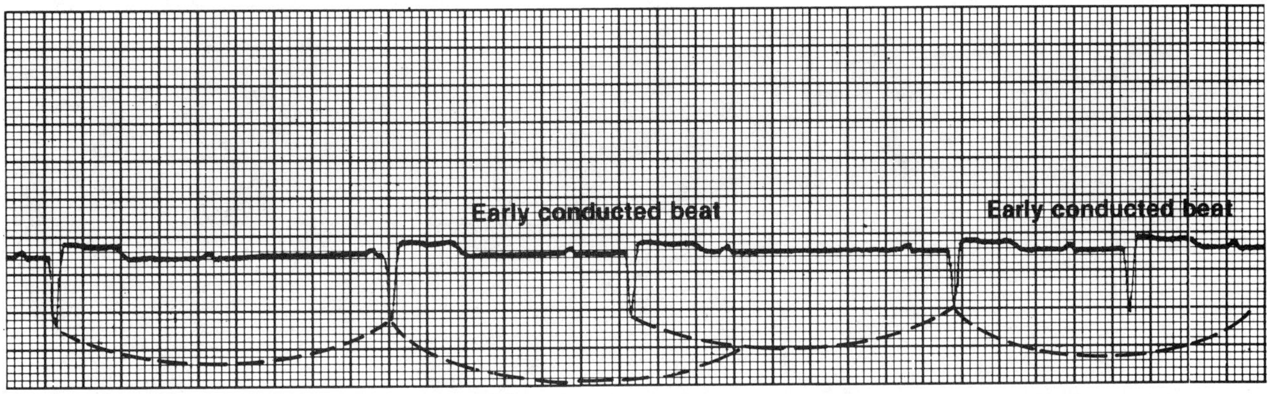

Answer strip 5-19

RHYTHM: *Atrial, slightly irregular; ventricular, irregular*

RATE: *Sinus, 63; ventricular, 30–40*

P WAVES: *Present—conducted occasionally*

PR INTERVAL: *0.34*

QRS COMPLEX: *0.10*

INTERPRETATION: *NSR with high-grade AV block*

THERAPY: *Atropine; isoproterenol; pacemaker*

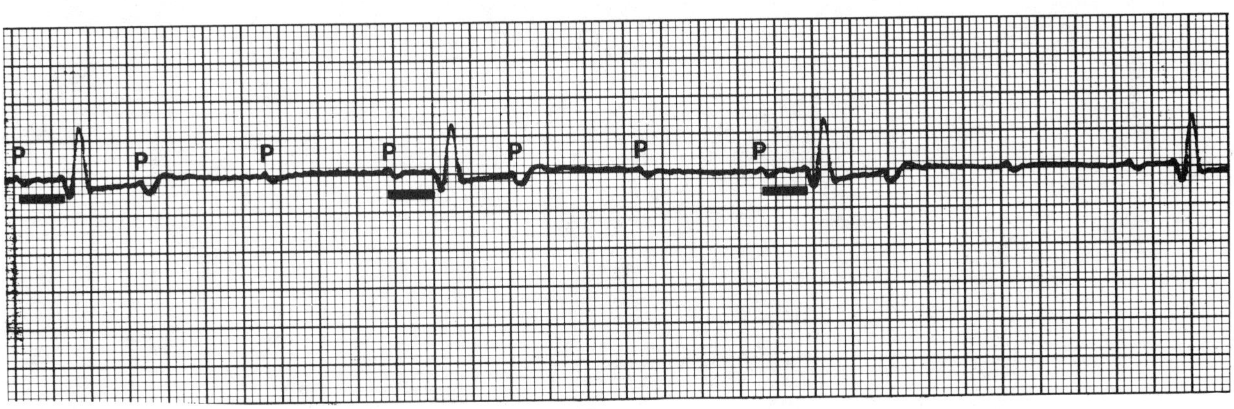

Answer strip 5-20

RHYTHM: *Atrial, regular; ventricular, regular*

RATE: *Sinus, 90; ventricular, 30*

P WAVES: *Present—only one out of three conducted*

PR INTERVAL: *0.26—constant*

QRS COMPLEX: *0.16*

INTERPRETATION: *NSR with 2° AV block, type II 3:1 conduction and bundle branch block*

THERAPY: *Atropine; isoproterenol; pacemaker*

6

DYSRHYTHMIAS RESULTING FROM IRRITABILITY

IRRITABILITY

In this chapter, we will discuss all the dysrhythmias that result from irritability of the myocardium, which produces enhanced automaticity and altered conductivity.

THE CAUSES AND EFFECTS OF IRRITABILITY

A detailed description of the causes of irritability and its effect on the heart is provided in Chapter 4. But, as a brief review, some of the factors that generate irritability are increased sympathetic tone, decreased vagal tone, ischemia or injury of the myocardium, hypokalemia, heat, myocardial stretch, hypoxia and acidosis, and drugs.

Even though the causes of irritability are varied, their effects on the electrical activity of the heart remain similar. If irritability affects the automaticity, it will accelerate the spontaneous discharge cycle (SDC) of ectopic pacing foci, usurping the pacing activity from the sinoatrial (SA) node and producing early beats that arrive before the next sinus beat is expected, or fast rhythms. The specific dysrhythmias produced by increased automaticity include accelerated junctional and ventricular rhythms, premature atrial contractions (PAC), premature junctional contractions (PJC), premature ventricular contractions (PVC), fusion beats, and the tachycardias. If the conductivity of the heart is affected, you may see the mechanism of depolarization change into flutter or fibrillation, or aberrant ventricular conduction. The specific dysrhythmias produced by altered conductivity include atrial or ventricular flutter, atrial or ventricular fibrillation, or aberrant ventricular conduction of supraventricular impulses. Another way that altered conductivity can cause irritability dysrhythmias is through the reentry mechanism.

REENTRY MECHANISM

Reentry occurs when a circuit is set up somewhere in the heart, which allows the propagation of repeated circulation of an electrical wavefront.

The circuit must have two fibers, (A and B), with unequal refractory periods. In this diagram, fiber A has a longer refractory period than does fiber B.

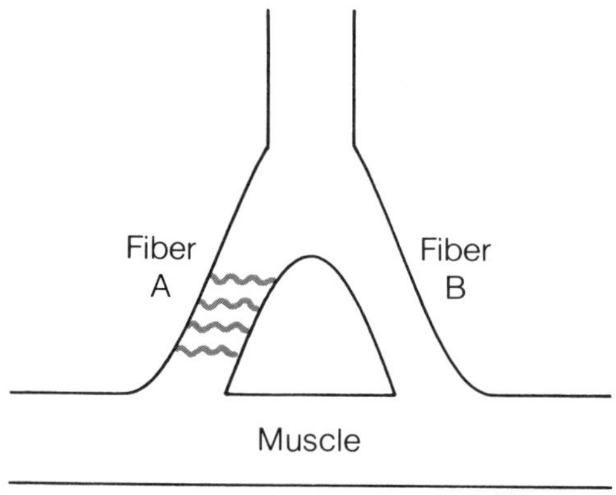

The impulse comes down from above, and when it reaches the fork where fibers A and B divide, it cannot move down fiber A because fiber A is still in the refractory period. It can proceed down fiber B in the normal fashion.

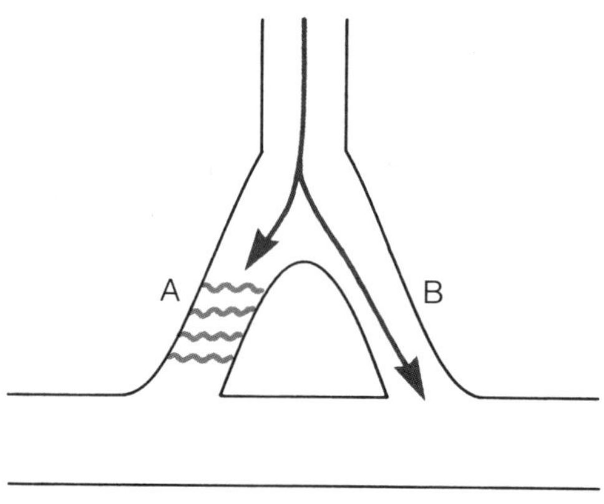

The impulse spreads through the muscle, and when it reaches the distal end of fiber A, the impulse can get back up fiber A in a retrograde fashion because fiber A has had time to recover.

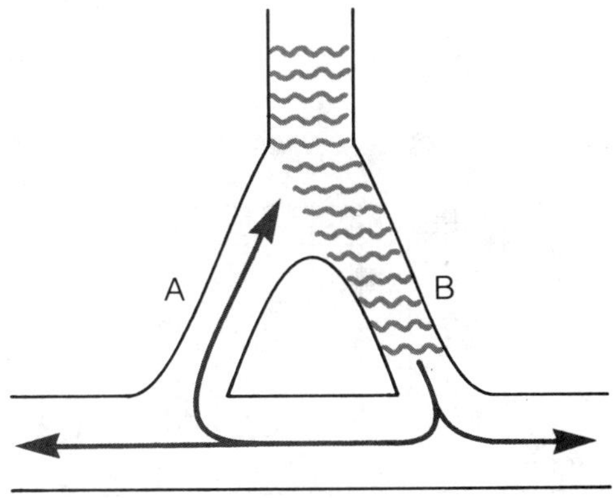

By the time the electrical impulse reaches the bifurcation of fiber B in the retrograde fashion, fiber B has recovered, so the impulse starts around again, and the reentry circuit is complete. The impulse circles around the reentry circuit, and each time it does, it causes another premature beat.

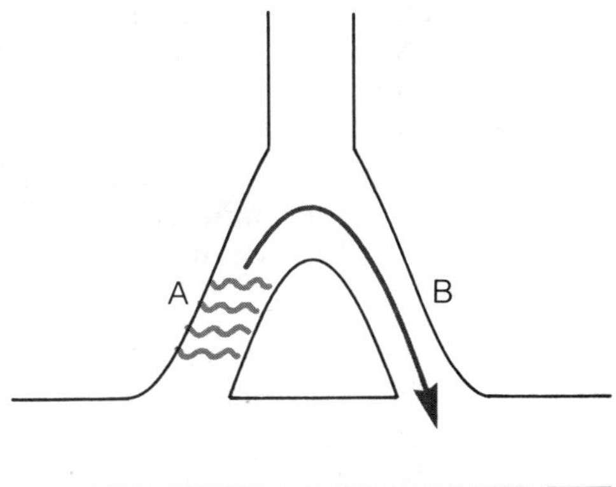

These reentry circuits can be located in the SA node, atria, atrioventricular (AV) node, His bundle, or in the Purkinje fibers and ventricular myocardium. They may cause premature beats in any of these locations. Two tachycardias commonly produced by reentry are known as the Wolff-Parkinson-White (WPW) syndrome and the Lown-Ganong-Levine (LGL) syndrome.

THE EARLY BEATS

When irritability speeds the SDC of an ectopic pacing focus or a reentry circuit begins, the result can be a premature beat that arrives earlier than the next sinus beat is expected. You can determine the site of origin of the early beat by comparing its configuration with that of the sinus beat. At times, early beats may have a wide, bizarre QRS complex. It may be difficult to determine the site of origin of these funny looking beats (FLBs), but with careful attention to the criteria, you should be able to reach a correct interpretation.

PREMATURE ATRIAL CONTRACTIONS

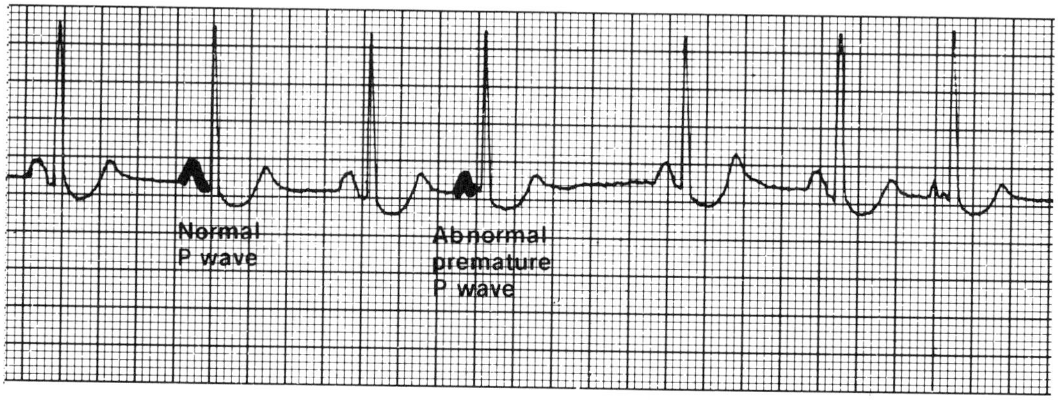

PACs occur when the irritable focus that fires off before the SA node does, or the reentry circuit, is located in the atrial myocardium. The main distinguishing characteristic of a PAC is an *abnormal, premature* P wave. The shape of this atrial P wave will differ from that of the sinus P wave in the same lead. The PR interval will also differ from that of the sinus PR, but will still be within normal limits.

The QRS complex of a PAC may be affected in one of three ways by the prematurity of the beat, and the refractoriness of the bundle branches. They may be normal, aberrantly conducted, or absent.

Normal QRS Complexes

The QRS of the PAC may be absolutely normal and be identical in configuration to the sinus QRSs. A normal QRS can occur only when the bundle branches have repolarized completely before the wave of depolarization from the PAC reaches them, allowing normal depolarization of the ventricles.

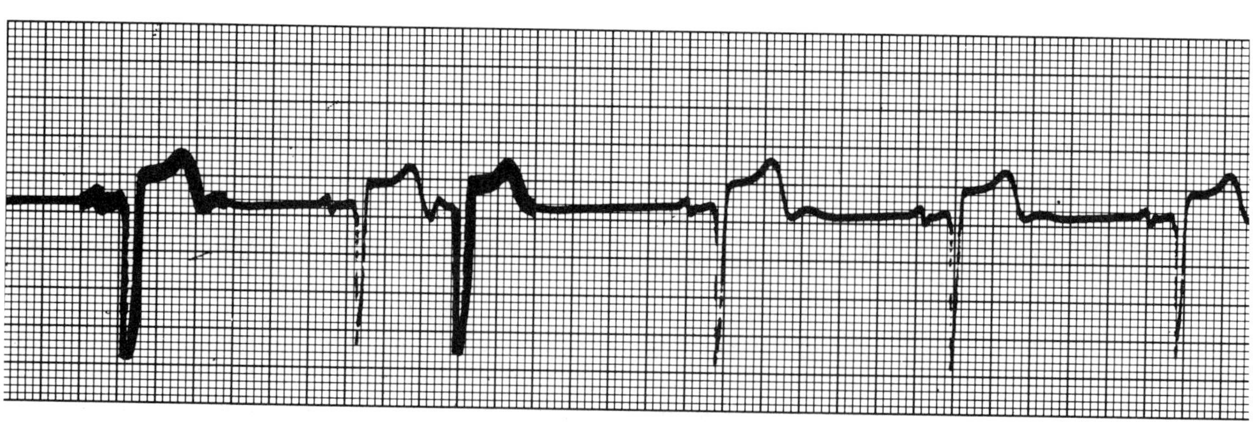

Aberrant QRS Complexes

When the wave of electrical activity from the PAC reaches the bundle branches before they have had time to completely repolarize from the preceding sinus beat, depolarization of the ventricles must proceed abnormally. Thus, the QRS complex will change shape and differ in configuration from the sinus QRS. The change in shape may be nothing more than the loss of an R wave or Q wave, or it could cause the QRS to resemble a ventricular beat. The earlier in the bundle branches' partial refractory period that the premature impulse arrives, the wider and more bizarre the QRS complex will be. Aberration is caused entirely by the prematurity of the beat, and not by any pathologic changes in the condition of the bundle branches.

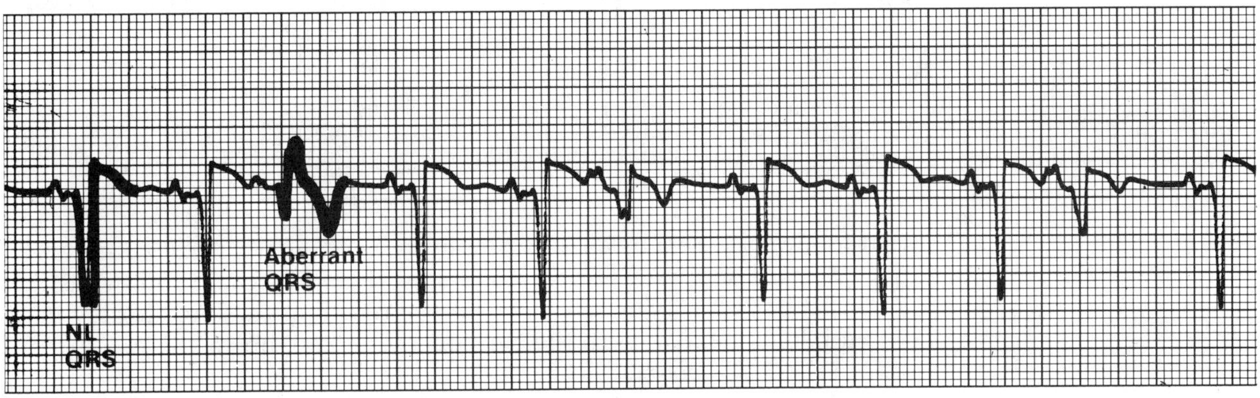

Absent QRS Complexes

If the premature impulses reach the AV node or bundle branches during the absolute refractory period, there will be no QRS complex at all. This is called a nonconducted PAC. It will appear as an abnormal premature P wave with no QRS following. This puts a pause in the underlying rhythm.

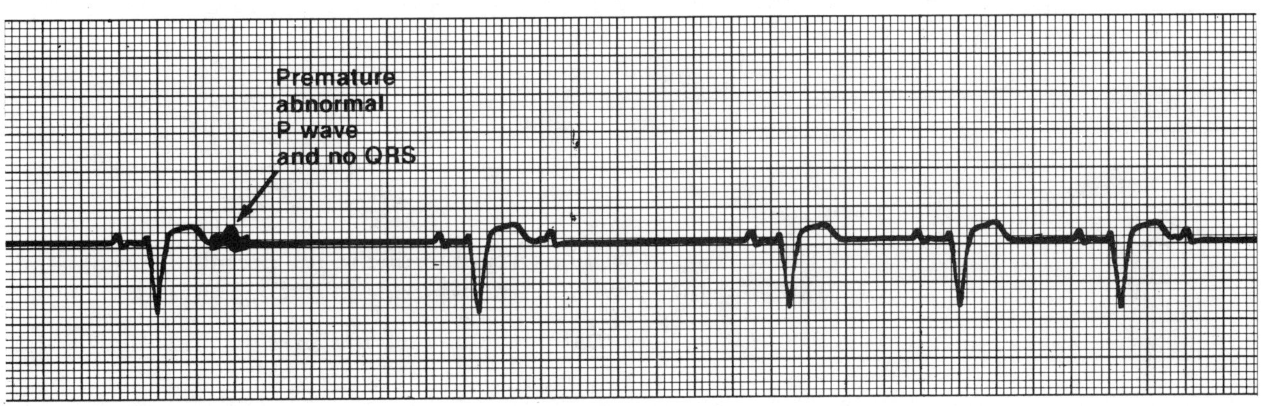

The Timing of PACs

PACs are, of course, premature, but they also will have certain effects on the underlying sinus rhythm. This occurs because the PAC arises in the atria, and the resulting wave of depolarization affects the SDC of the SA node. The PAC may "reset" the SA node, and the next sinus beat

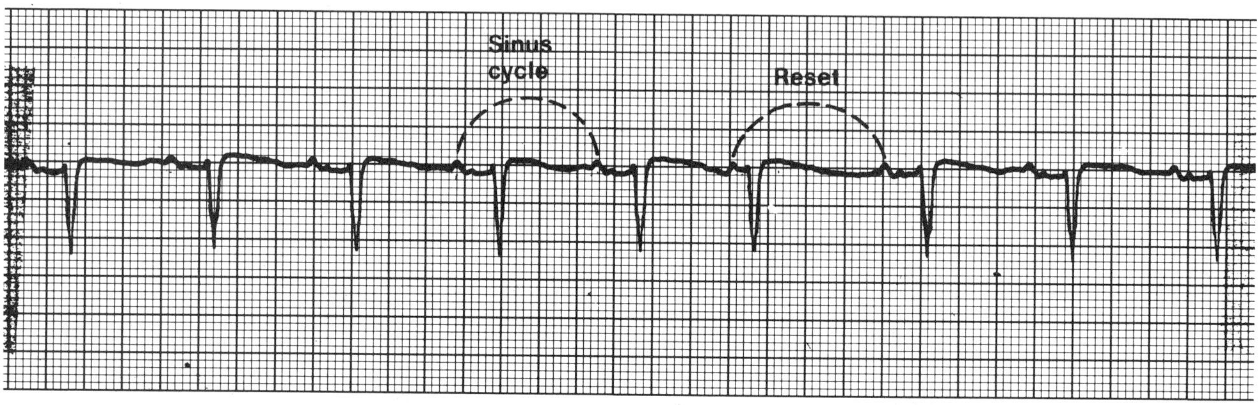

that follows the PAC by exactly one sinus cycle length. Most commonly, the PAC will suppress the SA node, and the sinus beats following the PAC will be at a slower rate than those preceding the PAC. It may take several sinus beats before the SA node gets back up to the rate it had before the PAC occurred.

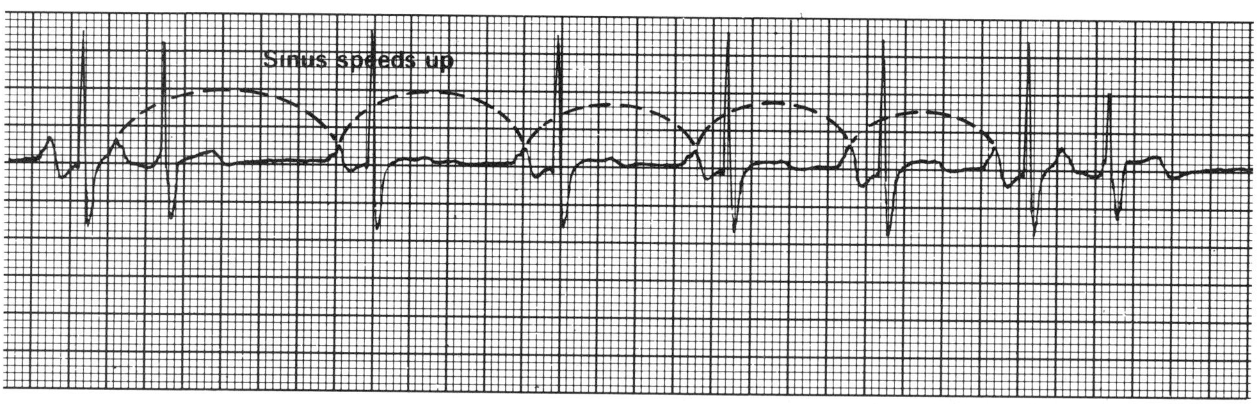

Criteria

RHYTHM: The rhythm will be irregular, due to the premature beats and the pauses, and the slowing of the SA node following the PAC.

RATE: The rate will be that of the underlying rhythm, plus that of the PACs.

P WAVES: The P waves of the PAC will be premature and differ in shape from that of the sinus P wave—*a premature, abnormal P wave!*

PR INTERVAL: The PR interval of the PAC will differ from that of the sinus beat, but probably will still be within normal limits.

QRS COMPLEX: The QRS complexes of a PAC will either be normal, wide and bizarre (aberrant), or missing (nonconducted).

Hemodynamic and Clinical Considerations

PACs are not considered to be a dangerous dysrhythmia, and very rarely require treatment. However, they should be taken as a warning of increasing atrial irritability, and the cause of this irritability should be determined. Some of the common causes of PACs include digitalis toxicity, atrial stretch resulting from early congestive heart failure, and changes in tissue oxygenation or electrolyte imbalances—all conditions far more serious than the dysrhythmia itself.

Therapy

Usually, no treatment is required but, if the PACs are causing runs of atrial tachycardia, digitalis, quinidine, procainamide, disopyramide, or propranolol can be used to suppress these beats.

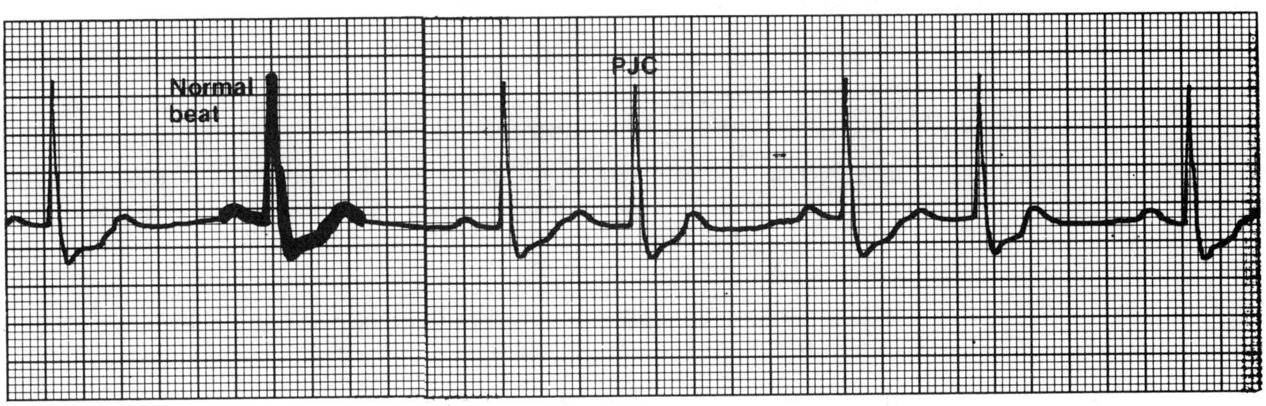

PREMATURE JUNCTIONAL CONTRACTIONS

PJCs occur when the irritable focus that fires off before the SA node can, or the reentry circuit, is located in the AV junction, probably in the bundle of His. PJCs have all the characteristics of any junctional beat. The most important characteristic is the presence of a *normal QRS complex*. Because the impulse arises within the conduction system, the wave of depolarization will go through the bundle branches and Purkinje fibers in the normal manner, producing a normal QRS.

Either there will be no P wave visible or, if retrograde conduction of the junctional impulse occurs, there will be an inverted P wave in front of or behind the QRS complex. If the inverted P wave is positioned in front of the QRS, the PR interval will be less than 0.12 second.

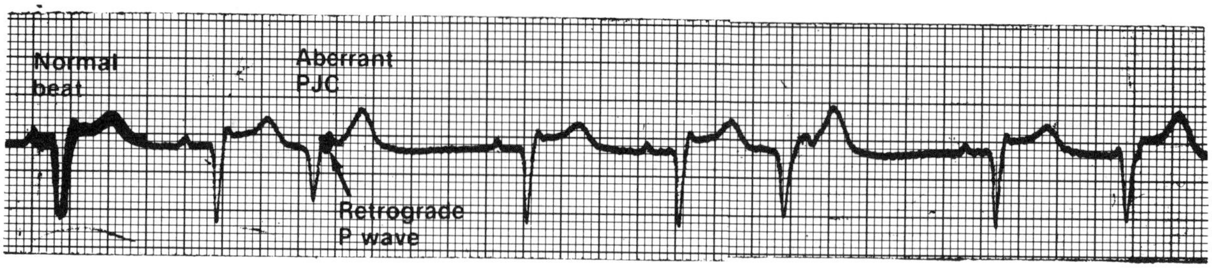

PJCs may also be aberrantly conducted in the same manner as PACs, but if they become really wide and bizarre and have no visible P wave, it is impossible to distinguish them from PVCs. An aberrantly conducted PJC may have a different-shaped QRS, but it must have a QRS duration of 0.06 to 0.12 second to be able to prove that it is, in fact, junctional in origin.

Criteria

RHYTHM: The rhythm will be irregular because of the premature beats. There will be pauses after the premature beats until the next sinus beat comes along.

RATE: The rate will be the rate of the underlying rhythm plus the PJCs.

P WAVES: There may be no visible P waves, or there may be retrograde P waves in front of or behind the QRS complex.

PR INTERVAL: There will be no PR interval if no P wave is visible or if the retrograde P is positioned behind the QRS. If a retrograde P is present in front of the QRS, the PR interval will be less than 0.12 second.

QRS COMPLEX: The QRS will probably be normal, but the configuration may differ from the sinus QRS.

Hemodynamic and Clinical Considerations

PJCs alone are considered a benign dysrhythmia unless they trigger runs of junctional tachycardia.

Therapy

Usually, no therapy is required, but this dysrhythmia will respond to any of the same drugs used to treat PACs. They also may be suppressed by lidocaine.

PREMATURE VENTRICULAR CONTRACTIONS

When the irritable ectopic focus that fires itself off before the SA node, or the reentry circuit, is located in the ventricle, a PVC occurs.

The most distinctive feature of a PVC is the wide, bizarre QRS complex that has all the footprints of any beat arising in the ventricles.

The QRS duration will be greater than 0.12 second. The ST segment and T wave will go in the opposite direction of the main QRS deflection.

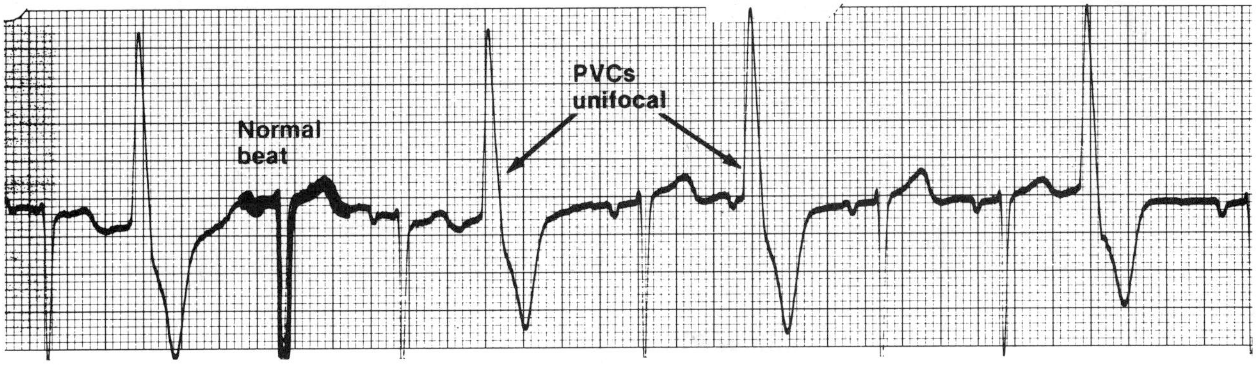

If the same irritable focus, or reentry circuit, causes all of the PVCs in a rhythm strip, all of the wide, bizarre QRS complexes will be identical in configuration, and are said to be unifocal or uniform PVCs. When more than one irritable focus or reentry circuit produces the PVCs, their shape will change with each different ectopic pacemaker. When the PVCs have different configurations, they are said to be multifocal or multiform.

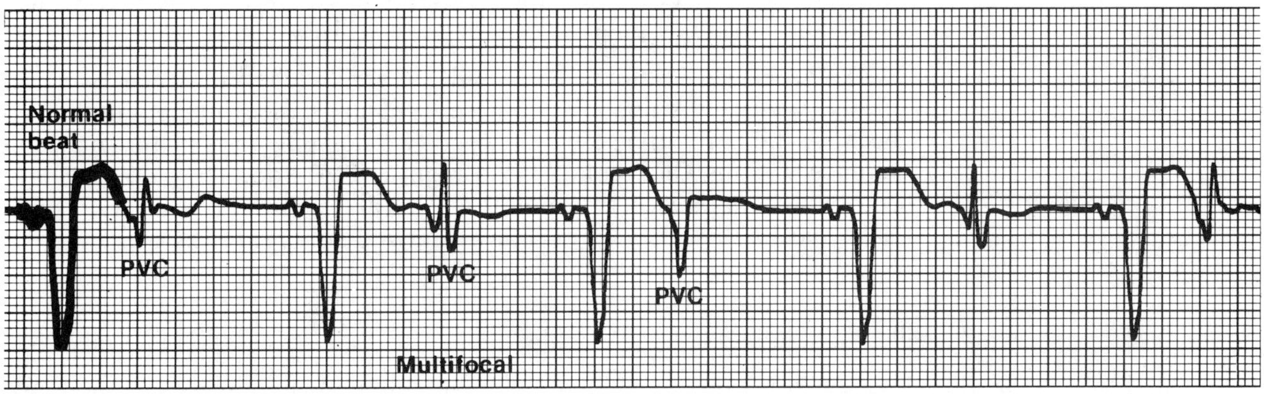

There will probably be no P wave associated with the QRS complex. Ventricular complexes don't usually have retrograde conduction into the atria, although it is possible for this to happen. This means that the SDC of the SA node is unaffected by the early ventricular beat, and atrial depolarization with its normal P wave occurs at the time it was expected. The sinus P wave probably will be buried in the QRS of the PVC, but at times it will be visible on the ST segment or in the T wave of the PVC.

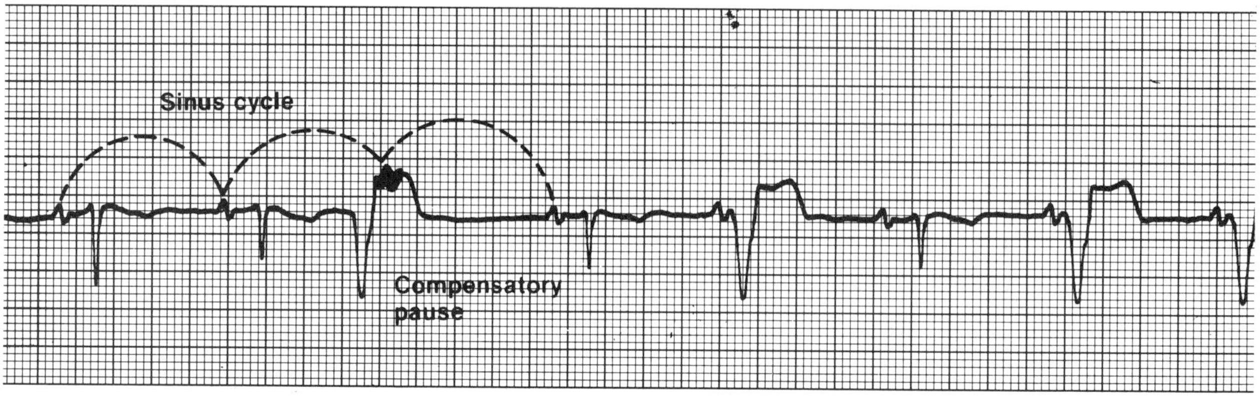

The Timing of PVCs

COMPENSATORY PAUSES PVCs will, of course, be premature, arriving before the next sinus beat is expected. The ventricles are depolarized early, but the atria are depolarized on time. Because the cycle of the SA node is not upset, there will be a pause in the rhythm after the PVC, but the next sinus beat occurs exactly when it is due. The pause following the PVC is called a compensatory pause when you can clock the P-to-P interval right through the PVC. The interval between the sinus beat preceding the PVC and the sinus beat following should measure exactly two sinus cycles in length. Most PVCs are followed by compensatory pauses, but it is not a law that they must. Some PVCs will have less than compensatory pauses, but they are still PVCs.

INTERPOLATED PVCs Some PVCs will be sandwiched between two normally conducted sinus beats. These PVCs are called interpolated beats because they are interposed between two normal sinus beats and don't replace a sinus QRS complex as regular PVCs do. They do not have compensatory pauses. Interpolated PVCs are commonly seen with sinus bradycardia, but they can occur at normal sinus rates as well.

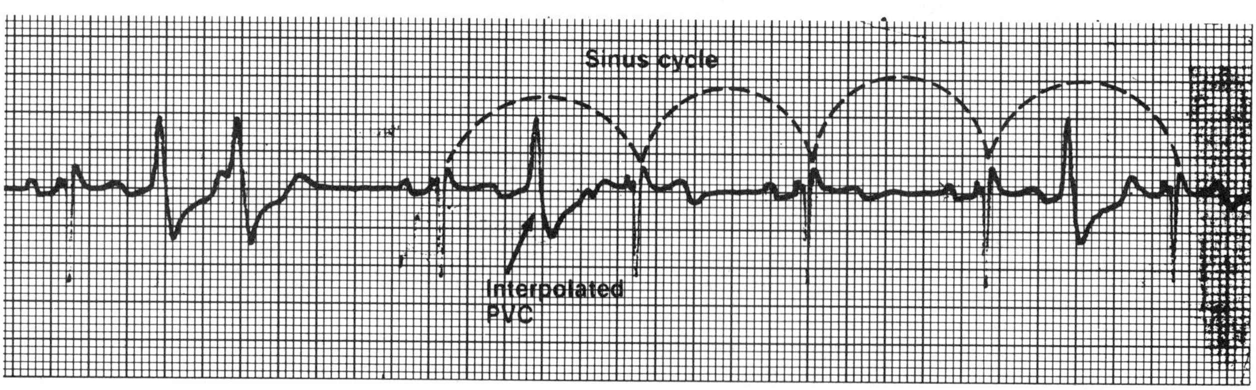

VENTRICULAR BIGEMINY At times, PVCs will occur in a repeating pattern, when every other beat or every third or fourth beat is a PVC. When

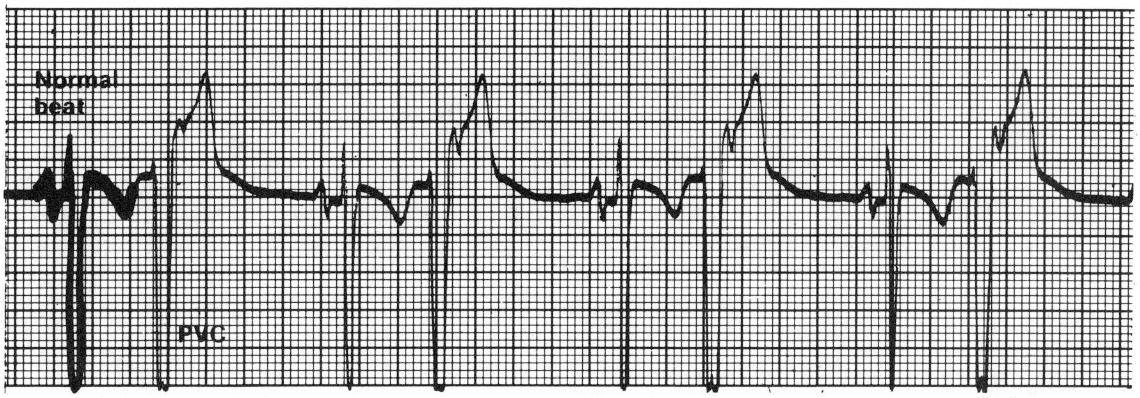

every other beat is a PVC, the rhythm is called ventricular bigeminy. When every third beat is premature, the correct terminology is ven-

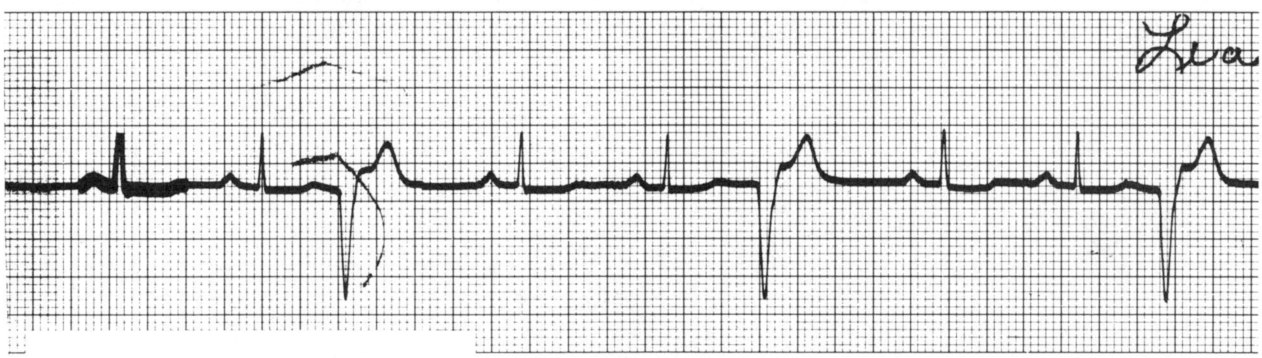

tricular trigeminy, and every fourth beat is called quadrigeminy. Many times, ventricular bi-, tri-, or quadrigeminy is caused by digitalis toxicity.

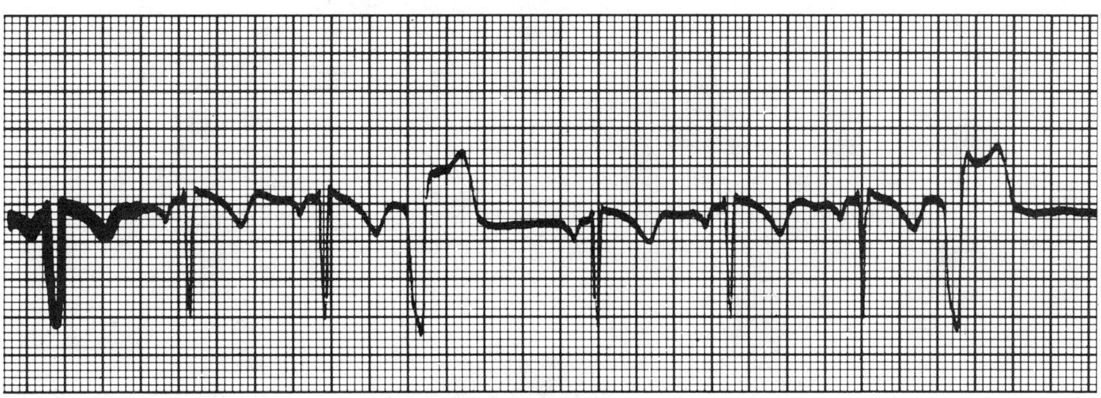

COUPLING INTERVALS The interval measured from the start of the QRS complex preceding the PVC to the first deflection of the PVC is called the coupling interval. This coupling interval is actually the SDC length of the ectopic focus or the timing of the reentry circuit causing the PVC. All PVCs arising from one ectopic focus, unifocal PVCs, should have the same coupling interval, and are then said to be fixed-coupled. Each separate focus will have a different coupling interval since every separate ectopic pacemaker will have a slightly different SDC length or reentry time. Thus, multifocal PVCs will have a different coupling interval each time the shape of the QRS complex changes.

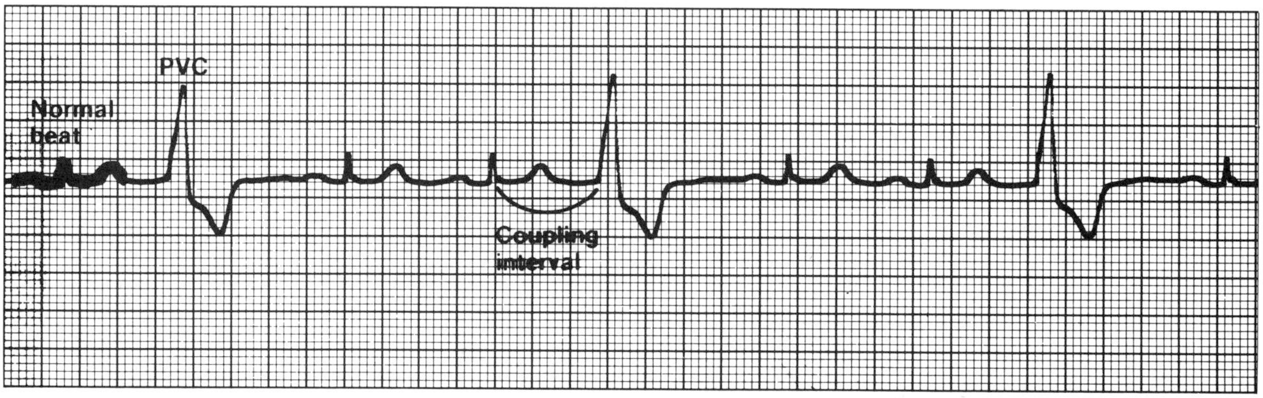

PAIRING When two PVCs occur one right after the other, they are said to be paired, or back-to-back. Three PVCs in a row are a short run of ventricular tachycardia.

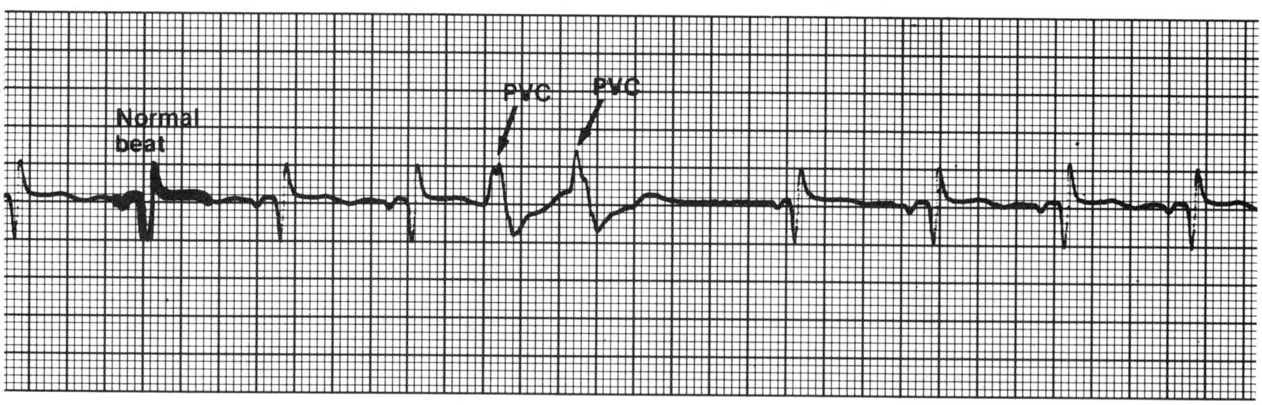

Criteria

RHYTHM: The rhythm is irregular because of the premature beats.

RATE: The rate is the rate of the underlying rhythm, plus the PVCs.

P WAVES: No P waves are associated with the PVCs, but the sinus P wave may be visible on the ST segment of the PVC.

PR INTERVAL: There are no PR intervals.

QRS COMPLEX: Wide, bizarre ventricular QRSs with the ST segment and T wave going in the opposite direction of the main QRS deflection.

Hemodynamic and Clinical Considerations

Everyone has PVCs at one time or another. If you are overly tired, stressed, have smoked too many cigarettes, or consumed too much coffee, you may well have PVCs. In the normal heart, these premature beats, although annoying, are not considered significant or dangerous. But, in the presence of ischemic heart disease or electrolyte imbalance, PVCs are considered dangerous beats that warn of the presence of ventricular irritability that can lead to the serious and lethal rhythms of ventricular tachycardia or ventricular fibrillation.

The PVCs themselves have no real hemodynamic significance, but the rhythms that can be initiated by the PVC most certainly do. If the QRS complex of the PVC hits during the vulnerable period of the cardiac cycle that occurs during repolarization and is represented on the ECG by the peak of the T wave, it can trigger repetitive firing (ventric-

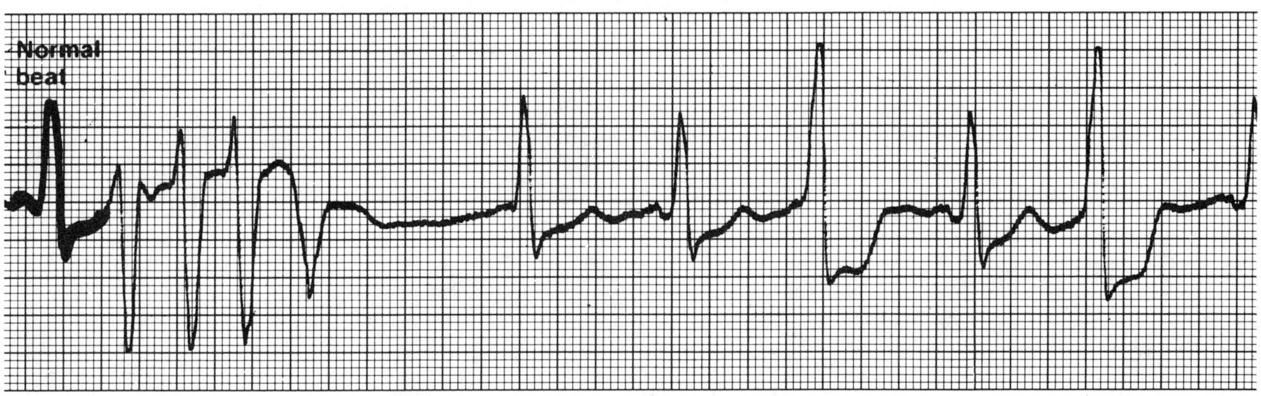

ular tachycardia) or chaotic firing (ventricular fibrillation). This is known as the R on T phenomenon.

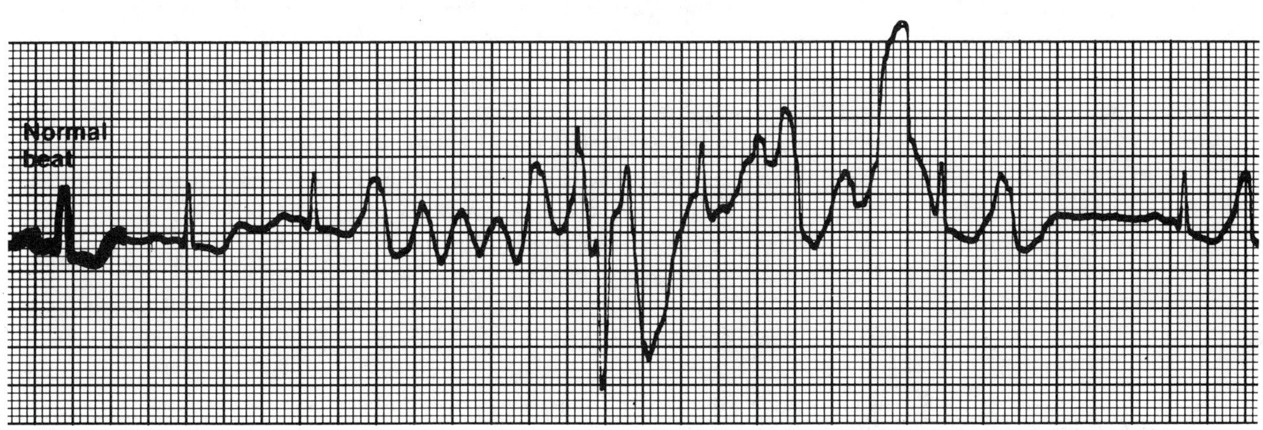

Therapy

After acute myocardial infarction (MI), a large majority of patients will have PVCs, because the damage to the ventricular muscle sets up the ideal conditions for ventricular irritability to arise. The injury and ischemia to the tissue promote increased automaticity, or the unequal refractoriness that causes reentry, and thus initiate PVCs. The theory behind therapy is that if the warning dysrhythmia, the PVCs, are abolished, the lethal dysrhythmias, ventricular tachycardia or fibrillation, will be prevented.

Many coronary intensive care units (CICUs) have protocols for therapy that standarize the treatment of PVCs. A typical protocol calls for therapy if the PVCs become more frequent than six per minute, multifocal, paired, closely coupled to the preceding T wave, or if short runs of ventricular tachycardia occur. However, protocols for therapy may not be the best way of handling PVCs, since it only takes one to produce ventricular tachycardia or ventricular fibrillation.

The first-line drug used to treat PVCs is lidocaine, given initially as an IV bolus dose that brings up the blood level rapidly to suppress the ventricular irritability, followed by an IV drip to maintain the blood level in the therapeutic range. If lidocaine is ineffective, other drugs that might be used are procainamide, propranolol, quinidine, bretylium tosylate, or phenytoin. Because low serum potassium generates ventricular irritability, some PVCs will respond to potassium infusions when other drug therapy is not effective. PVCs produced by digitalis toxicity may respond well to phenytoin.

FUSION BEATS

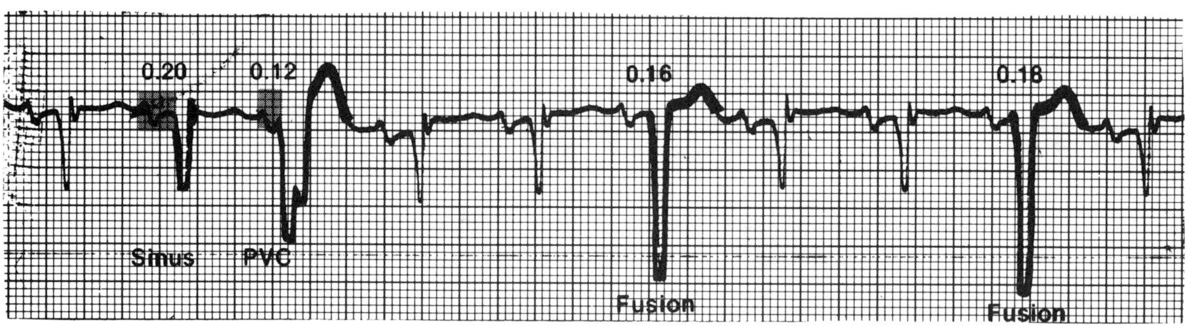

The final type of early beat is a fusion beat. These beats have also been called Dressler beats, summation beats, or end-diastolic PVCs. They are a combination of a sinus beat and a PVC, and occur when a PVC fires off just after the sinus P wave. The ventricular myocardium is depolarized, partly by the sinus impulse being conducted from above, and partly by the ectopic ventricular impulse from the PVC. The two impulses meet or fuse somewhere in the ventricles.

The main characteristics of this type of PVC, making identification easy, are that the P wave will be on time but the QRS complex will be premature. The P wave is on time because it is the sinus P wave, and you can clock the P-to-P interval across the strip. The QRS of the fusion beat will be early, thus shortening the PR interval of the fusion beat. The configuration of the QRS complex of the fusion beat will be somewhere in between the shape of the sinus QRS and the shape of the PVC. The PR interval of the fusion beat controls the change in shape of the QRS. The closer the fusion beat PR interval is to the PR measurement of the sinus beat, the more the fusion QRS will resemble the sinus QRS configuration. The shorter the fusion PR interval becomes, the wider and more bizarre the QRS will be. This is true because the longer the PR interval becomes, the greater the amount of time that is available for the sinus impulse to penetrate the ventricular conduction system. If the fusion of impulses occurs low in the ventricles, more of the ventricular myocardium is depolarized by the sinus impulse, making the fusion QRS more nearly like the sinus QRS. With shorter PR intervals, the impulse from the PVC depolarizes more of the ventricular myocardium in an abnormal manner. The fusion then occurs high in the ventricles, and the QRS of the fusion will look more like the QRS of the PVC.

The PR interval may be too short to allow time for the sinus impulse to depolarize any of the ventricular myocardium. If the PR interval of what appears to be a fusion beat is shorter than 0.06 second less than the sinus PR interval, no fusion can occur, and you have a sinus P wave followed by an end-diastolic PVC. For example, if the PR interval of the sinus beat is 0.20 second, fusion can only happen when the PR interval of the fusion beat is between 0.14 second and 0.20 second.

0.20 second	(sinus PR interval)
−0.06 second	
0.14 second	(shortest PR interval at which fusion can still occur)

In this example, any beat with a PR interval less than 0.14 second is not fusion, and the QRS is purely a PVC sitting just behind a sinus P wave.

Criteria

RHYTHM: The atrial rhythm will be regular sinus rhythm. The ventricular rhythm will be slightly irregular because of the early QRS complexes of the fusion beats.

RATE: The rate will be the sinus rate.

P WAVES: The P waves will be normal sinus P waves that clock all the way across the strip.

PR INTERVAL: The PR interval of the fusion beat must be somewhere in between the sinus PR measurement and 0.06 second less than the sinus PR, or it isn't fusion.

QRS COMPLEX: The fusion QRS complex will have a configuration somewhere between the sinus QRS and the PVC.

Hemodynamic and Clinical Considerations

Fusion beats should be considered the same as PVCs. They indicate ventricular irritability. They actually can be viewed as being more of a potential problem than PVCs, because they can be overlooked very easily. Since they are preceded by a normal sinus P wave, and because the QRS complex may be only slightly premature or bizarre in configuration, they can be missed entirely.

Therapy

The treatment for fusion beats is the same as that of PVCs.

IRRITABILITY DYSRHYTHMIAS AT NORMAL RATES

The following rhythms will occur if a lower pacing focus has an SDC faster than that of the SA node, not because the SA node is slowed, but because the rate of the lower pacer has been accelerated because of irritability. These rhythms also may be seen in the face of complete AV block, when the sinus impulse cannot reach the ventricles.

ACCELERATED JUNCTIONAL RHYTHM

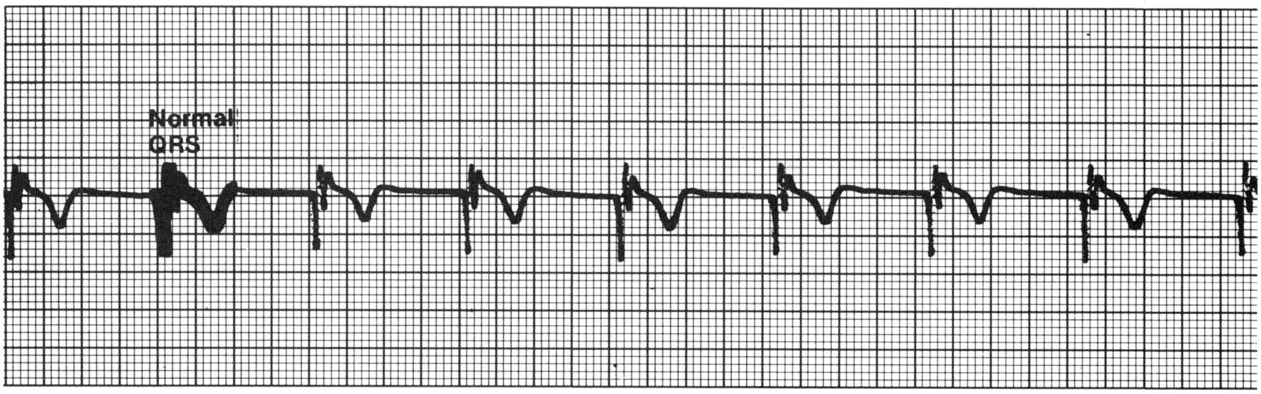

When a somewhat irritable focus located in the AV junction develops an SDC shorter than that of the normal SA nodal rate, or if a third-degree AV block exists, a junctional rhythm may result. But, this junctional rhythm is running at a rate faster than that usually seen coming from a junctional focus. The rate inherent in junctional tissue is normally 40 to 60 beats per minute, but this focus is firing at a rate of 60 to 100 times a minute. This rhythm is not a result of the escape mechanism seen with suppression of the SA node, but it is the increased automaticity that causes the ectopic pacemaker to usurp the pacing function from the SA node. This particular dysrhythmia has been called different things—e.g., non-paroxysmal junctional tachycardia and slow junctional tachycardia—but a rate of 60 to 100, though admittedly faster than that inherent in junctional tissue, is still not a tachycardia. I feel the interpretation best describing this rhythm is accelerated junctional rhythm.

Criteria

RHYTHM: The rhythm will be regular, plus or minus three small squares.

RATE: The rate will be between 60 to 100 beats per minute.

P WAVES: The P waves will have the same criteria as any other junctional beat. No visible P wave, or retrograde P waves will be present, either behind or in front of the QRS complex.

PR INTERVAL: There is no PR interval, or it is less than 0.12 second if the retrograde P wave is sitting in front of the QRS complex.

QRS COMPLEX: The QRS complex will be normal for the patient in the lead being monitored.

Hemodynamic and Clinical Considerations

This rhythm is very likely to cause no problems for the patient, and if seen in the face of a third-degree AV block, it is actually the desired rhythm since the rate is well within normal limits, rather than the 40 to 60 rate usually seen coming from a junctional pacer. The only thing that might pose a problem would be the absence of a P wave before the QRS complex, which would cause a loss of atrial kick. A patient with marginal ventricular contractility could conceivably be thrown into acute left ventricular failure without atrial kick to maximize the contractility of the ventricular myocardium.

Therapy

This particular dysrhythmia usually requires no therapy. Its rate is within normal limits and, unless the loss of atrial kick is a problem, the patient's cardiac output probably is normal. If there is no third-degree AV block, and the junctional pacer slows or stops, the SA node is still capable of firing at a normal rate. If therapy is required, drugs such as quinidine, procainamide, or perhaps lidocaine might be used. By using these suppressive drugs to slow the rate of the junctional focus, the SA node can regain control of the rhythm and the resulting AV synchrony adds atrial kick and the cardiac output will increase.

ACCELERATED VENTRICULAR RHYTHM

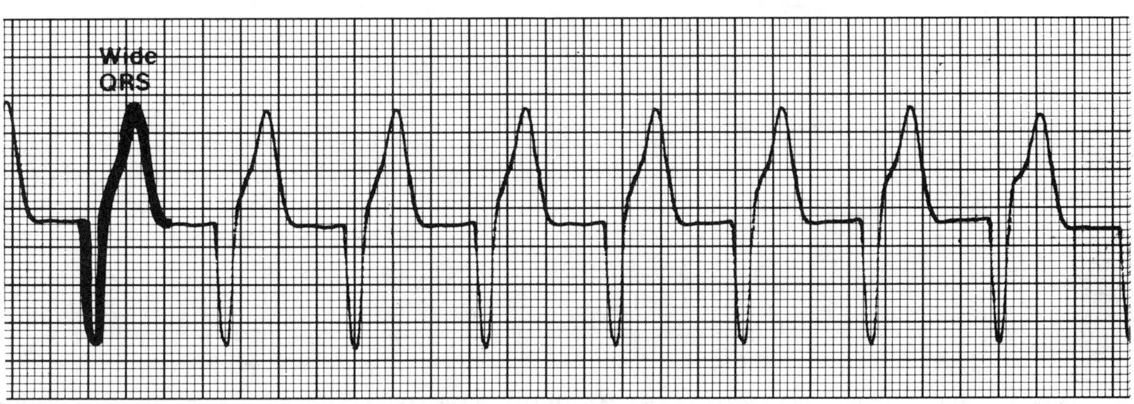

The mechanism for accelerated ventricular rhythm is the same as that of accelerated junctional rhythm. Irritability affects a pacing focus in the ventricles, and the ventricular focus fires at a rate of 40 to 100 beats per minute.

This rhythm may also occur during third-degree AV block, and is much better hemodynamically for the patient, since the ventricular rate is much closer to normal than the 20 to 40 beats per minute usually seen in an idioventricular rhythm.

The terminology for this rhythm is also somewhat confusing. Sometimes called slow ventricular tachycardia, it is best described as accelerated ventricular rhythm.

Criteria

RATE: The ventricular rhythm may be regular, or slightly irregular, since we are dealing with an undependable ventricular focus.

RATE: The ventricular rate will be between 40 to 100 beats per minute.

P WAVES: There will be no P waves associated with the QRS complexes.

PR INTERVAL: There is no PR interval.

QRS COMPLEX: Wide, bizarre ventricular complexes are present, with the ST segment and T wave going in the opposite direction from the main QRS deflection.

Hemodynamic and Clinical Considerations

This rhythm could conceivably cause problems for the patient if the rate of pacing focus is at the bradycardic end of the rate limits of 40 to 100 beats. Also, since related P waves are absent, there is a loss of atrial kick. Either slow rates or decreased ventricular contractility resulting from loss of atrial kick could cause the cardiac output to drop and the patient to become symptomatic.

Therapy

Treatment for this rhythm would be needed only at the slow end of the rate range, and would be the same as that of idioventricular rhythm.

ACCELERATED VENTRICULAR RHYTHM COMPETING WITH NORMAL SINUS RHYTHM

Many times, particularly in the first few hours after acute MI, an irritable focus in the ventricles develops an SDC within 10 beats per minute of the SA node's rate. Because there is usually no retrograde conduction into the atria from ventricular foci, the SA node retains control of atrial depolarization but the two pacing foci, the SA node and ventricular focus, begin to compete for control of ventricular depolarization. You will see the site of the pacemaker pass from the SA node to the ventricles and back. When the pacing site is in the SA node, there will be a sinus rhythm showing on the ECG. When the ventricular focus starts firing before the sinus impulse can get to the ventricles, you will see an accelerated ventricular rhythm. However, you will see the sinus P waves running underneath, but not related to the ventricular complexes. The pacing site shifts every time one focus speeds up or the other slows down. You may see a fusion beat occur as the pacer shifts from the

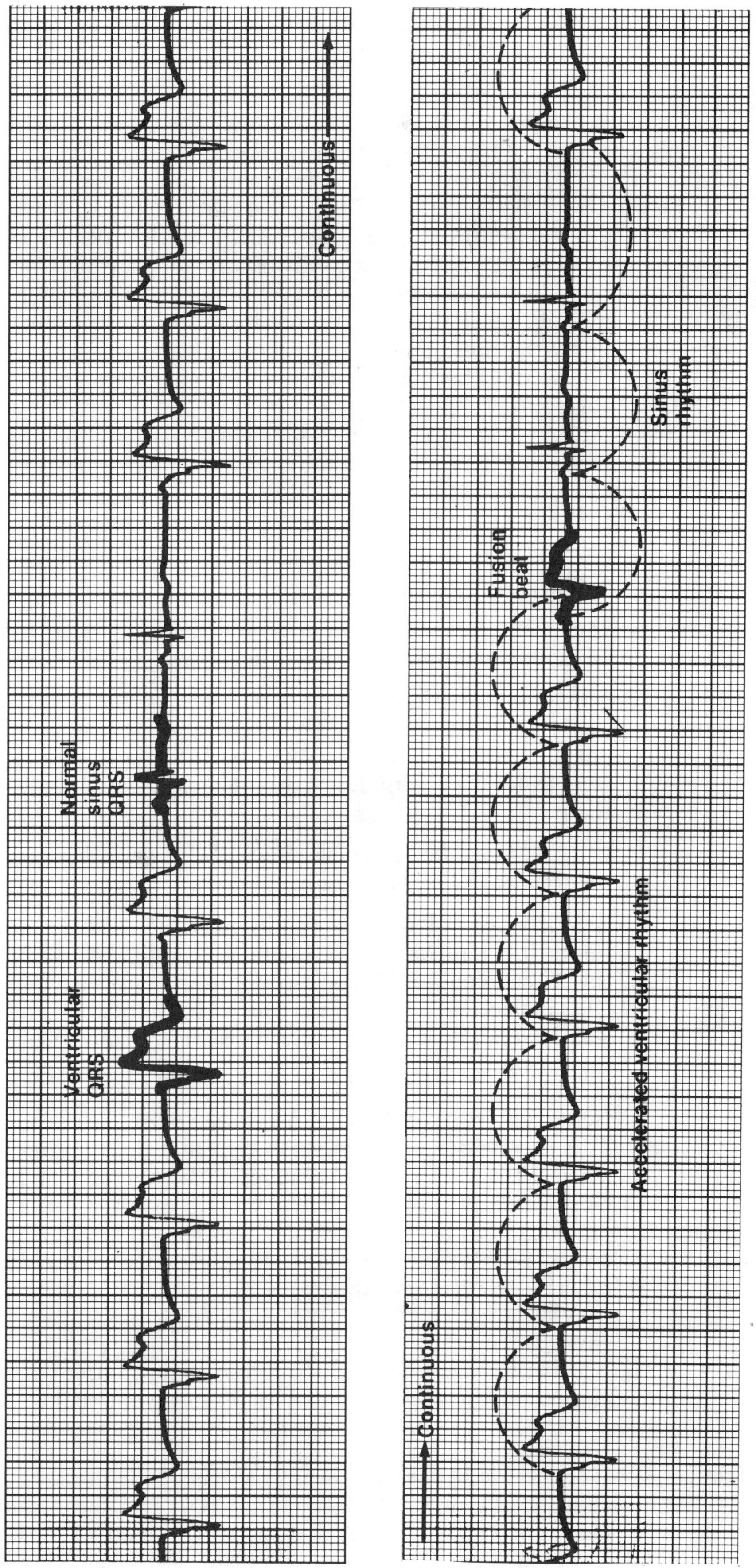

Ventricular QRS
Normal sinus QRS
Continuous
Continuous
Accelerated ventricular rhythm
Fusion beat
Sinus rhythm

ventricles to the SA node or back. The pacemaker that fires first will control ventricular depolarization.

This dysrhythmia is frequently called AV dissociation, and it is true that the atria and ventricles are, at times, being run by two separate pacemakers. But, this same situation occurs in third-degree AV block, and also during ventricular tachycardia. These three rhythms are widely dissimilar in degree of seriousness and type of therapy required. I feel that AV dissociation is a "junk term" that will fit too many rhythms, not unlike supraventricular tachycardia, and thus should not be used because it can lead to misunderstanding and perhaps incorrect therapy. It is much more logical and precise to call this rhythm the way you see it: accelerated ventricular rhythm competing with normal sinus rhythm which, after all, describes exactly what is happening.

Criteria

RHYTHM: Both the sinus and ventricular rhythms may be regular or slightly irregular as their rates change.

RATE: The rates of the SA node and the ventricular focus will be within 10 beats per minute of each other.

P WAVES: The P waves will be present and conducted in the sinus sections of this rhythm. They will also be present in the ventricular parts of this rhythm, but they will not be associated with the wide ventricular QRS complexes, and they will march independently through them.

PR INTERVAL: The PR intervals will be normal and constant in the sinus sections of the dysrhythmia.

QRS COMPLEX: The sinus-conducted QRS will be normal for that patient. The ventricular QRS complexes will be wide and bizarre, with the ST segment and T wave going in the opposite direction of the main QRS deflection. You also may have fusion beats whose QRS complexes will have a shape somewhere between the sinus QRS and the ventricular QRS.

Hemodynamic and Clinical Considerations

This is considered a benign rhythm that does not require therapy. The rate will be within normal limits. The ventricular focus's SDC is too close in rate to that of the SA node, so there cannot be an R on T phenomenon. If the ventricular focus stops firing, the SA node still operates. So, all the dangers usually associated with ventricular dysrhythmias do not apply in this case.

Therapy

No therapy is needed, but of course the patient must be monitored closely for the appearance of increasing ventricular irritability.

THE FAST RHYTHMS

If the irritability in the heart increases, the dominant pacemaker will begin to fire at a rate faster than 100 beats per minute, and a tachycardia occurs. If the SA node is still in control, but is firing at a fast rate, a sinus tachycardia is present. But when irritability shortens the SDC of an ectopic pacemaker, that focus usurps the pacing function from the SA node. Depending upon the location of the ectopic pacing focus, you will see either atrial, junctional, or ventricular tachycardia.

Sometimes these tachydysrhythmias are caused by a reentry mechanism, rather than by increased automaticity.

SINUS TACHYCARDIA

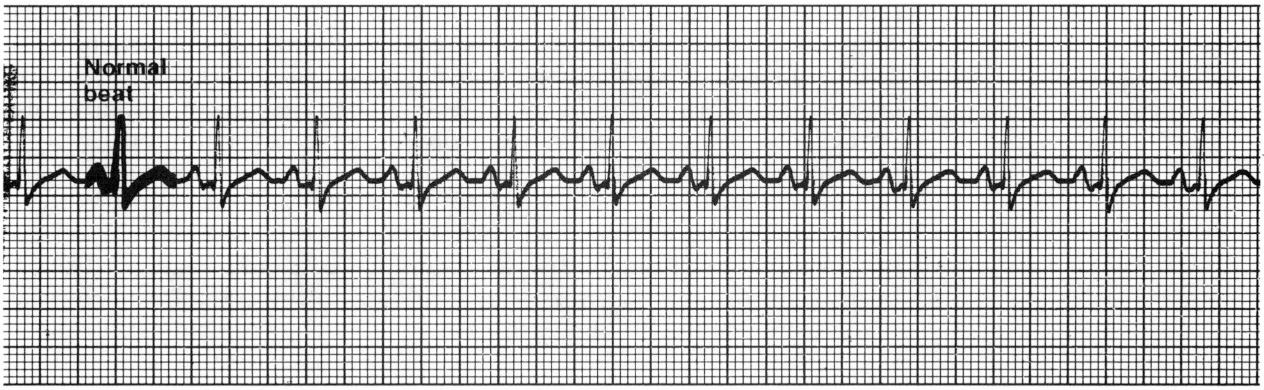

Whenever an outside influence increases sympathetic tone, the SA node will develop a shorter SDC and begin to fire at a rate that is faster than 100 beats a minute. Some of these outside influences are exercise, stress, fear, fever, hypotension, and congestive heart failure. On ECG, you will see sinus beats, but they will be occurring at a much faster rate than normal.

Criteria

RHYTHM: The rhythm in sinus tachycardia will be very regular. When the rate is fast, there is no room for a three small square variation in regularity. Each beat should clock exactly.

RATE: The rate will be greater than 100 beats per minute.

P WAVES: The P waves will be present and normal, with a P wave in front of each QRS complex. At faster rates, the beats are much closer together, and the P wave will move into the T wave of the preceding beat, thus becoming difficult to identify. If the P wave is superimposed on the preceding T wave, the shape of that T wave will be altered. By comparing the ST segment and T wave configuration of the patient's sinus beat at a normal rate with that of a tachycardic beat, the presence of a hidden P wave can be determined.

PR INTERVAL: The PR interval will be within the normal limits of 0.12 to 0.20 second if no AV block is present. However, at faster rates the PR interval may shorten.

QRS COMPLEX: The QRS complexes may be normal in duration, with identical configurations throughout the strip. But, at faster rates the

QRS complexes may widen and change shape. This change in configuration from the patient's normal QRS is caused by the bundle branches' inability to repolarize in time to conduct these rapid sinus impulses normally.

Hemodynamic and Clinical Considerations

Sinus tachycardia in the healthy heart is a normal physiological response to increased metabolic demands for more oxygenated blood and nutrients. However, in the damaged, ischemic heart with coronary artery disease, which limits the supply of oxygen to the myocardium, a simple sinus tachycardia can cause real problems for the patient.

As increased sympathetic tone increases the heart rate, it also increases the contractility of the muscle. Ventricles that are contracting harder and faster need more oxygenated blood. If the oxygen supply is limited by obstruction in the coronary arteries and cannot meet the increased demand, the muscle becomes ischemic and angina or even infarction can result.

Another problem may occur when the ventricular contractility has been compromised by damage or ischemia to the cells. If the contractility is marginal, the increase in rate with the resulting decrease in filling time and stroke volume, may cause a decrease in contractility, which will drop the cardiac output, the blood pressure, and coronary artery perfusion.

Therapy

In normal hearts no therapy is needed. But in the diseased heart it is usually in the patient's best interest to keep the heart rate within a normal range. Treatment for sinus tachycardia is aimed at removing the cause of the irritability. If the cause is anxiety, tranquilizers should be used. Antipyretics may be needed if the patient has a fever.

ATRIAL TACHYCARDIA

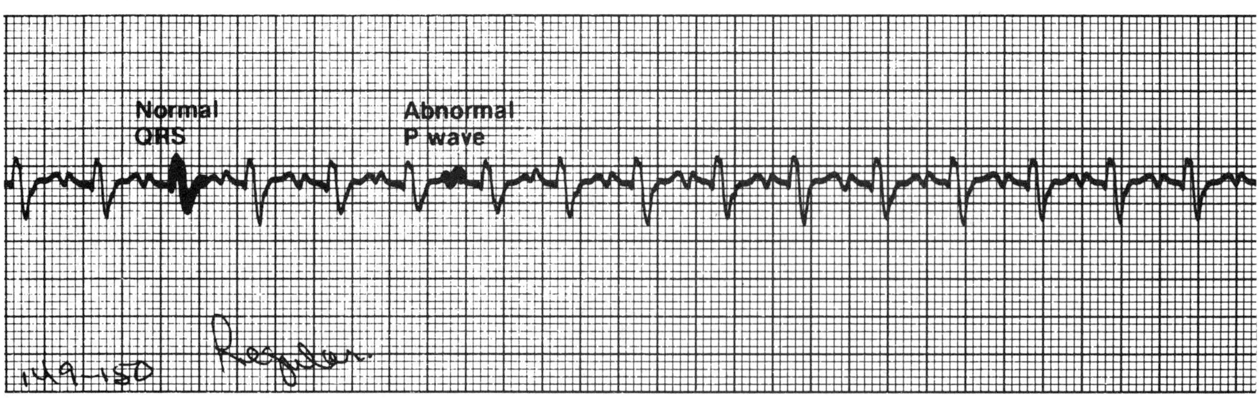

If the irritability is affecting the atrial myocardium, an ectopic pacemaker may be allowed to take over and dominate the rhythm. This ectopic focus, in certain circumstances, will only usurp the pacing function from the SA node for a single beat, and the result is a PAC. But if this irritable focus begins to fire repeatedly, an atrial tachycardia begins. Three or more PACs in a row is considered to be a short run of atrial tachycardia.

Criteria

RHYTHM: The rhythm in atrial tachycardia will be absolutely regular with no variations.

RATE: The rate limits set for atrial tachycardia are 150 to 250 beats per minute.

P WAVES: There will be P waves present in front of each QRS complex, but these P waves will be abnormal in configuration and different in shape than the sinus P wave. Of course, as the rate increases and the beats get closer together, the abnormal P wave will move into the preceding T wave, which can make the interpretation of this rhythm quite difficult.

QRS COMPLEX: The QRS complex may be the same as the sinus QRS, since the abnormality is in the atria, not the ventricles. But at faster rates, aberrant ventricular conduction can begin, and the QRS may widen and become bizarre in shape.

VARIATIONS OF ATRIAL TACHYCARDIA

There are two common variations on the theme that may occur with atrial tachycardia: paroxysmal atrial tachycardia (PAT) and atrial tachycardia with block.

Paroxysmal Atrial Tachycardia

Although this may be an exercise in semantics, the P in PAT stands for paroxysmal, which means suddenly or abruptly. Therefore, in order to have PAT, this tachycardia must begin abruptly with a PAC. PAT may end just as suddenly as it started. The criteria for this variation are just the same as that of atrial tachycardia, with the exception that with a PAT, you see it begin abruptly.

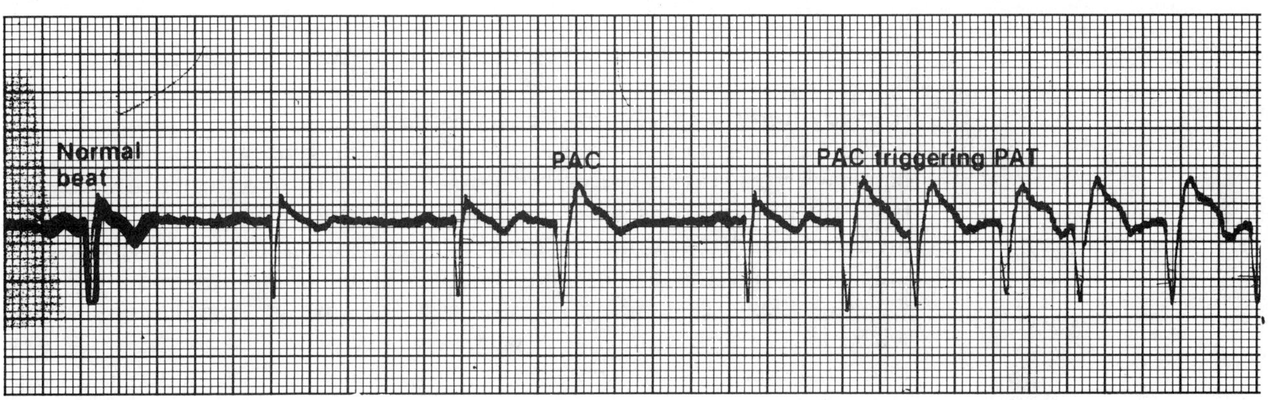

Atrial Tachycardia with Block

In atrial tachycardia with block, the AV node is doing what it is supposed to do, namely, to protect the ventricles from rapid atrial stimuli. The AV node provides a physiologic block which limits the number of rapid atrial stimuli that reach the ventricular conducting system.

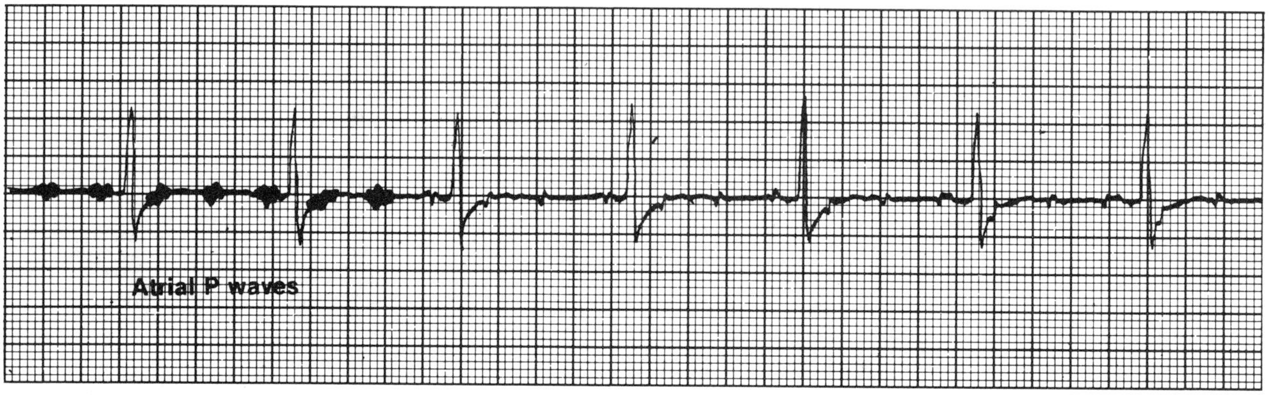

Criteria

RHYTHM: The atrial rhythm will be absolutely regular. The ventricular rhythm will be either regular or irregular, depending on the type of physiologic block at the AV node.

RATE: The atrial rate will be between 150 to 250 beats per minute. The ventricular rate will be less than the atrial.

P WAVES: There will be abnormal atrial P waves present, but not all of them are conducted to the ventricles.

PR INTERVAL: The PR interval can be within normal limits, but it may vary, depending on the type of block at the AV node. If a regular, fixed-ratio kind of block is present, the PR intervals will be constant. If a Wenckebach kind of conduction exists, the PR intervals will increase until a beat is dropped. If the physiologic block at the AV node is complete, the PR intervals will vary with each beat.

QRS COMPLEX: The QRSs will be present, but there will not be QRSs after every P wave. There may be a regular block, in a 2:1, 3:1, or 4:1 pattern, or there may be irregular QRSs in Wenckebach groups.

Hemodynamic and Clinical Considerations

Atrial tachycardia will produce all of the hemodynamic alterations that occur with any fast rate dysrhythmia. PAT is a dysrhythmia that occurs frequently in persons with normal hearts, and is caused by stress or anxiety. Usually, it does not cause any real problems in these individuals, although the person may become short of breath and may feel weak or dizzy, depending on how fast the rate is. Atrial tachycardia with block is a rhythm that is very typically produced by digitalis toxicity, although it can occur in people who are not taking any digitalis preparation.

Therapy

The therapy for atrial tachycardia is aimed at controlling the ventricular rate and converting the patient back to NSR. The course of the therapy depends on the patient's hemodynamic response to the tachycardia. If the patient is dropping his blood pressure or showing signs of acute left ventricular failure, immediate intervention is needed, most likely in the form of synchronized countershock. It is hoped that cardioversion will abolish the ectopic focus, and allow the SA node to regain control of the rhythm.

If the patient's clinical picture is not one of deteriorating hemodynamic status, medical therapy will be used first. Traditional drug therapy includes the use of digitalis to block down the AV node to control the ventricular rate. This may also break up the tachycardic mechanism and allow conversion to normal sinus rhythm (NSR). Other drugs that may accomplish the same thing include quinidine, procainamide, or propranolol. Edriphonium HCl or vasopressors also may be used. Some of these drugs work by increasing vagal tone, and slow down the rate by decreasing conduction through the AV node.

Many times, some form of vagal maneuver may be attempted before drug therapy is instituted. Common procedures such as Valsalva's maneuver or carotid sinus massage may be used to try to increase the vagal tone and stop the tachycardia.

The calcium antagonist, verapamil, is rapidly becoming the drug of choice in the treatment of atrial tachycardia, particularly PAT. It works by blocking down the AV node. It seems to work effectively and predictably with few of the side effects found with the more conventional drugs. It is particularly effective in converting reentry tachycardias to NSR by breaking up the reentry circuit.

JUNCTIONAL TACHYCARDIA

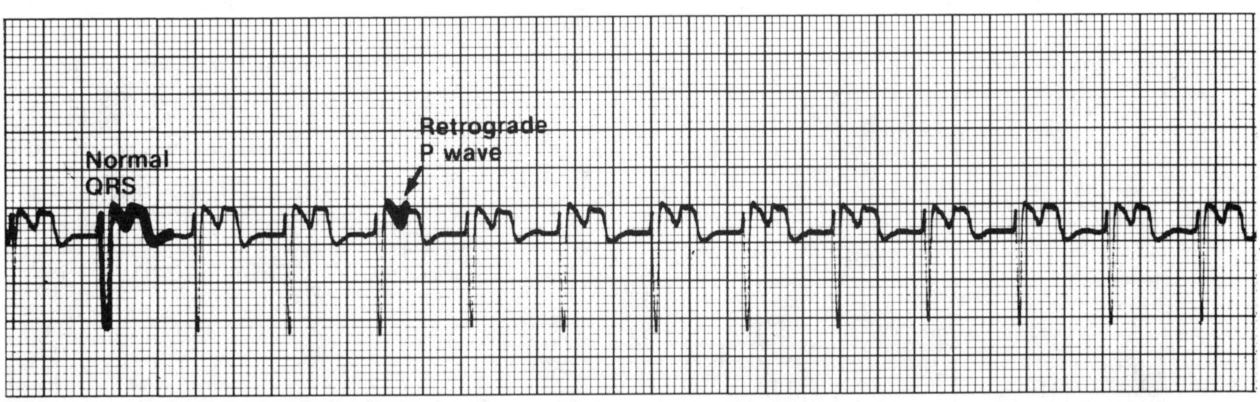

Junctional tachycardia begins when an irritable focus or a reentry circuit is found in the AV junction. This same irritability may have produced single PJCs preceding the tachycardia. These beats arising in the AV junction will meet all the criteria as any other junctional complex. Three or more PJCs in a row are considered to be a short run of junctional tachycardia.

Criteria

RHYTHM: The rhythm in junctional tachycardia is absolutely regular with no room for the three small square variation.

RATE: Junctional tachycardia commonly has rate limits from 100 to 200 beats per minute.

P WAVES: The P waves in junctional tachycardia are the same as any junctional complex. There may be no P waves, or retrograde P waves may be present before or after the QRS complex.

PR INTERVAL: The PR interval, if a retrograde P wave is positioned in front of the QRS complex, will be less than 0.12 second.

QRS COMPLEX: The QRS complex in junctional tachycardia should be identical to the sinus QRS. But at faster rates, aberration may cause a junctional QRS to widen and change shape.

Hemodynamic and Clinical Considerations

Junctional tachycardia has all the same problems inherent in atrial tachycardia. Junctional tachycardia also may prove troublesome for the patient if the retrograde atrial activity is not positioned in front of the ventricular contraction and atrial kick is lost. This could be enough to throw the patient into acute left ventricular failure, if his contractility is marginal from the start.

Therapy

All of the same therapies used to treat atrial tachycardia can be applied to junctional tachycardia, with an additional drug that may have some effect on junctional irritability. Lidocaine will sometimes abolish junctional tachycardia.

SUPRAVENTRICULAR TACHYCARDIA

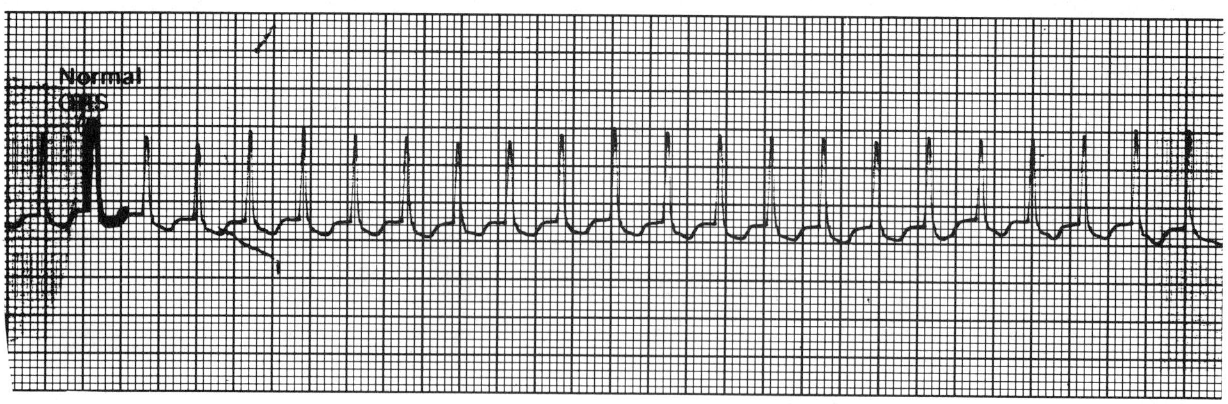

Supraventricular tachycardia (SVT) is a term used to describe a tachycardia that is being generated somewhere above the ventricles. It should only be used when it is impossible to say where the tachycardia is coming from, and it is then needed to differentiate this rhythm from ventricular tachycardia. SVT could be sinus or atrial tachycardia with the P wave hidden in the preceding T wave. It could be junctional tachycardia, with no visible P wave. Or, it even could be atrial flutter with 1:1 or 2:1 conduction that obscures the flutter waves.

Many times, the QRS complex remains narrow and normal, in which case differentiating these tachycardias from ventricular tachycardia is not difficult. However, if the QRS complex in a SVT widens

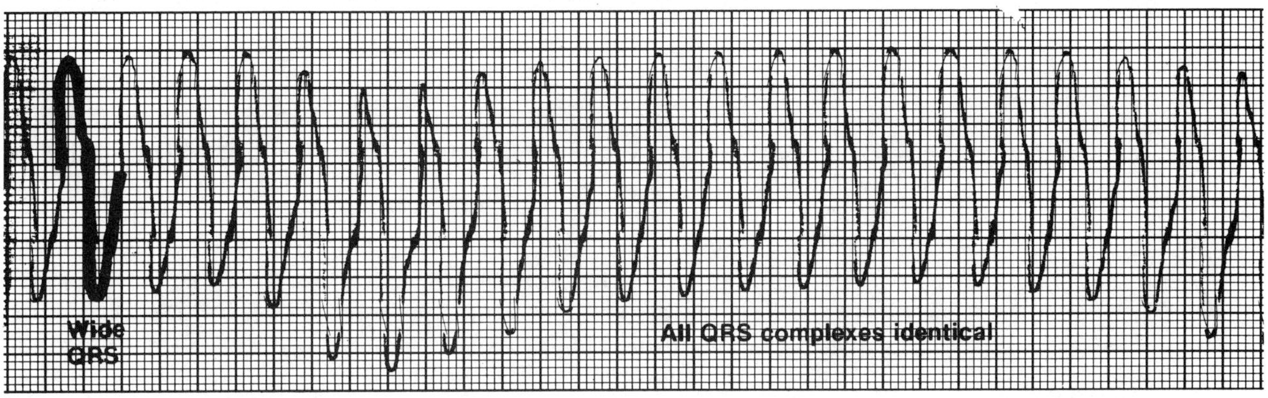

SVT with aberrant ventricular conduction

because the fast rate produces aberrant ventricular conduction, then distinguishing this rhythm from ventricular tachycardia can really be difficult. There are a few characteristics that are typical of SVT that may help you to make the correct interpretation.

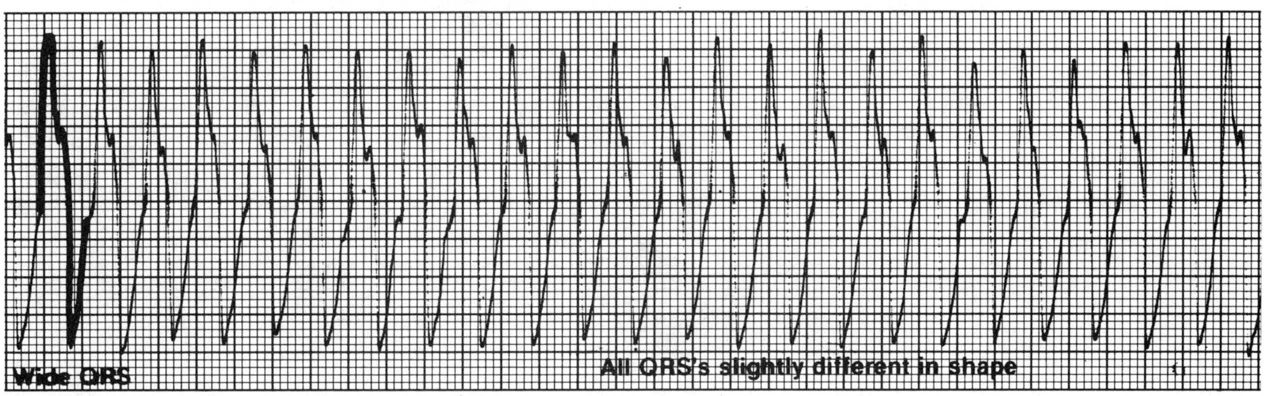

Ventricular tachycardia

Criteria

RHYTHM: The rhythm in SVT is absolutely, monotonously regular.

RATE: The rate will be faster than 100 beats per minute.

P WAVES: The atrial activity is probably present, but is not visible.

PR INTERVAL: The PR interval is not measurable.

QRS COMPLEX: The QRS complex may be narrow and normal, or wide and bizarre, but each QRS is identical to all of the others. This monotonously regular rhythm has identical QRS complexes, because the atrial activity, although not readily seen, is positioned in the same place in relation to each QRS. This is because the atrial activity is causing each QRS complex.

Hemodynamic and Clinical Considerations

The hemodynamic and clinical considerations are the same as those for atrial tachycardia.

Therapy

The therapy for SVT is essentially the same as that for atrial tachycardia. Some form of vagal maneuver may be the initial therapy in SVT. Carotid sinus massage or Valsalva's maneuver may break up the reentry circuit or suppress the irritable focus, and convert the patient to NSR. Another use for increased vagal tone in SVT is to block down the AV node, and slow the ventricular response. This can uncover the exact atrial activity that is causing the tachycardia. By decreasing the number of QRS complexes, you then may be able to see the abnormal P waves of atrial tachycardia, the normal P waves of sinus tachycardia, the retrograde P waves of junctional tachycardia, if present, or the sawtooth waveforms produced by atrial flutter.

VENTRICULAR TACHYCARDIA

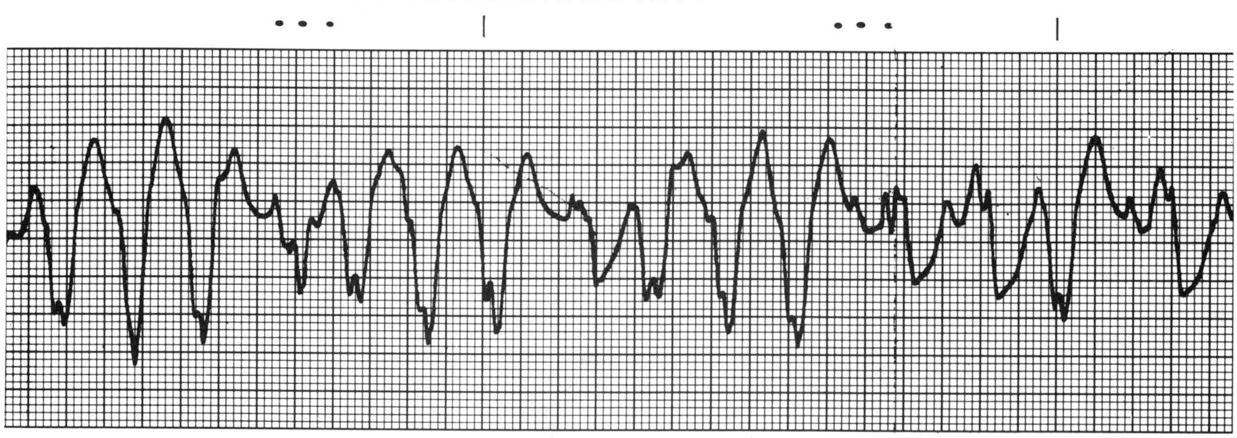

Ventricular tachycardia is produced when irritability in the ventricular myocardium accelerates the SDC of an ectopic focus or sets up a reentry circuit, either of which begins depolarizing at a rate faster than that of the SA node. Control of ventricular depolarization is usurped by the ventricular focus but, since there usually is no retrograde conduction to the atria from ventricular pacemakers, control of atrial depolarization is still maintained by the SA node. There are two separate pacemakers running the heart, one in the atria and one in the ventricles. But, the two separate rhythms produced are not related to each other.

Criteria

RHYTHM: The rhythm may be regular or slightly irregular since ventricular pacing foci are not particularly dependable.

RATE: The rate will be between 100 and 250 beats per minute in the ventricles. The atrial rate probably will not be measurable.

P WAVES: P waves are present, but they will not be readily visible. They are totally independent of the ventricular rhythm.

PR INTERVAL: There are no PR intervals.

QRS COMPLEX: The QRS complexes will be wide and bizarre. Each QRS will have a slightly different shape than all of the others. The shifting configuration is caused by the P wave, marching independently through the QRS complexes and deforming their shape.

Hemodynamic and Clinical Considerations

Ventricular tachycardia can produce all the same hemodynamic alterations caused by any tachycardia. But ventricular tachycardia has the added attraction of frequently turning into ventricular fibrillation. The patient may be merely short of breath, restless, and complaining of chest pain, or he may be unresponsive and pulseless.

Therapy

The therapy for ventricular tachycardia depends entirely upon the clinical picture of the patient. If the patient is awake and alert, with some symptoms of decreasing cardiac output but no life-threatening hemodynamic alterations, the therapy consists of a lidocaine bolus and drip. If the lidocaine doesn't suppress the tachycardia, elective cardioversion is indicated. If, however, the patient is pulseless and unresponsive, a different treatment is in order. The Advanced Cardiac Life Support (ACLS) standards recommend the following protocol in the case of a monitored patient. A precordial thump should be performed, with a synchronized countershock delivered as soon as possible. If the cardioverter is not immediately available, cardiopulmonary resuscitation (CPR) should be performed until the countershock is available. Lidocaine should also be given as an IV bolus and drip.

THE FLUTTERS AND FIBRILLATION

If the irritability of the myocardium increases, a different mechanism of depolarization can occur.

There may be an electrical circuit generated in which a wave of depolarization circles around a chamber, followed by a wave of repolarization. This "circus movement" of electrical activity is self-perpetuating, and produces the characteristic saw-tooth or zig-zag waveforms known as flutter waves. When this circus movement is above the AV node, atrial flutter results. If it is below the AV node, ventricular flutter is present.

When irritability becomes even more pronounced, chaotic, continuous depolarization of random fibers throughout a chamber can begin, and fibrillation occurs—either atrial or ventricular fibrillation, depending on the chamber involved. Fibrillation also produces characteristic waveforms that can be either coarse or fine wavy irregular undulations of the baseline.

ATRIAL FLUTTER

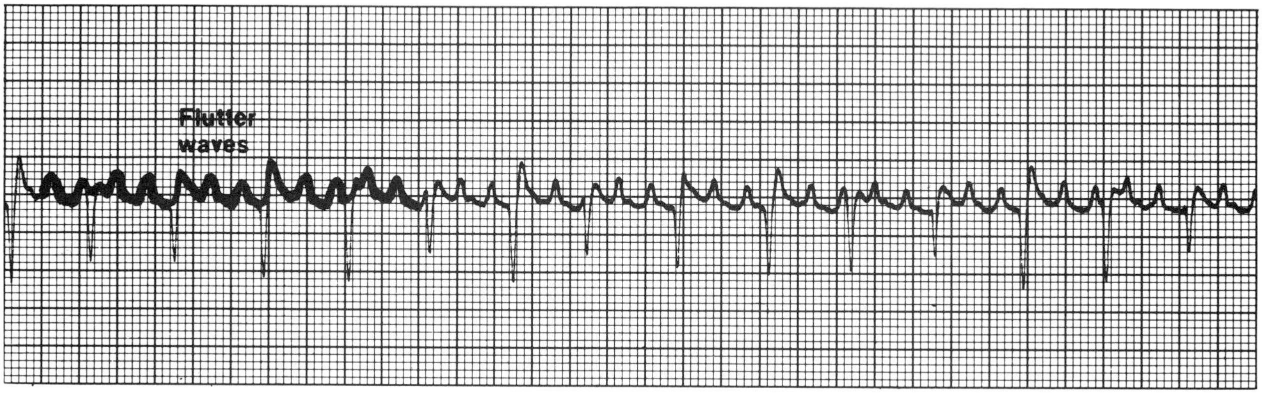

When the flutter mechanism is present in the atria, the distinctive pattern of atrial flutter is seen on the ECG.

Criteria

RHYTHM: The atrial rhythm is absolutely regular. The ventricular rhythm may be regular or irregular depending on the conduction pattern through the AV node.

RATE: The atrial rate will be between 250 and 350 beats per minute, and is commonly seen around 300. One would hope that the ventricular rate will be less than the atrial rate, if the AV node is supplying the physiologic block it should, protecting the ventricles from rapid atrial stimulation.

P WAVES: There are no P waves present in atrial flutter. Instead, you have regular saw-tooth waveforms called flutter waves. These waveforms are regular and identical in shape. Since the circus movement producing the flutter waves goes around the atria continuously, there will be no isoelectric line between beats.

PR INTERVAL: Since there is no P wave, there won't be a PR interval.

QRS COMPLEXES: The QRSs will be normal for the patient in the lead that you are monitoring since the abnormality is in the atria, and conduction from the AV junction through the ventricles should be normal. However, with rapid ventricular response, ventricular aberration can occur. The ventricular rate may be fast or normal, depending upon the amount of physiologic block provided by the AV node. Generally speaking, untreated atrial flutter will have two flutter waves for every QRS, 2:1 conduction. Assuming that the atrial rate is around 300 beats per minute, the ventricular response with 2:1 conduction would be around 150 beats per minute. After therapy is initiated, the physiologic block at the AV node increases, and the conduction rate will drop to a 4:1 pattern. This gives you a ventricular response around 75 beats per minute, a much more effective rate for the patient.

The ventricular rhythm will be regular if there is a regular conduction ratio: 2:1, 4:1, etc. However, if there is a varying physiologic block at the AV node, the conduction pattern becomes irregular and the RR interval varies. When making your interpretation, the conduction ratio should be included, *i.e.*, atrial flutter with varying conduction, or 2:1 conduction, etc. Most of the time, a regular conduction pattern will even be numbered, 2:1, 4:1 and so on, but odd-numbered ratios can and do occur.

Hemodynamic and Clinical Considerations

The presence of atrial flutter is usually indicative of some pathologic process in the heart, although it also can occur as a result of emotional stress. Flutter also may be found as a transient rhythm in response to pulmonary embolization or thyroid storm.

Flutter can cause problems for the patient in two different ways. First, if the ventricular response is rapid, the filling time decreases and the output drops, just as it can with any tachycardia. Second, since the atria are fluttering, there is a loss of atrial kick that can cause a decrease in contractility of the ventricular myocardium, which also results in a decrease in cardiac output and a back-up in ventricular volume and pressures, producing acute left ventricular failure.

Therapy

Atrial flutter is difficult to treat with pharmacologic agents. However, flutter usually responds quickly to synchronized countershock and at a low watt-second setting. However, countershock is a painful and sometimes dangerous procedure, so drug therapy is more likely to be used initially, unless the patient is symptomatic from this dysrhythmia.

Since untreated flutter usually has a fast ventricular response, initial therapy is aimed at increasing the amount of block at the AV node. A vagal maneuver may be attempted but, traditionally, the first-line drug to be used would be digitalis, which blocks down the AV node to control the ventricular rate, and which may allow conversion to NSR. Digitalis, at high doses, may have the effect of changing the flutter to fibrillation, which is fairly easy to convert to NSR pharmacologically. After digitalization is achieved, a Class I preparation such as quinidine or procainamide will be used, to stop the atrial irritability and convert to NSR. These Class I drugs should never be given before the AV node is sufficiently blocked because as they slow down the atrial rate 1:1 conduction may begin at a rate of about 180 to 200 beats per minute, which will greatly increase the ventricular rate.

As with other fast supraventricular rhythms, Verapamil is becoming an important agent in blocking down the AV node and controlling the ventricular rate during initial therapy.

ATRIAL FIBRILLATION

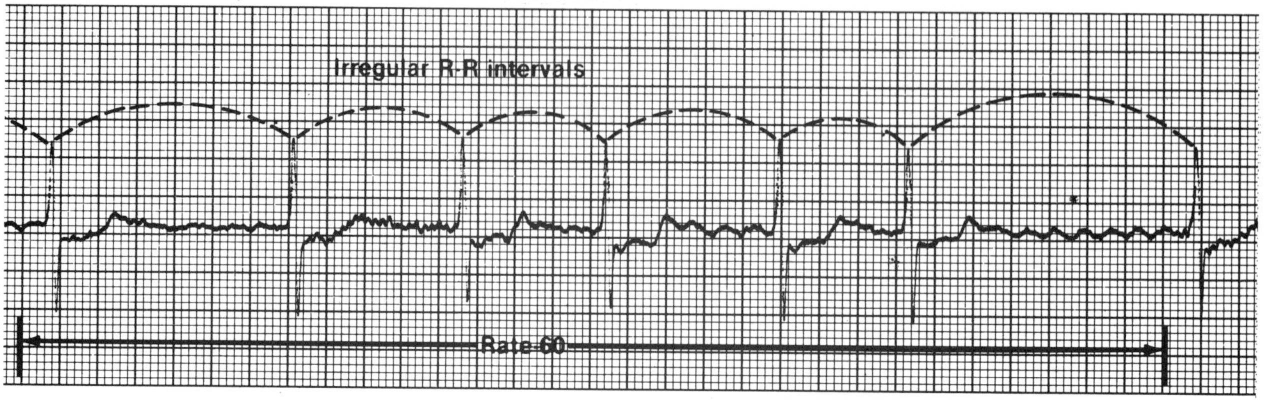

When this mechanism of continuous chaotic depolarization of random atrial fibers begins, everything about the patient's rhythm becomes irregular. In fact, it is this total lack of any regular pattern that becomes the tip-off that atrial fibrillation is occurring.

Criteria

RHYTHM: The rhythm in atrial fibrillation is totally and completely irregular. The atria are depolarizing chaotically, and the ventricles are responding whenever an impulse can make it through the AV node and into the ventricular conduction system.

RATE: The atrial rate is uncountable but, as a point of interest, the AV node is being bombarded with irregular atrial stimuli anywhere from 350 to 700 or 800 times per minute. The ventricular rate will again depend upon the amount of physiologic block present in the AV node. Generally, untreated atrial fibrillation will have a ventricular response greater than 100 beats per minute, and is called uncontrolled atrial

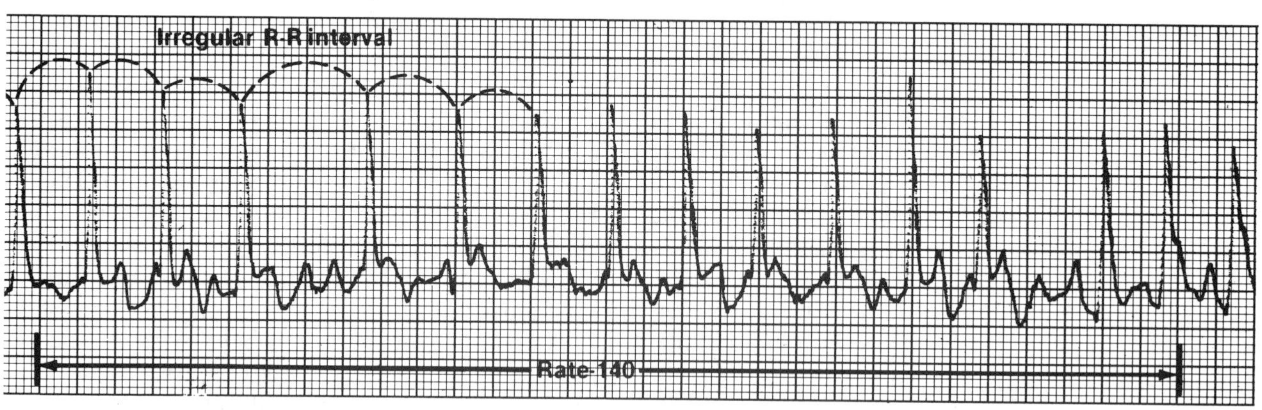

fibrillation. When treatment has been initiated, the AV node blocks down, slowing the ventricular response to less than 100 beats per minute, and this is called controlled atrial fibrillation.

P WAVES: Again, there are no P waves present, and because of the continuous chaotic atrial depolarization, there will be no isoelectric line between beats. Instead of P waves, there will be irregular spikes, dips, or undulations of the baseline that are called fibrillation waves. These fibrillation waves may be very coarse waveforms that may nearly

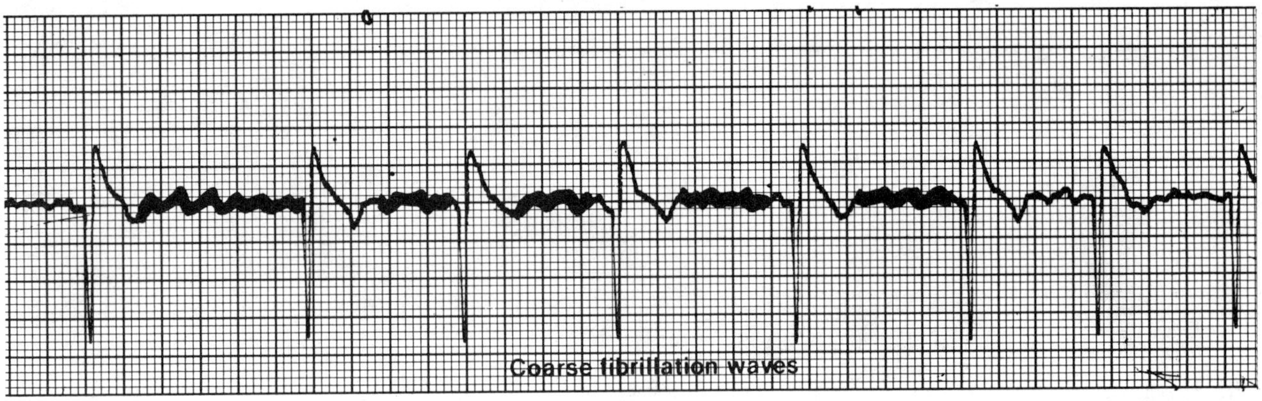

resemble flutter waves. They may be the typical wormy undulations frequently seen in atrial fibrillation. Unfortunately, these waves may be so fast and so fine that the electrical activity is not picked up at all

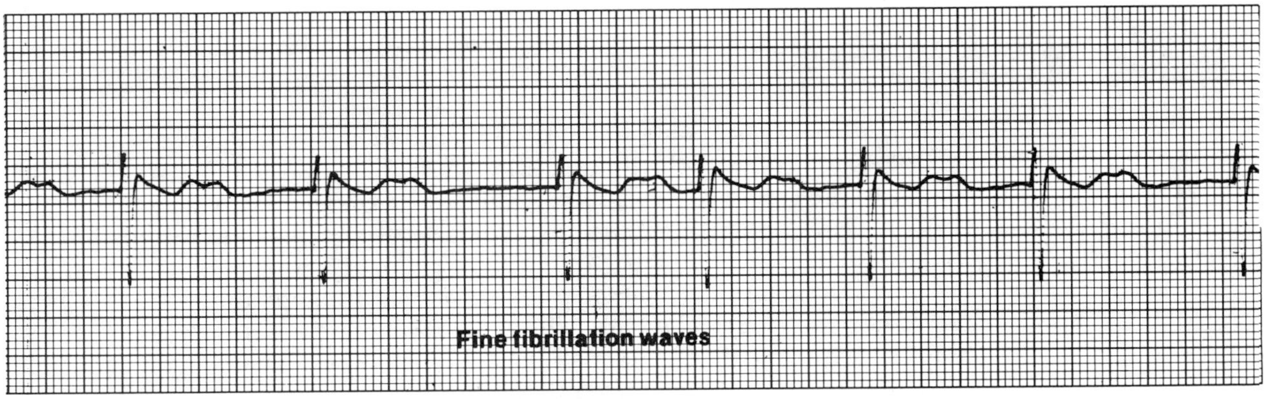

by conventional monitoring leads. Thus, what you see on the rhythm strip is a straight line. When the fibrillation waves are coarse, they are sometimes called fib-flutter waves. When they are so rapid and small in amplitude that they can't be seen, they are called fine or straight line atrial fibrillation.

PR INTERVAL: There are no PR intervals.

QRS COMPLEX: The QRS complexes will be the patient's normal ones, since conduction through the ventricles, although irregular, is normal. At times, in this very irregular rhythm, if a long RR interval is followed by a very short RR interval, the QRS ending the short interval may become wide and bizarre because of aberrant ventricular conduction. This long-short RR interval aberration is called the Ashman phenomenon. The wide FLBs, known as Ashman beats, produced by this mecha-

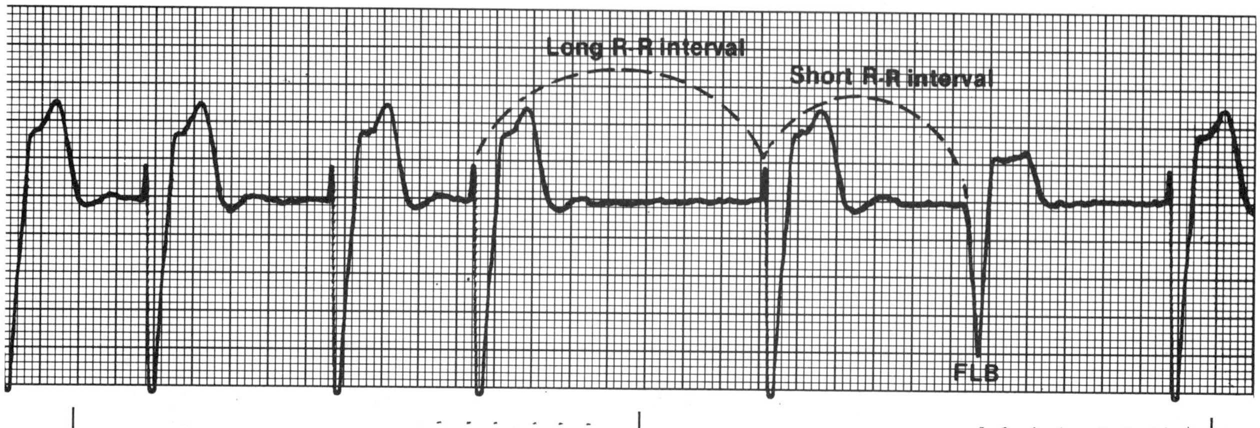

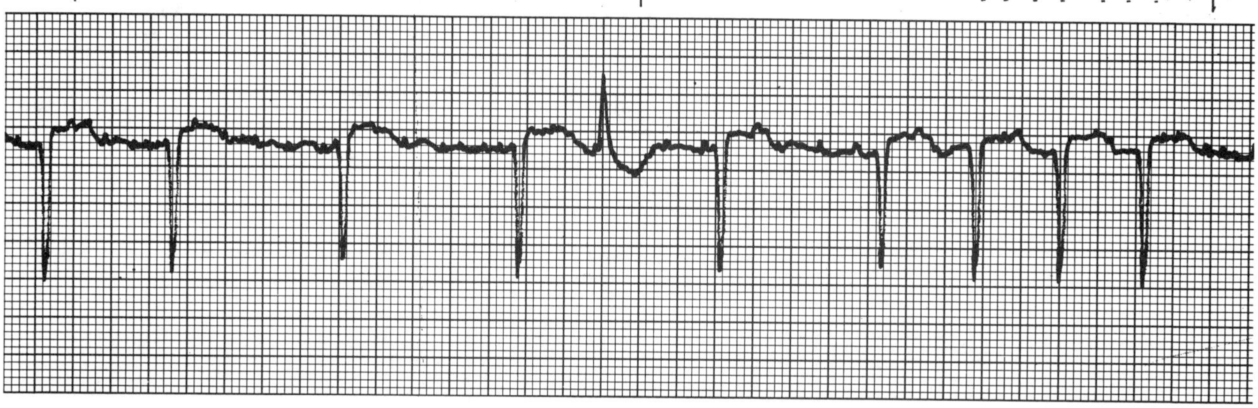

nism can greatly resemble PVCs. Because there are no P waves or regular intervals in atrial fibrillation, it may be nearly impossible to tell if these FLBs are generated by SV aberration or by ventricular ectopy.

Now, from the preceding criteria, it seems as if atrial fibrillation would be a fairly straightforward rhythm to interpret, but actually atrial fibrillation is one of the hardest rhythms for the novice to find. When the ventricular rate is fast, the QRS complexes close together, or when the fibrillation waves are so fine as to be invisible, you can't tell what the atrial mechanism is. This, coupled with the total lack of any pattern, causes considerable confusion for the neophyte. After awhile, you will begin to pick up the total lack of any regular pattern as the clue to the correct interpretation of this dysrhythmia.

Hemodynamic and Clinical Considerations

Atrial fibrillation is even more likely to be produced by pathologic conditions in the heart than atrial tachycardia or atrial flutter. Valvular disease or congestive heart failure, with the resulting back-up of pressures, puts stretch on the atrial myocardium, which in turn produces irritability. The hemodynamic alterations produced by atrial fibrillation are the same as those caused by atrial flutter.

Because the atrial myocardium is fibrillating, it is not contracting, but squirming and quivering; blood flow through the atria stagnates; and thrombus formation can occur. When the patient is converted to NSR, the resulting atrial contraction may cause embolization. If the clot is in the right atrium, a pulmonary embolus will result. If the clot is in the left atrium, the patient could suffer a cardiovascular accident, MI, or any other problem produced by blocked circulation.

Therapy

The treatment of atrial fibrillation is much the same as that of atrial flutter. Digitalis will increase the physiologic block in the AV node and control the ventricular rate. Class I drugs may convert the rhythm to NSR. Verapamil is used frequently instead of digitalis to control the ventricular rate. If the patient is symptomatic because of the fast ventricular rate or loss of atrial kick, cardioversion will be the treatment of choice.

If the patient is chronically in atrial fibrillation, conversion to NSR is probably pointless, because chronic atrial fibrillation usually is caused by some structural abnormality in the heart such as mitral stenosis. You may get rid of the fibrillation for a while, but since the underlying cause has not been resolved, they are very likely to go right back into fibrillation. Patients in chronic fibrillation are also likely to have a good chance of embolization as well.

VENTRICULAR FLUTTER

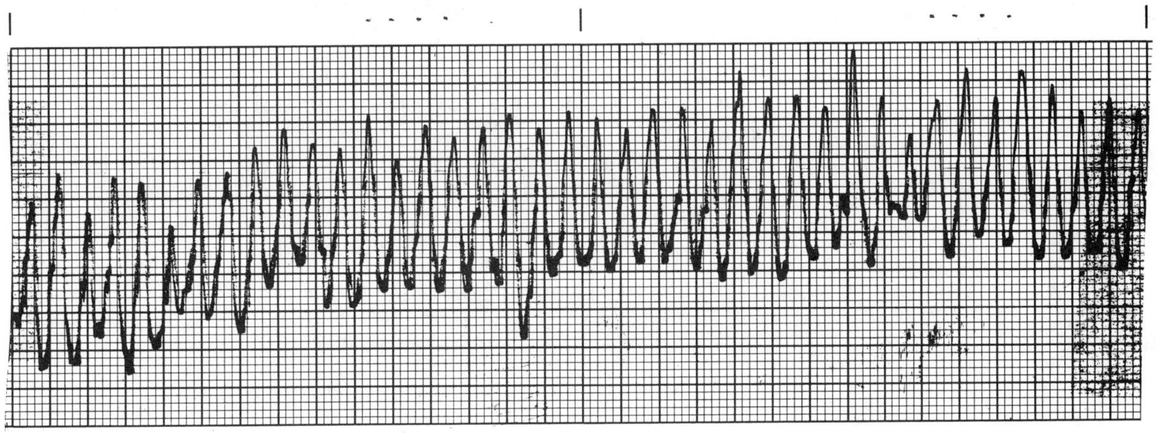

The mechanism for ventricular flutter is the same as that of atrial flutter, but in this case the ventricular chambers are involved.

Criteria

RHYTHM: The rhythm is regular.

RATE: The ventricular rate is between 250 and 350 beats per minute. The atrial rate is not obtainable.

P WAVES: No P waves are visible.

PR INTERVAL: PR intervals are not measurable.

QRS COMPLEX: There is no real QRS, but rather a wide zig-zag pattern produced by the circus movement in the ventricles.

Hemodynamic and Clinical Considerations

As in atrial flutter, ventricular flutter does not allow an effective contraction. The patient in ventricular flutter has no pulse, no cardiac output, and is clinically in just as precarious a situation as he would be in ventricular fibrillation.

Therapy

Therapy is the same as that for ventricular fibrillation.

VENTRICULAR FIBRILLATION

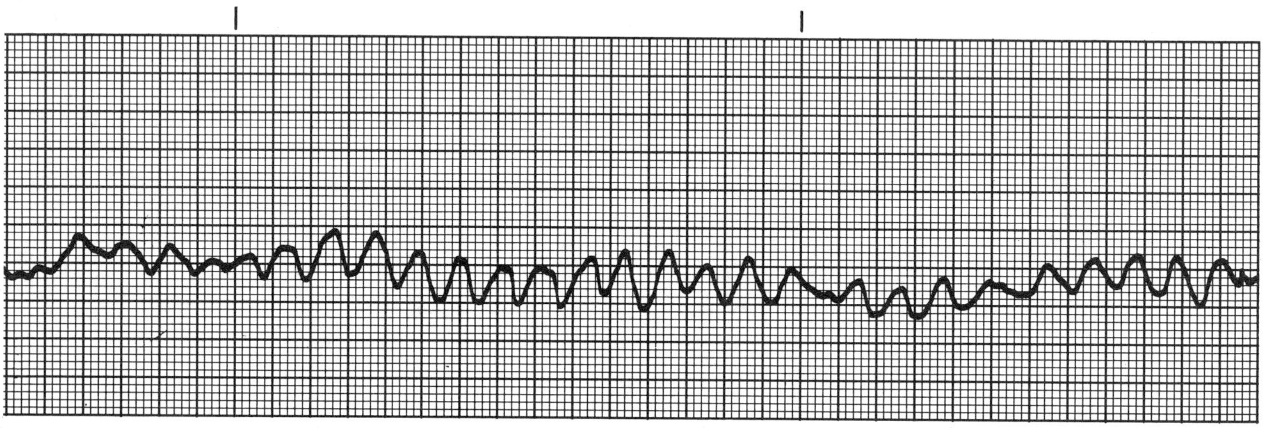

Ventricular fibrillation is the same mechanism as atrial fibrillation, but ventricular fibrillation is, of course, a lethal dysrhythmia, incompatible with life.

Criteria

RHYTHM: The rhythm is totally irregular.

RATE: The rate is unmeasurable.

P WAVES: P waves are unrecognizable.

PR INTERVAL: The PR intervals are not measurable.

QRS COMPLEX: There are no QRS complexes, only chaotic spikes and dips of the baseline.

Hemodynamic and Clinical Considerations

The ventricular muscle is quivering, and no blood is being pumped from the heart. The patient is pulseless and breathless, and clinically dead. If therapy is not instituted within two to three minutes, the chance for the patient's survival is very slim. Irreversible brain death begins within four to six minutes after the heart arrests.

Therapy

The treatment for ventricular fibrillation consists of immediate defibrillation, and of course, CPR until defibrillation can be accomplished. This is Code Blue time, and a standard protocol for therapy in the arrest situation has been established by the American Heart Association in the Advanced Cardiac Life Support course being given all over the country.

SUMMARY CHART OF DYSRHYTHMIAS

DYSRHYTHMIA	RHYTHM	RATE (beats/minute)	P WAVES	PR INTERVAL	QRS COMPLEX	COMMENTS
Normal Rates						
Normal sinus rhythm	Regular (± 3 mm)	60–100	Normal, one preceding each QRS, same in configuration	Normal	Normal	A normal P wave is the hallmark of sinus rhythms.
Sinus arrhythmia	Irregular—cyclic slowing and speeding with respirations	60–100, may be below 60	Normal	Normal	Normal	Irregularity caused by ↑ and ↓ in vagal tone due to respirations causing the SA node to depolarize faster then slower in a cycle.
Accelerated junctional rhythm	Regular	60–100	None, or retrograde before or after QRS	None, or less than 0.12 second	Normal	Occurs when a focus in the junction with a faster rate than the SA node becomes the pacemaker.
Accelerated ventricular rhythm	Regular to slightly irregular	40–100	None associated with the ventricular complexes	None	Wide, bizarre ventricular complexes	May occur when the sinus and ventricular pacemaker rates are nearly the same. When the ventricular focus is depolarizing faster than the sinus, it is in command. The pacemaker will shift back and forth from the sinus to the ventricle (two pacemakers competing for control of the heart).
Bradycardias						
Sinus bradycardia First-degree SA block	Regular	↓ 60	Normal	Normal	Normal	Normal physiologic response to sleep. Unable to determine this rhythm on the surface ECG.

(*Continued*)

DYSRHYTHMIA	RHYTHM	RATE (beats/minute)	P WAVES	PR INTERVAL	QRS COMPLEX	COMMENTS
Second-degree SA block, type 1 (Sinus Wenckebach)	Irregular P-to-P; shortens progressively until the pause which will be less than two of the sinus cycles preceding the pause	Same as underlying rhythm	Present and normal, but absent during the pause	Normal	Normal but missing during pause	This rhythm is frequently interpreted as sinus arrhythmia, but sinus arrhythmia slows and then speeds in cycles.
Second-degree SA block, type 2 (Exit Block)	Regular with pauses that are two, three, four, or more sinus cycles in length	↓ 60 because of pauses	Normal	Normal	Normal but missing during pause unless escape beats are present	
Third-degree SA block (Sinus Arrest)	Regular with pauses that are *not* multiples of the sinus cycle length	↓ 60 because of pauses	Present and normal but missing during pause	Normal	Normal but missing during pauses	This rhythm is indistinguishable from an actual sinus arrest on the surface ECG.
Wandering atrial pacemaker (WAP)		Usually ↓ 60 may be normal	Change in configuration, one preceding each QRS	Normal; may change as the configuration of the P wave changes	Normal	There may be two or more different P waves as the atrial focus changes.
Junctional rhythm	Regular	40–60	None or retrograde before or after QRS	None or less than 0.12 second	Normal	Occurs when the SA node fails, allowing the junction to take over as pacemaker. An escape rhythm.
Ventricular rhythm	Regular to slightly irregular	20–40	None associated with QRS	None	Wide, bizarre ventricular complexes	Occurs when all higher pacemakers fail or are blocked. An escape rhythm.
Tachycardias						
Sinus tachycardia	Regular	↑ 100	Normal	Normal	Normal but may widen at faster rates	
Atrial tachycardia	Regular	150–250	Present, but abnormal in configuration; may be buried in preceding P wave	May not be measurable	Normal but may be widened at faster rates due to aberrant conduction through the ventricles	May have missing QRSs in a regular pattern (*i.e.*, 2:1, 3:1) due to a physiologic blocking by the AV node (atrial tachycardia with block).

Paroxysmal atrial tachycardia (PAT)	Regular	150–250	Present but abnormal in configuration; may be buried in preceding P wave	May not be measurable	Normal but may be widened	Begins abruptly with a PAC. A run of PACs.
Junctional tachycardia	Regular	↑ 100	None or retrograde before or after QRS	None or less than 0.12 second	Normal or widened	Occurs when an irritable focus in the junction depolarizes faster than the SA node and becomes the pacemaker.
Supraventricular tachycardia	Regular	100–250	Unable to see. Buried in preceding T wave	Unmeasurable	Normal or widened; each QRS is identical in configuration.	Junk term—when the rapid rate makes the visualization of P waves impossible, which would tell whether the tachycardia is originating in the SA node, atria, or junction.
Ventricular tachycardia	Slightly irregular	100–250	None associated with the ventricular complexes. The sinus P wave may be visible in QRS.	None	Wide, bizarre QRS. Each is slightly different due to the sinus P wave marching independently through the QRSs.	Ventricular tachycardia is triggered by a PVC. May see fusion beats associated with the ventricular tachycardia.
Escape Beats						
Atrial escape beats	Irregular due to pauses. Escape beat is late.	Underlying rate is slow	Present but abnormal. Differs in configuration from sinus P wave.	Normal but may differ from sinus PR	Normal	Escape beats are always *late*.
Junctional escape beats	Irregular due to the pauses. Escape beat is late.	Underlying rate is usually slow	None or retrograde before or after QRS	None or less than 0.12 second	Normal	The junctional beats occur after a long pause. They are *NOT* premature!
Ventricular escape beats	Irregular due to pauses. Escape beat is late.	Underlying rate is slow	None preceding escape beat	None	Wide, bizarre ventricular complex	Occurs when a pause in the underlying rhythm becomes long enough and no higher pacemaker escapes.

(*Continued*)

DYSRHYTHMIA	RHYTHM	RATE (beats/minute)	P WAVES	PR INTERVAL	QRS COMPLEX	COMMENTS
Premature Beats						
Premature atrial contractions (PACs)	Irregular due to premature beats	Underlying rhythm plus PACs	P wave of premature beat is abnormal in configuration	Normal but may be different than the sinus PR	(1) Normal (2) Wide and bizarre due to aberrant conduction through the ventricles during partial refractory period. (3) Missing due to extreme prematurity of P wave falling during the absolute refractory period of the ventricles.	The amount of prematurity of the beat determines whether the QRS will be normal, aberrant, or absent.
Premature junctional contractions (PJCs)	Irregular due to premature beats	Underlying rhythm plus PJCs	Normal in underlying rhythm. Premature beat has: (1) No P wave visible. (2) Retrograde P wave preceding QRS. (3) Retrograde P wave following QRS.	None or less than 0.12 second with a retrograde P wave	Normal	The presence or absence of retrograde P waves is caused by a difference in conduction velocity through the AV node. This placement of P waves is true in all junctional rhythms.
Premature ventricular contractions (PVCs)	Irregular due to premature beats	Underlying rhythm plus PVCs	None preceding PVC	None	Wide and bizarre	(1) May have compensatory pause following PVC. (2) May be interpolated.
Fusion beats	*Atrial*—regular; *Ventricular*—slightly irregular	Underlying rhythm plus fusion beats	Normal but PP interval regular	PR interval of fusion beat is less than the normal beat	Varies from slightly widened to wide, bizarre complex. RR interval is early on the fusion beat	Results from the combination of the sinus impulse and a PVC occurring at nearly the same time.
AV Blocks						
First-degree AV block			Normal and all are conducted	Greater than 0.20 second and constant	None missing	The AV node is fatigued and delays the impulse longer than normal.

Second-degree AV block Mobitz I (Wenckebach)	*Atrial*—regular; *Ventricular*—irregular due to changing PR interval and dropped beat	Atrial more than ventricular	Normal but not all are conducted	Prolongs with each successive beat until a QRS is dropped	RR interval is irregular. One QRS is missing after last P wave	The AV node fatigues and the PR interval gradually prolongs until the AV node blocks out one impulse. During the pause that follows, the AV node recovers, and the next beat is normal and the Wenckebach progression begins again.
Second-degree AV block Mobitz II	*Atrial*—regular; *Ventricular*—regular	Ventricular less than atrial	Normal but not all are conducted	Normal or prolonged but is constant	Not every P wave is followed by a QRS.	The AV node is even more fatigued, and blocks out every other or two, or three P waves as they come down, until the node recovers and one is conducted.
Third-degree AV block or complete AV block	*Atrial*—regular; *Ventricular*—regular, but slower than the atria	*Atrial*—normal; *Ventricular*—slow	Normal, but not related to the QRS. None conducted.	Varies with each complex	Wide, slow, ventricular complexes, but may be normal if the ventricular pacemaker is in the atrioventricular junction	The AV node is completely fatigued and it blocks out all impulses from the SA node and won't conduct to the ventricles. The ventricles are paced by a focus in the ventricles.
Terminal Rhythms						
Primary ventricular standstill	Regular	*Atrial*—normal; *Ventricular*—none	Normal	None	None	The AV node blocks all impulses and no ventricular pacemaker escapes
Secondary standstill	*Ventricular*—regular; *Atrial*—none	*Atrial*—none; *Ventricular*—very slow	None	None	Wide, bizarre complexes	This is purely electrical, with no resulting contraction. Also called electromechanical dissociation (EMD).
Agonal rhythm	Irregular	Slow	None	None	Multifocal ventricular complexes	"Dying Heart"
Asystole						Straight line

(Continued)

DYSRHYTHMIA	RHYTHM	RATE (beats/minute)	P WAVES	PR INTERVAL	QRS COMPLEX	COMMENTS
Flutter and Fibrillation						
Atrial flutter	*Atrial*—regular; *Ventricular*—regular or irregular	*Atrial*—250–350; *Ventricular* varies less than atrial	None but "F" or flutter waves (regular saw-tooth wave-forms).	None	May be two, three, four or more "F" waves for each QRS	Ventricular rhythm may be regular if a constant (*i.e.*, 4:1) ratio of F waves to QRSs exists, but will be irregular if the ratio varies.
Atrial fibrillation	Totally irregular	*Atrial*— ↑ 350; *Ventricular*— ↑ 100 uncontrolled, ↓ 100 controlled	None but "f" or fibrillation waves (totally chaotic, irregular wave-forms). May vary from coarse (wormy baseline) to fine (straight-line fibrillation) waves.	None	Normal—totally irregular	The ventricular rhythm is irregular due to varying response of the AV node to constant irregular bombardment from the atria.
Ventricular flutter	Regular to slightly irregular	250–350	None	None	Rapíd zig-zag pattern of bizarre ventricular complexes	Has the same hemodynamic implications as ventricular fibrillation.
Ventricular fibrillation	Totally irregular, chaotic		None	None	None but irregular waveforms	

PRACTICE STRIPS

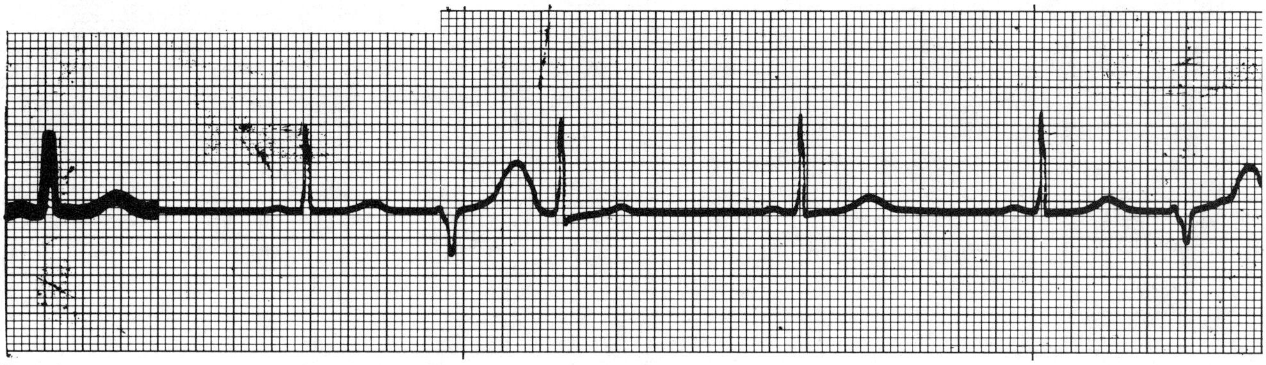

Practice strip 6-1

RHYTHM:

RATE:

P WAVES:

PR INTERVAL:

QRS COMPLEX:

INTERPRETATION:

THERAPY:

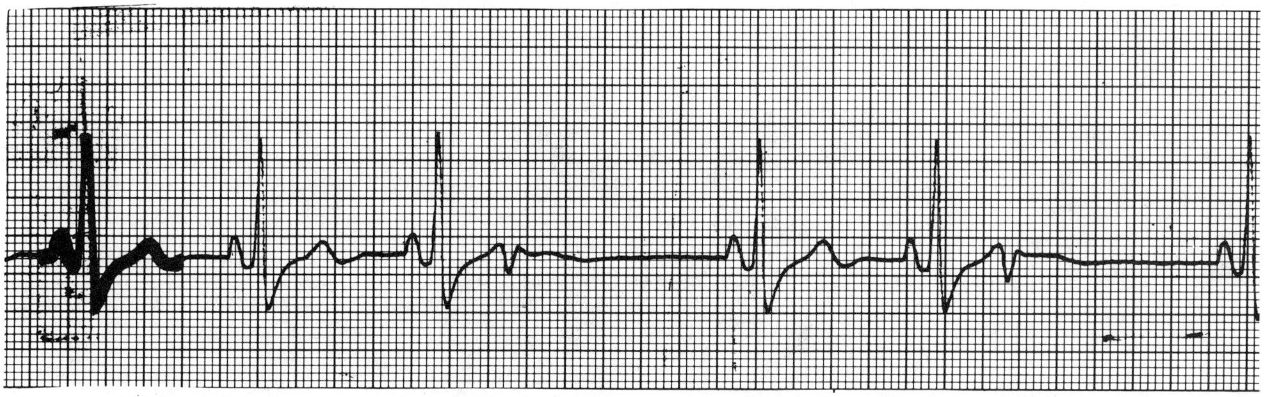

Practice strip 6-2

RHYTHM:

RATE:

P WAVES:

PR INTERVAL:

QRS COMPLEX:

INTERPRETATION:

THERAPY:

A normal beat is highlighted in each strip if one is present.

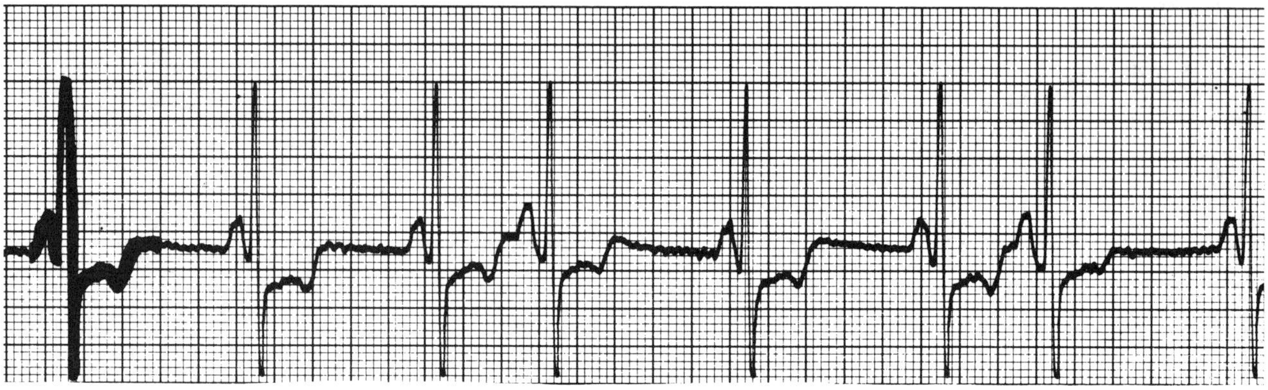

Practice strip 6-3

RHYTHM:

RATE:

P WAVES:

PR INTERVAL:

QRS COMPLEX:

INTERPRETATION:

THERAPY:

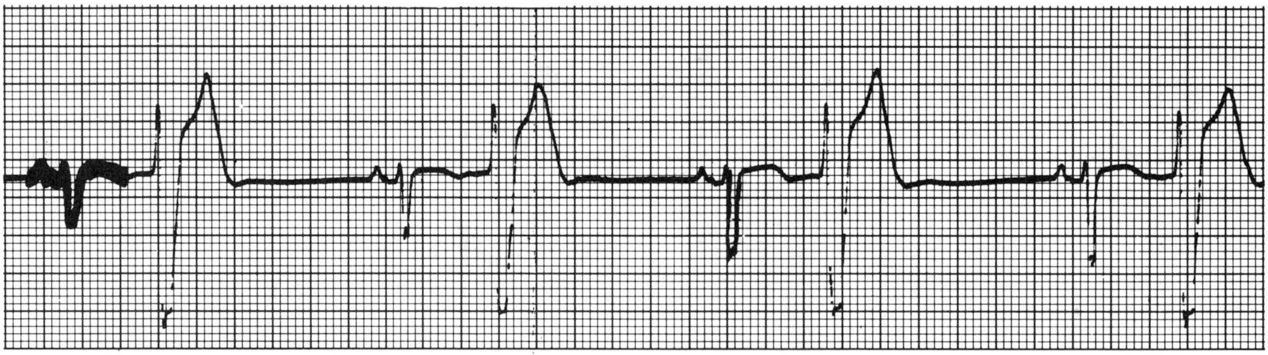

Practice strip 6-4

RHYTHM:

RATE:

P WAVES:

PR INTERVAL:

QRS COMPLEX:

INTERPRETATION:

THERAPY:

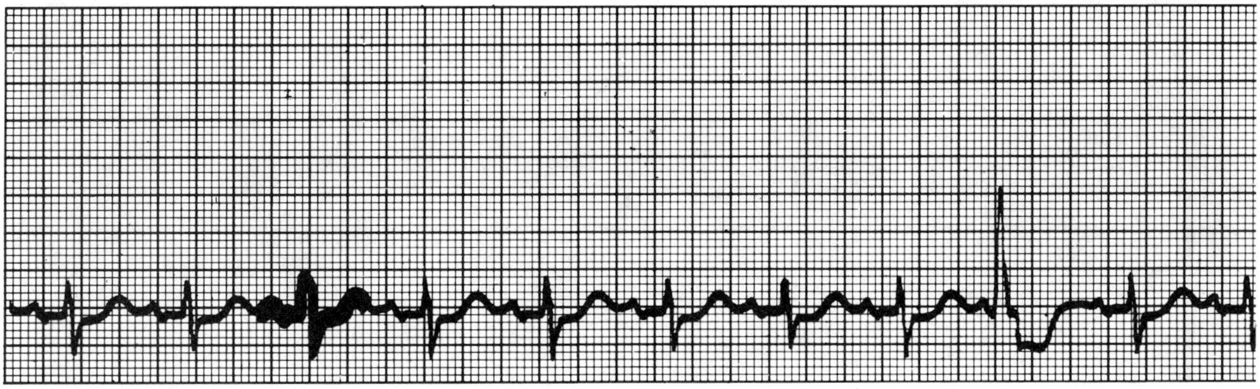

Practice strip 6-5

RHYTHM:

RATE:

P WAVES:

PR INTERVAL:

QRS COMPLEX:

INTERPRETATION:

THERAPY:

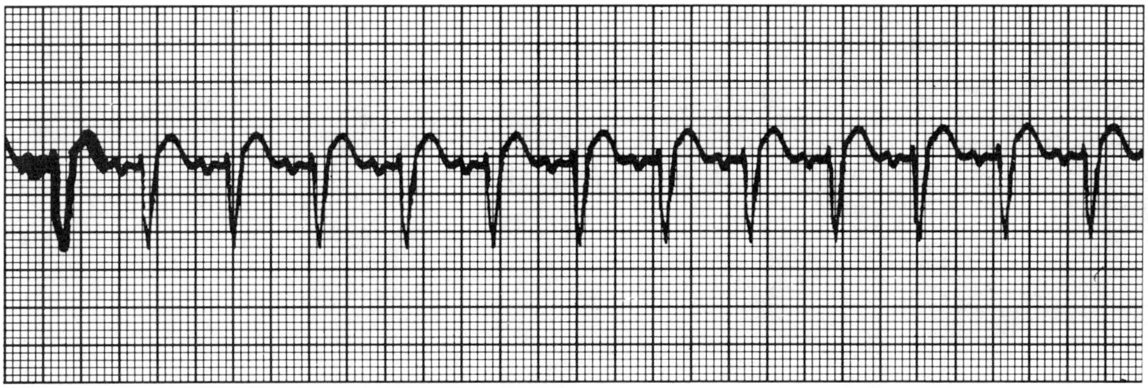

Practice strip 6-6

RHYTHM:

RATE:

P WAVES:

PR INTERVAL:

QRS COMPLEX:

INTERPRETATION:

THERAPY:

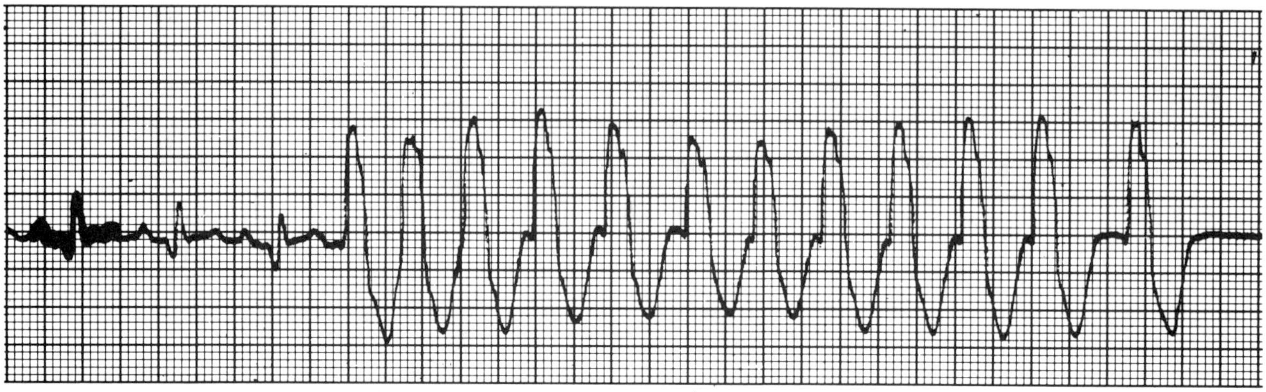

Practice strip 6-7

RHYTHM:

RATE:

P WAVES:

PR INTERVAL:

QRS COMPLEX:

INTERPRETATION:

THERAPY:

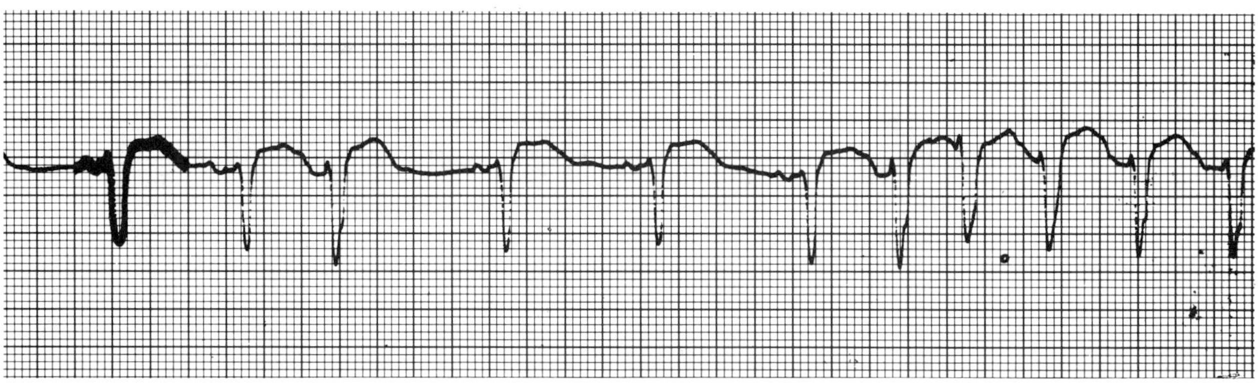

Practice strip 6-8

RHYTHM:

RATE:

P WAVES:

PR INTERVAL:

QRS COMPLEX:

INTERPRETATION:

THERAPY:

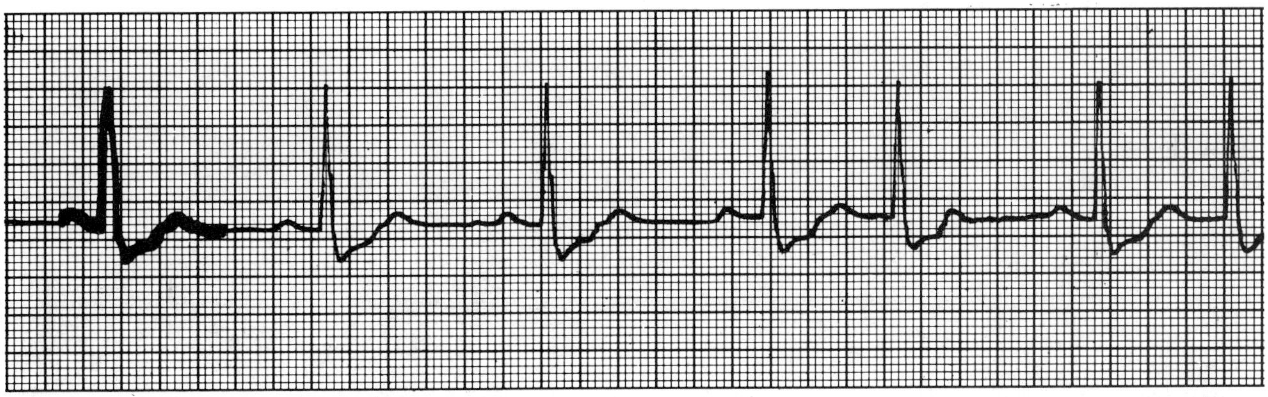

Practice strip 6-9

RHYTHM:

RATE:

P WAVES:

PR INTERVAL:

QRS COMPLEX:

INTERPRETATION:

THERAPY:

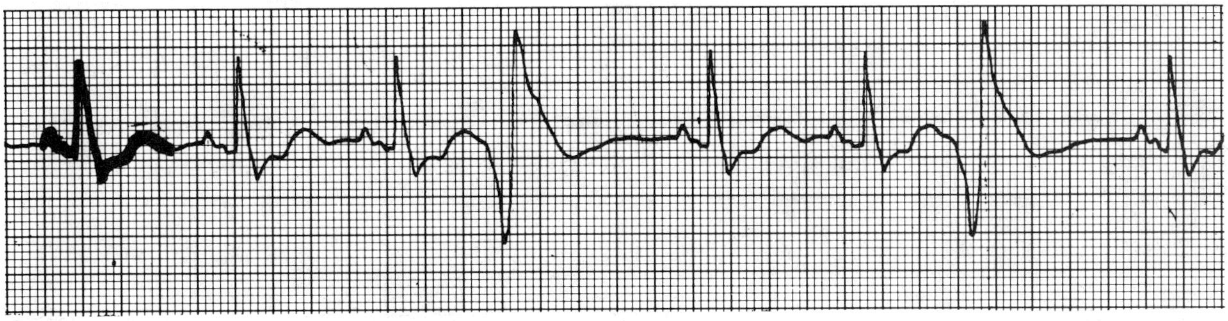

Practice strip 6-10

RHYTHM:

RATE:

P WAVES:

PR INTERVAL:

QRS COMPLEX:

INTERPRETATION:

THERAPY:

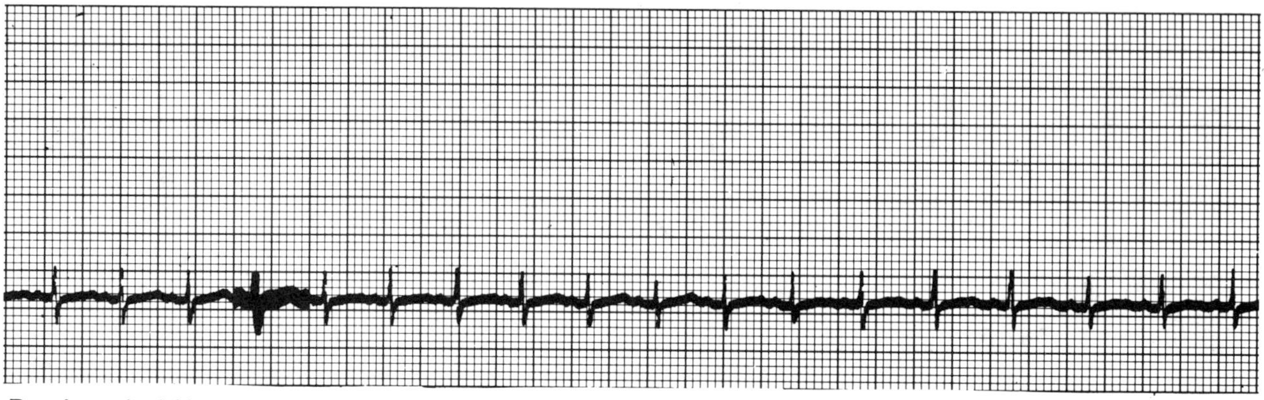

Practice strip 6-11

RHYTHM:

RATE:

P WAVES:

PR INTERVAL:

QRS COMPLEX:

INTERPRETATION:

THERAPY:

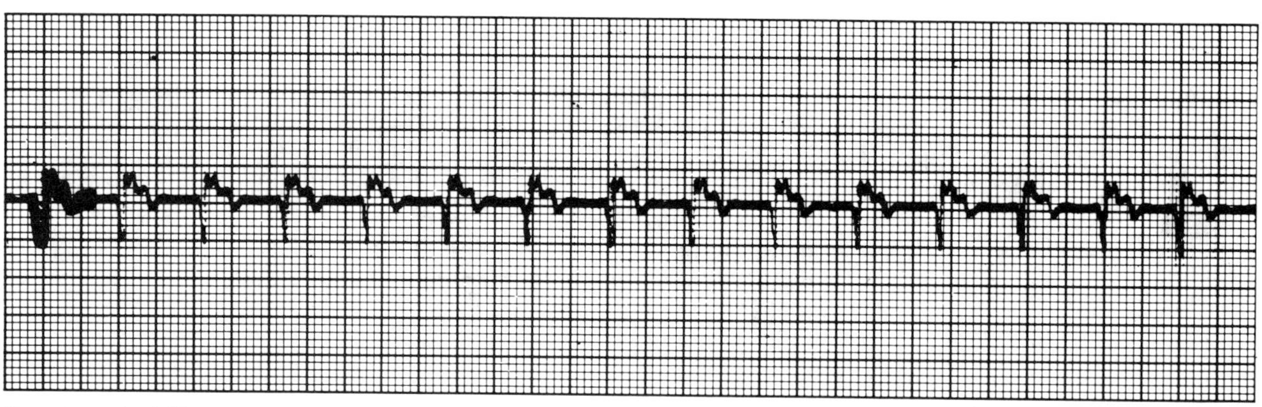

Practice strip 6-12

RHYTHM:

RATE:

P WAVES:

PR INTERVAL:

QRS COMPLEX:

INTERPRETATION:

THERAPY:

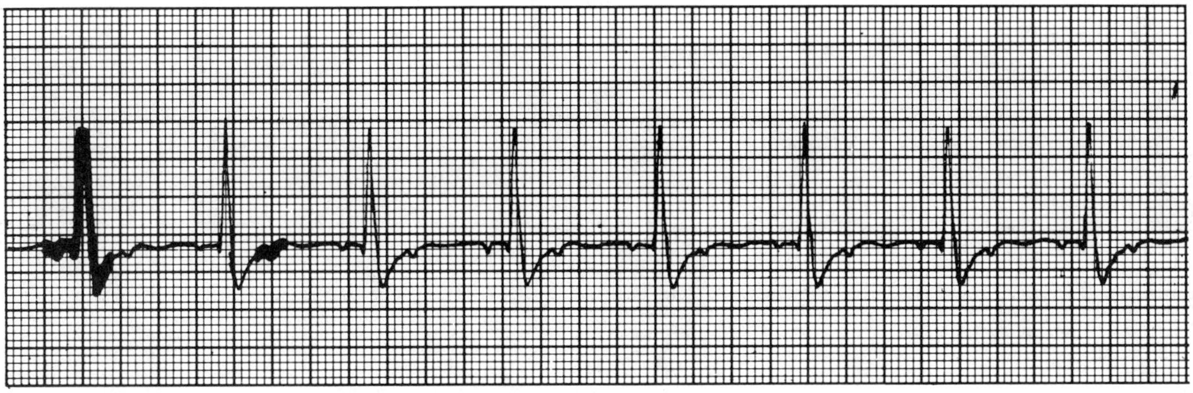

Practice strip 6-13

RHYTHM:

RATE:

P WAVES:

PR INTERVAL:

QRS COMPLEX:

INTERPRETATION:

THERAPY:

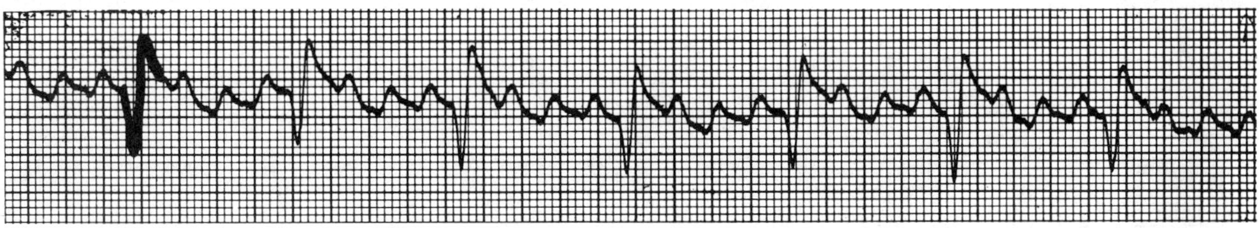

Practice strip 6-14

RHYTHM:

RATE:

P WAVES:

PR INTERVAL:

QRS COMPLEX:

INTERPRETATION:

THERAPY:

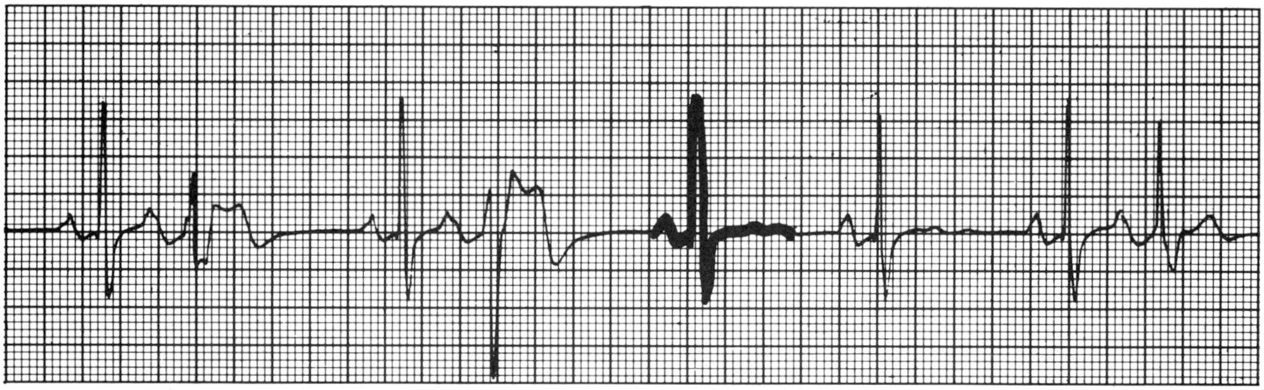

Practice strip 6-15

RHYTHM:

RATE:

P WAVES:

PR INTERVAL:

QRS COMPLEX:

INTERPRETATION:

THERAPY:

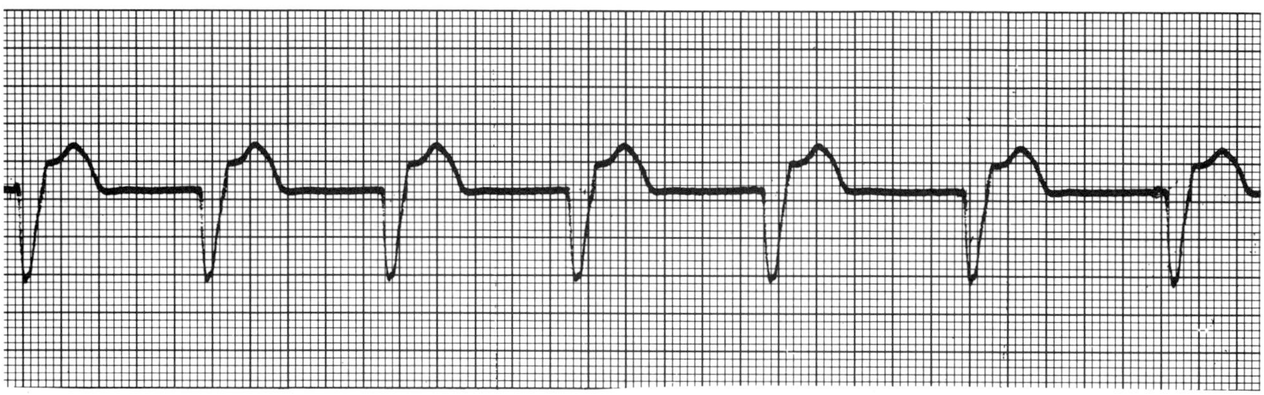

Practice strip 6-16

RHYTHM:

RATE:

P WAVES:

PR INTERVAL:

QRS COMPLEX:

INTERPRETATION:

THERAPY:

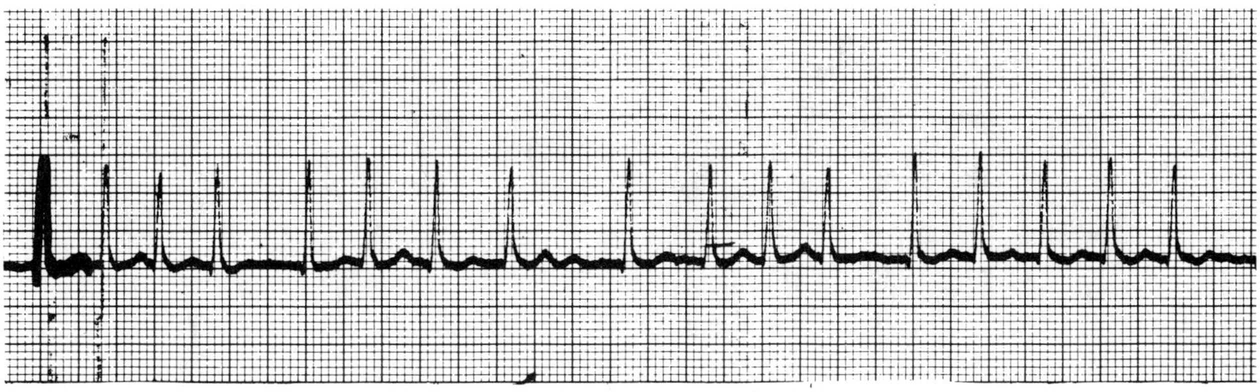

Practice strip 6-17

RHYTHM:

RATE:

P WAVES:

PR INTERVAL:

QRS COMPLEX:

INTERPRETATION:

THERAPY:

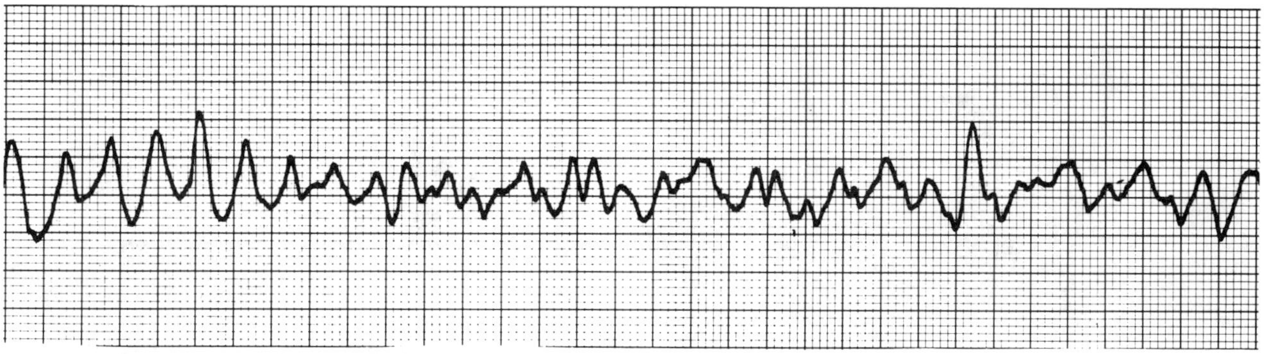

Practice strip 6-18

RHYTHM:

RATE:

P WAVES:

PR INTERVAL:

QRS COMPLEX:

INTERPRETATION:

THERAPY:

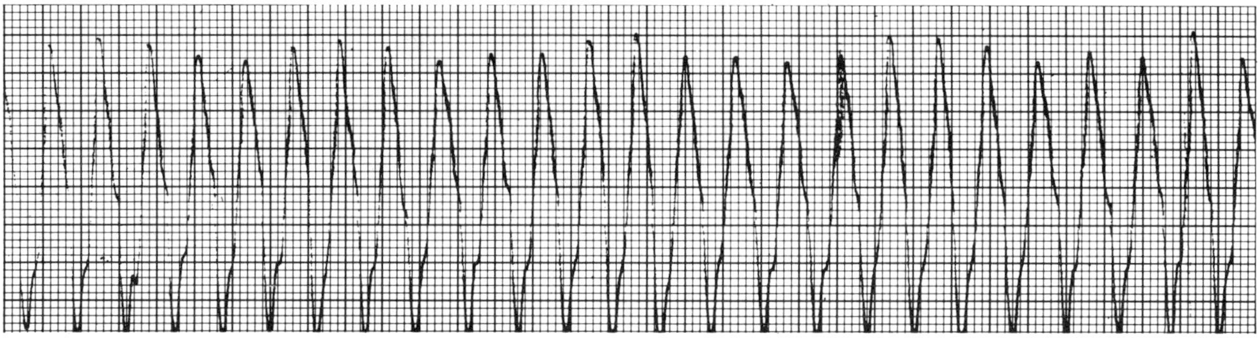

Practice strip 6-19

RHYTHM:
RATE:
P WAVES:
PR INTERVAL:
QRS COMPLEX:
INTERPRETATION:
THERAPY:

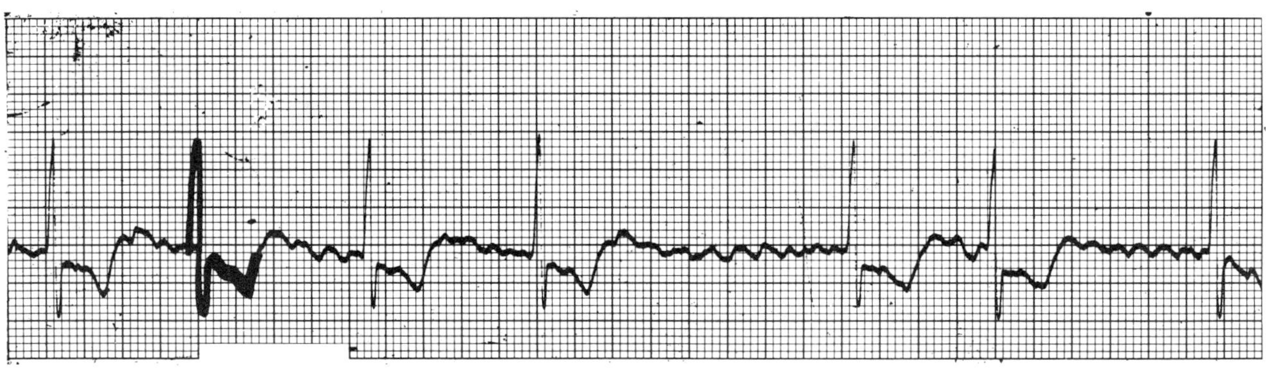

Practice strip 6-20

RHYTHM:
RATE:
P WAVES:
PR INTERVAL:
QRS COMPLEX:
INTERPRETATION:
THERAPY:

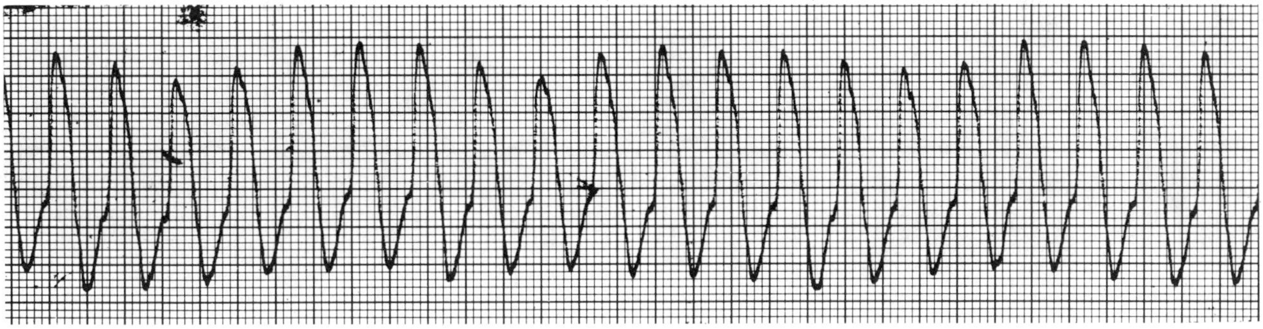

Practice strip 6-21

RHYTHM:

RATE:

P WAVES:

PR INTERVAL:

QRS COMPLEX:

INTERPRETATION:

THERAPY:

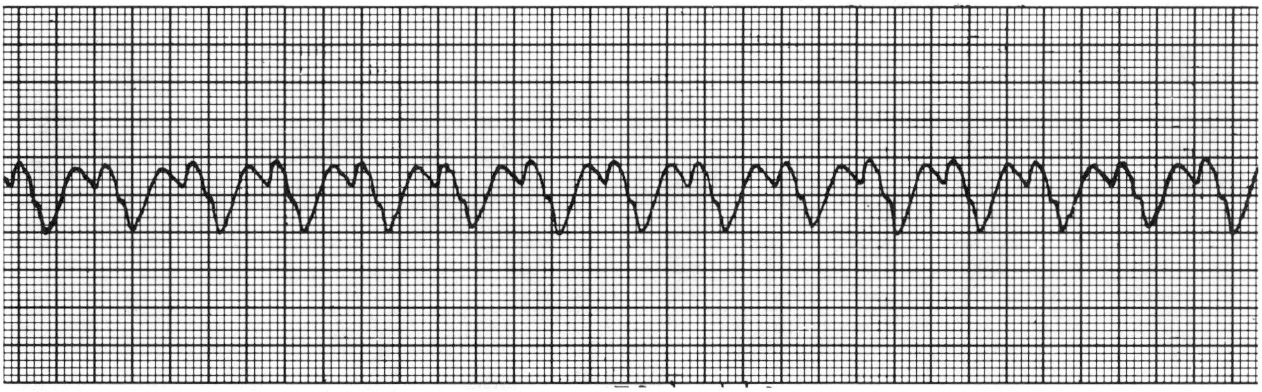

Practice strip 6-22

RHYTHM:

RATE:

P WAVES:

PR INTERVAL:

QRS COMPLEX:

INTERPRETATION:

THERAPY:

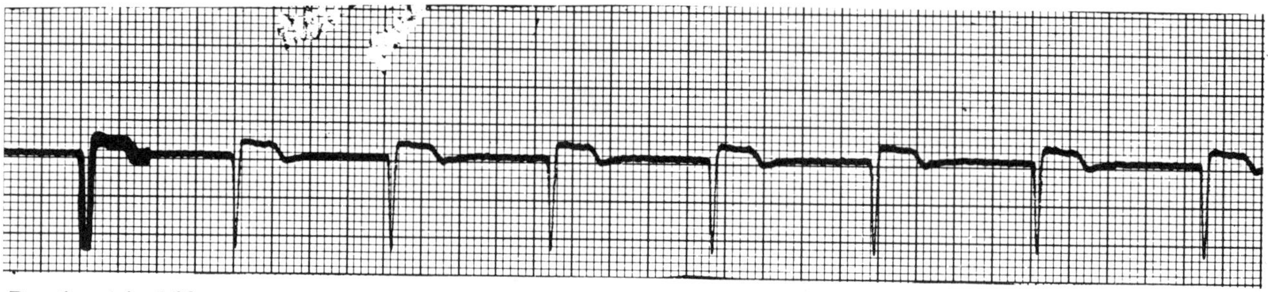

Practice strip 6-23

RHYTHM:
RATE:
P WAVES:
PR INTERVAL:
QRS COMPLEX:
INTERPRETATION:
THERAPY:

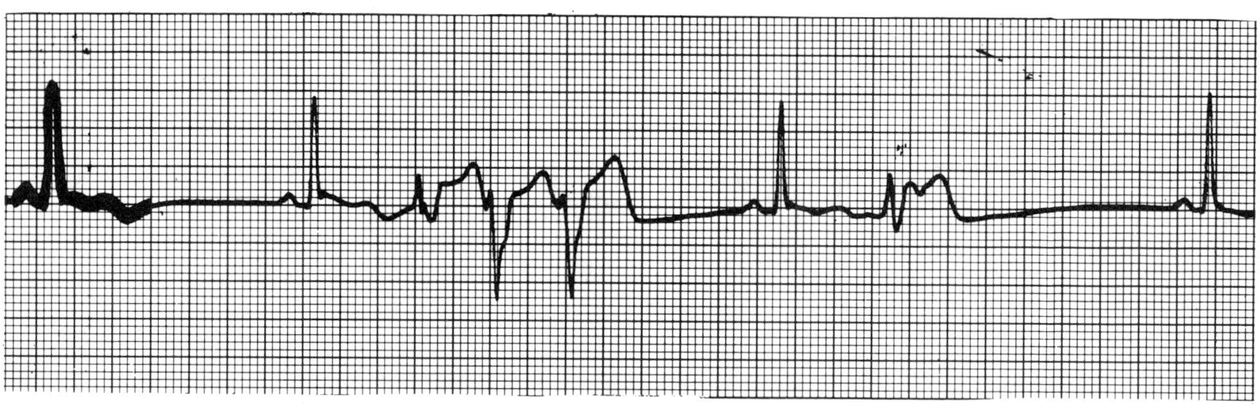

Practice strip 6-24

RHYTHM:
RATE:
P WAVES:
PR INTERVAL:
QRS COMPLEX:
INTERPRETATION:
THERAPY:

ANSWER STRIPS

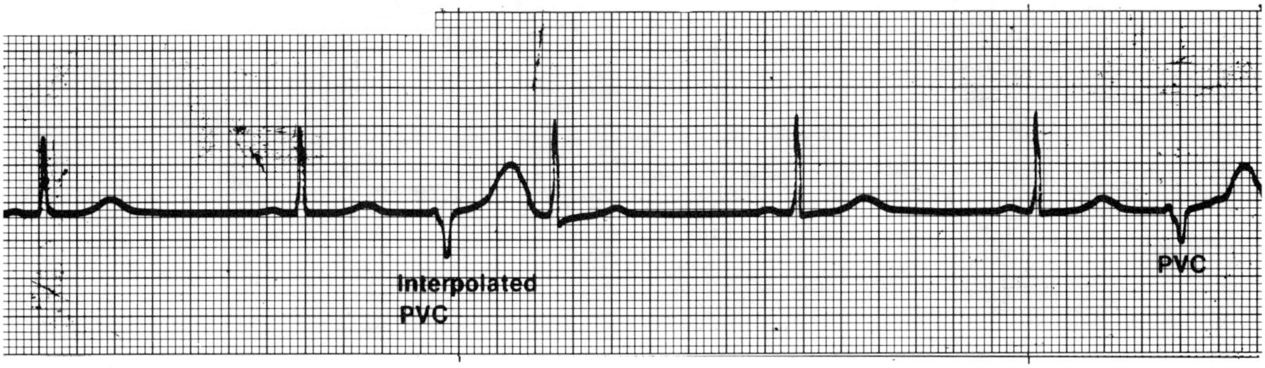

Answer strip 6-1

RHYTHM: *Irregular due to premature beats*

RATE: *Sinus, 45*

P WAVES: *Present—None with premature beats*

PR INTERVAL: *0.20 second*

QRS COMPLEX: *0.08 second; early beats; wide and bizarre*

INTERPRETATION: *Sinus bradycardia with unifocal PVCs (1 is interpolated)*

THERAPY: *Lidocaine*

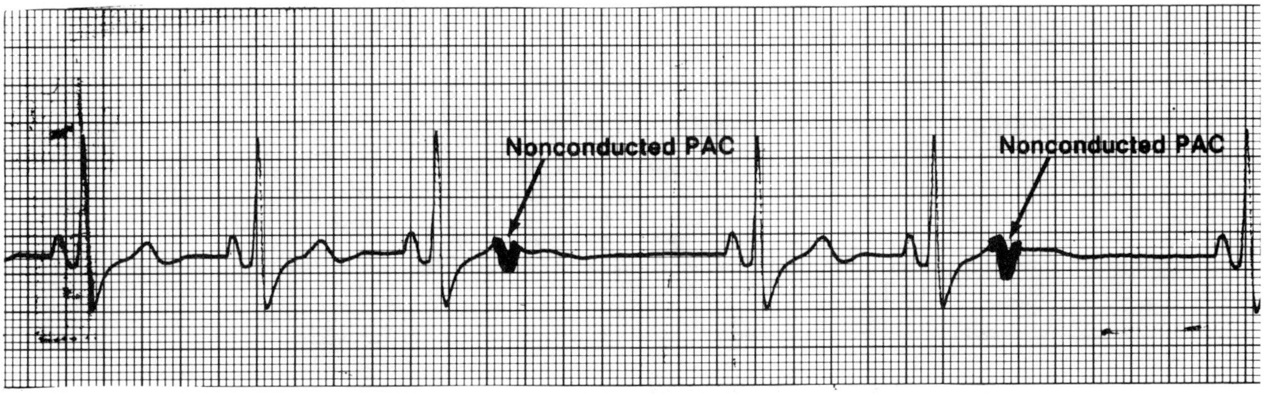

Answer strip 6-2

RHYTHM: *Irregular due to pauses*

RATE: *Sinus, 66*

P WAVES: *Normal—present before each pause, differs in shape*

PR INTERVAL: *0.14 second*

QRS COMPLEX: *0.16 second*

INTERPRETATION: *NSR with BBB and non-conducted PACs*

THERAPY: *None needed*

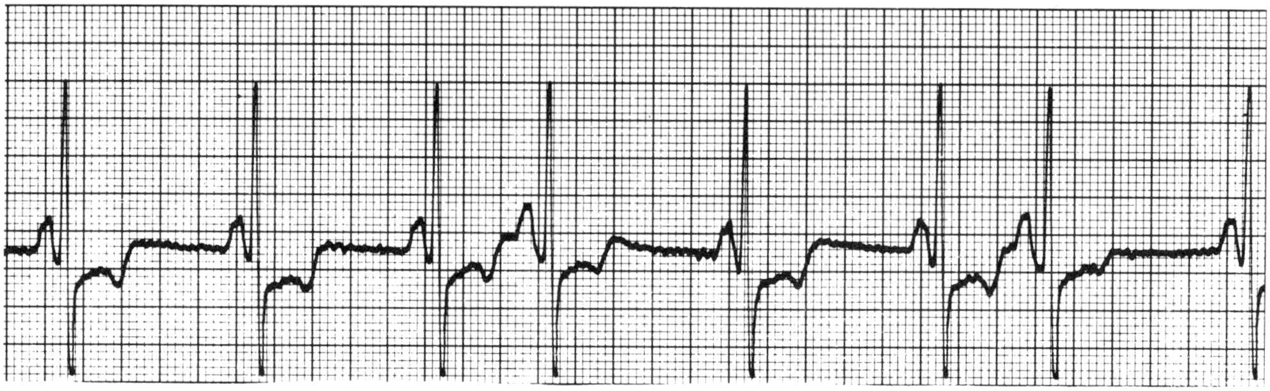

Answer strip 6-3

RHYTHM: *Irregular due to premature beats*

RATE: *65*

P WAVES: *Present—change in configuration in front of early beats*

PR INTERVAL: *0.14–0.16 second in early beat*

QRS COMPLEX: *0.10 second*

INTERPRETATION: *NSR with PACs*

THERAPY: *None. Observe patient*

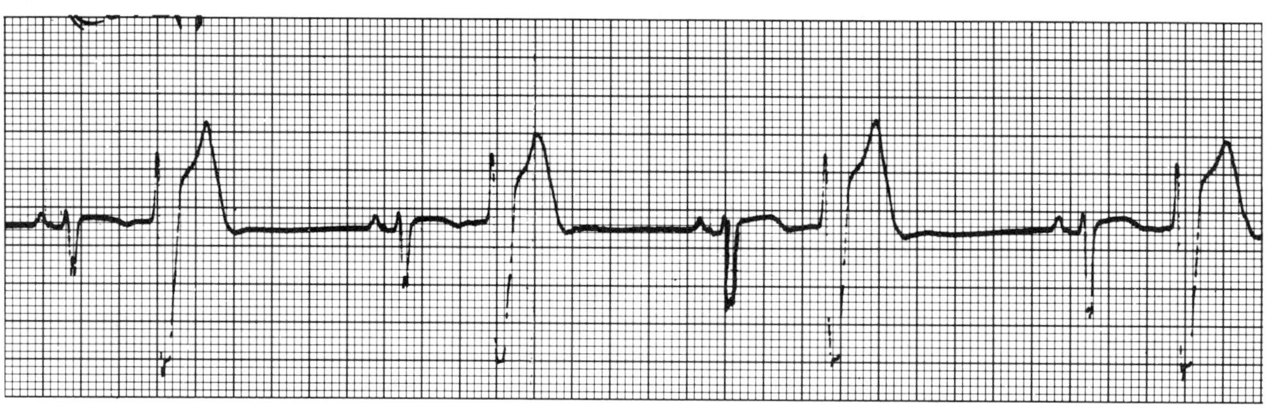

Answer strip 6-4

RHYTHM: *Regularly irregular, every other beat is early*

RATE: *80*

P WAVES: *Present in sinus beats; none in early beats*

PR INTERVAL: *0.16 second*

QRS COMPLEX: *0.10 second—early beats wide and bizarre*

INTERPRETATION: *Ventricular bigeminy*

THERAPY: *Check for digitalis toxicity; check potassium levels. Lidocaine; dilantin*

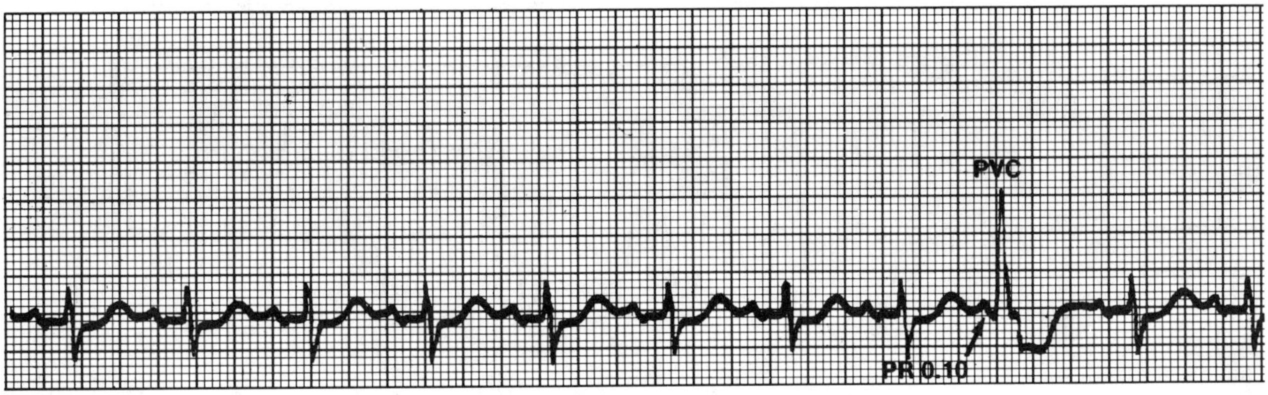

Answer strip 6-5

RHYTHM: *Irregular due to one early QRS*

RATE: *95*

P WAVES: *Present*

PR INTERVAL: *0.20 second*

QRS COMPLEX: *0.10 second; early QRS; wide and bizarre*

INTERPRETATION: *NSR with one PVC (This is not a fusion beat because the PR is too short.)*

THERAPY: *Lidocaine*

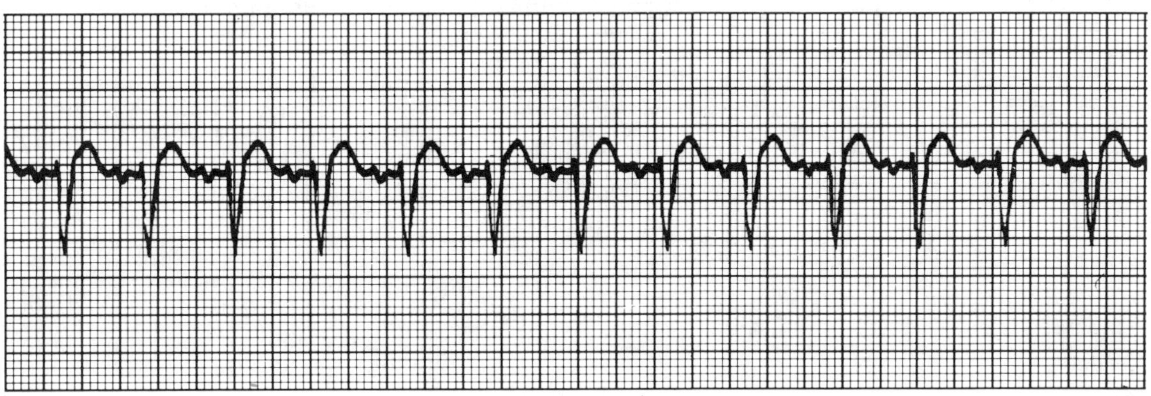

Answer strip 6-6

RHYTHM: *Regular*

RATE: *140*

P WAVES: *Normal*

PR INTERVAL: *0.18 second*

QRS COMPLEX: *0.11 second*

INTERPRETATION: *Sinus tachycardia*

THERAPY: *Find cause and remove if possible*

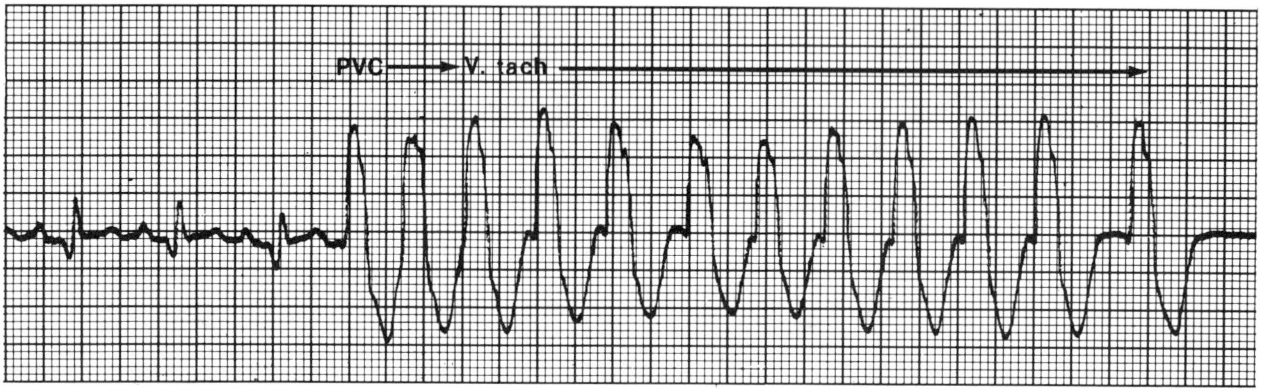

Answer strip 6-7

RHYTHM: *Regular → irregular*

RATE: *115 → 210*

P WAVES: *Present—none associated with wide QRSs*

PR INTERVAL: *0.18 second*

QRS COMPLEX: *0.10 second → wide and bizarre*

INTERPRETATION: *Sinus tachycardia → ventricular tachycardia*

THERAPY: *Lidocaine*

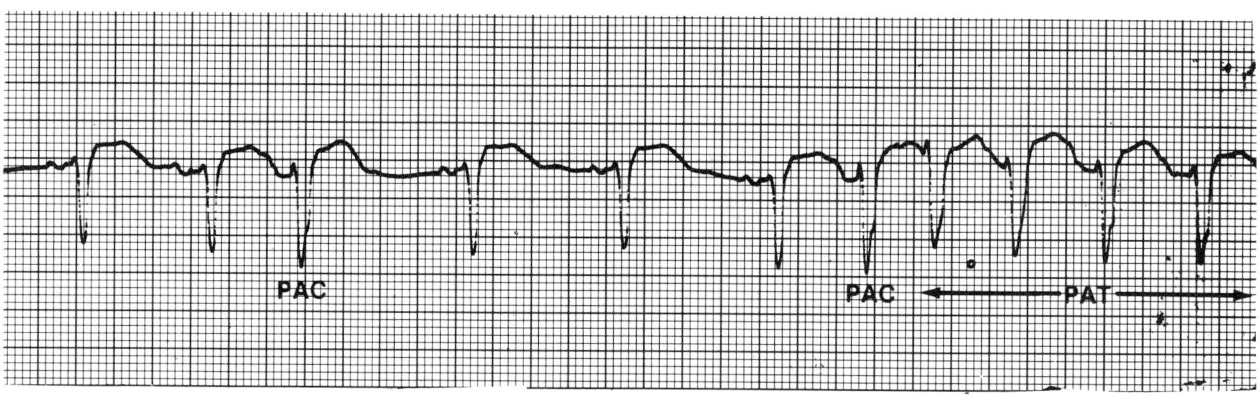

Answer strip 6-8

RHYTHM: *Irregular due to premature beats and tachycardia*

RATE: *Sinus, 75; tachycardia, 130–150*

P WAVES: *Normal—change in shape in early beats and tachycardia*

PR INTERVAL: *0.16 second*

QRS COMPLEX: *0.10 second; widens in tachycardia*

INTERPRETATION: *NSR with PACs → PAT*

THERAPY: *Verapamil or digitalis and a Class I agent; cardioversion if necessary*

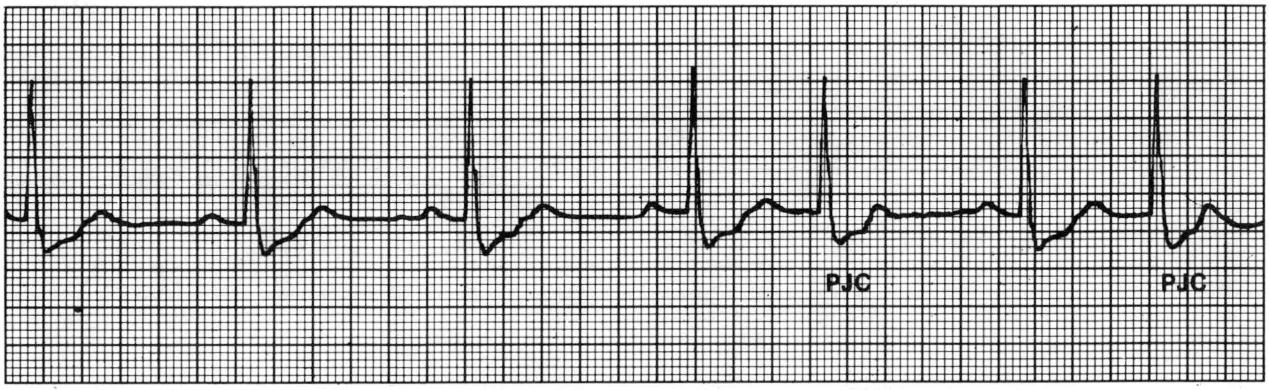

Answer strip 6-9

RHYTHM: *Irregular due to premature beats*

RATE: *52*

P WAVES: *Normal—none in premature beats*

PR INTERVAL: *0.24 second*

QRS COMPLEX: *0.12 second*

INTERPRETATION: *Sinus bradycardia with first-degree AV block and PJCs*

THERAPY: *Observe patient for ↑ block or slowing rate*

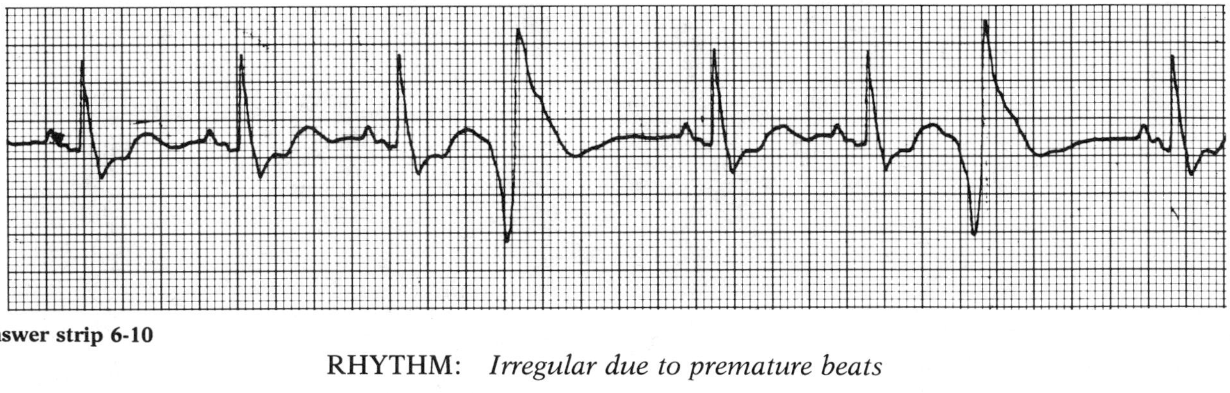

Answer strip 6-10

RHYTHM: *Irregular due to premature beats*

RATE: *72*

P WAVES: *Present—none with premature beat*

PR INTERVAL: *0.18 second*

QRS COMPLEX: *0.16 second. Wide and bizarre in premature beats.*

INTERPRETATION: *NSR with BBB and unifocal PVCs*

THERAPY: *Lidocaine*

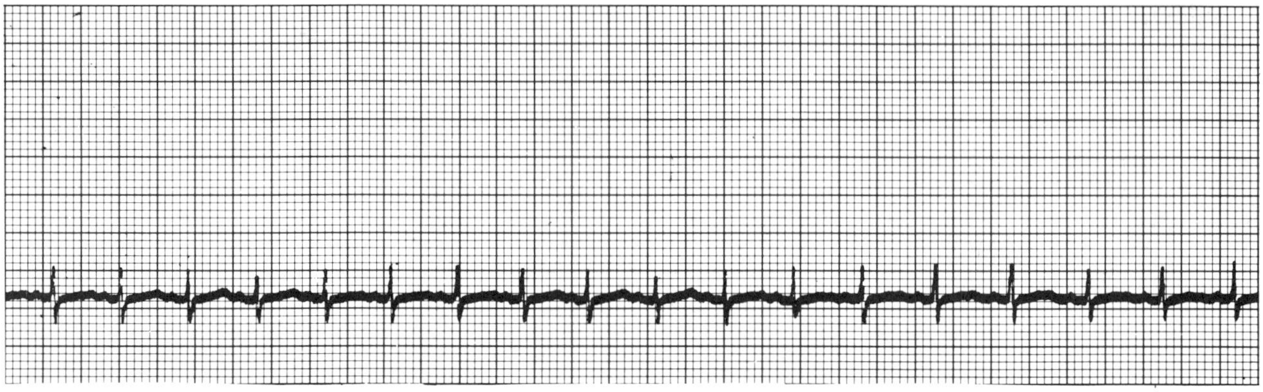

Answer strip 6-11

RHYTHM: *Regular*

RATE: *180*

P WAVES: *Present in front of QRS?*

PR INTERVAL: *?*

QRS COMPLEX: *0.06 second*

INTERPRETATION: *Supraventricular tachycardia, possibly atrial*

THERAPY: *Vagal stimulation; digitalis and a Class I agent, or verapamil; cardioversion*

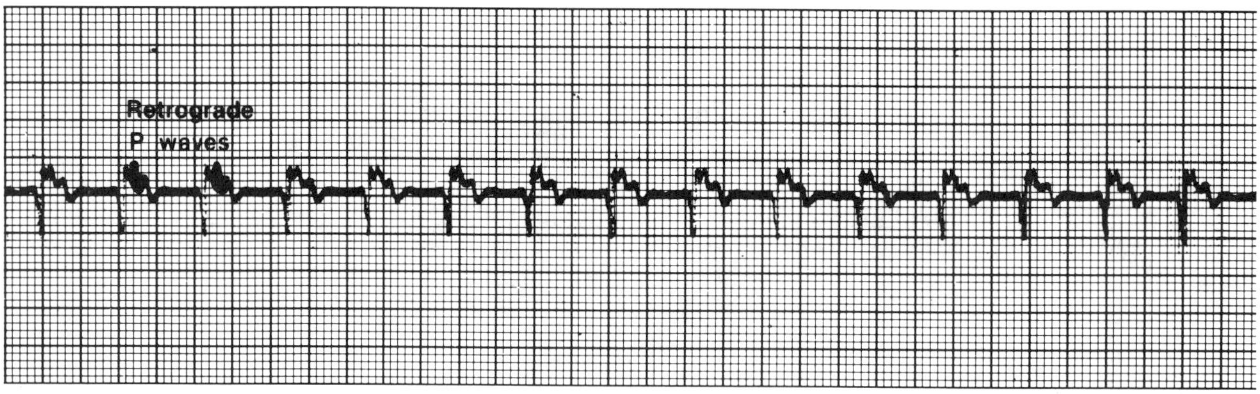

Answer strip 6-12

RHYTHM: *Regular*

RATE: *145*

P WAVES: *Retrograde following QRS*

PR INTERVAL: —

QRS COMPLEX: *0.08 second*

INTERPRETATION: *Junctional tachycardia*

THERAPY: *Vagal stimulation; digitalis and a Class I agent, or verapamil; cardioversion*

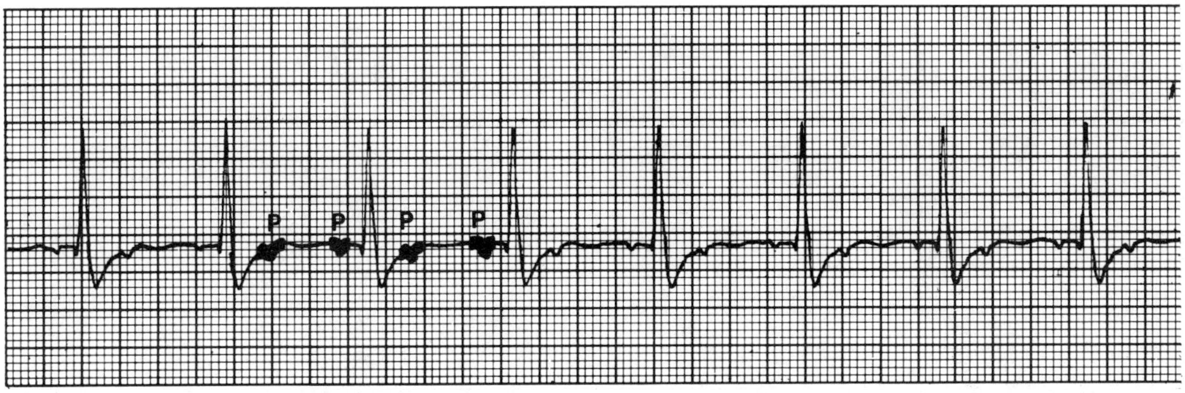

Answer strip 6-13

RHYTHM: *Regular*

RATE: *Atrial, 160; ventricular, 80*

P WAVES: *Present—every other one not conducted*

PR INTERVAL: *0.16 second*

QRS COMPLEX: *0.12 second*

INTERPRETATION: *Atrial tachycardia with 2:1 block*

THERAPY: *Check digitalis and K^+ levels; Dilantin*

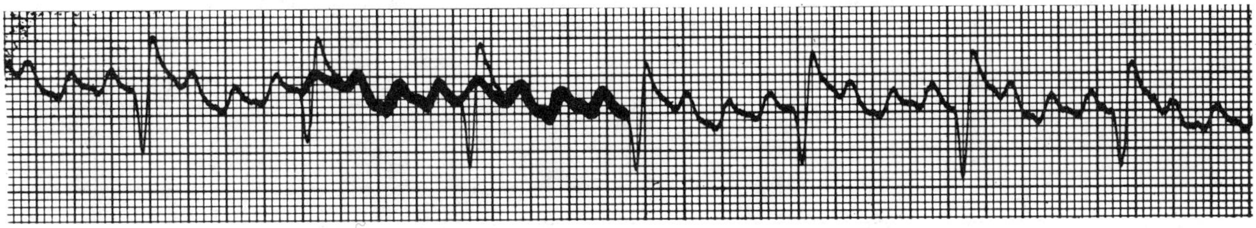

Answer strip 6-14

RHYTHM: *Regular*

RATE: *Atrial, 280; ventricular, 70*

P WAVES: *None—flutter waves*

PR INTERVAL: —

QRS COMPLEX: *0.10 second*

INTERPRETATION: *Atrial flutter with 4:1 conduction*

THERAPY: *Digitalis, then a Class I agent; cardioversion*

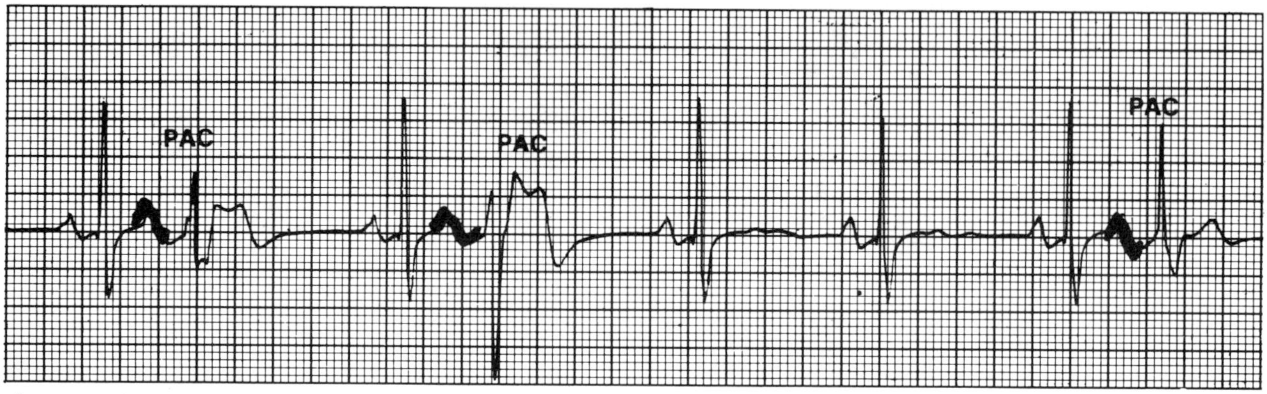

Answer strip 6-15

RHYTHM: *Irregular due to premature beats*

RATE: *63*

P WAVES: *Present—changes in configuration in early beats*

PR INTERVAL: *0.18 second*

QRS COMPLEX: *0.10 second. Changes in shape in premature beats*

INTERPRETATION: *NSR with PACs with aberrant ventricular conduction*

THERAPY: *Observe patient*

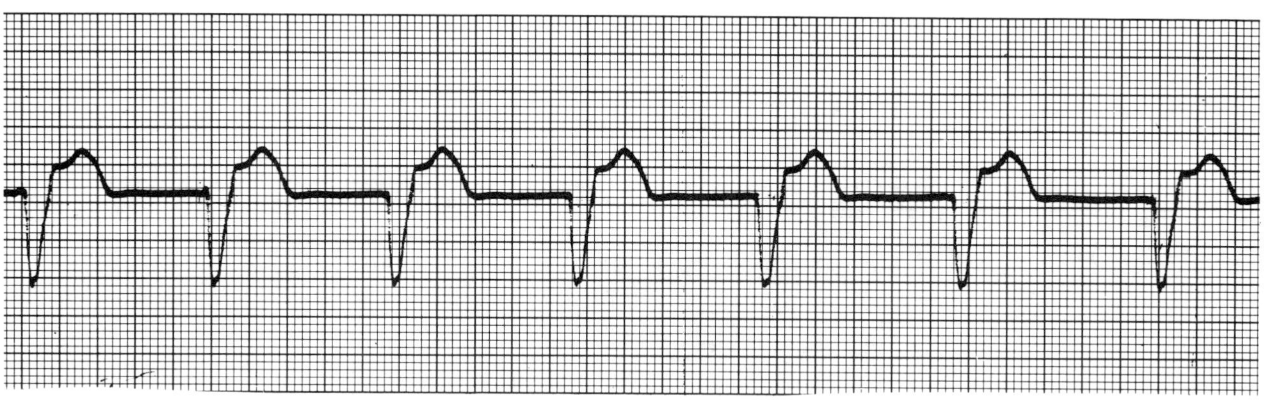

Answer strip 6-16

RHYTHM: *Regular, slowing*

RATE: *58*

P WAVES: *None*

PR INTERVAL: *None*

QRS COMPLEX: *0.16 second; wide and bizarre*

INTERPRETATION: *Accelerated ventricular rhythm*

THERAPY: *Check cause; if suppression, atropine; if irritability, none.*

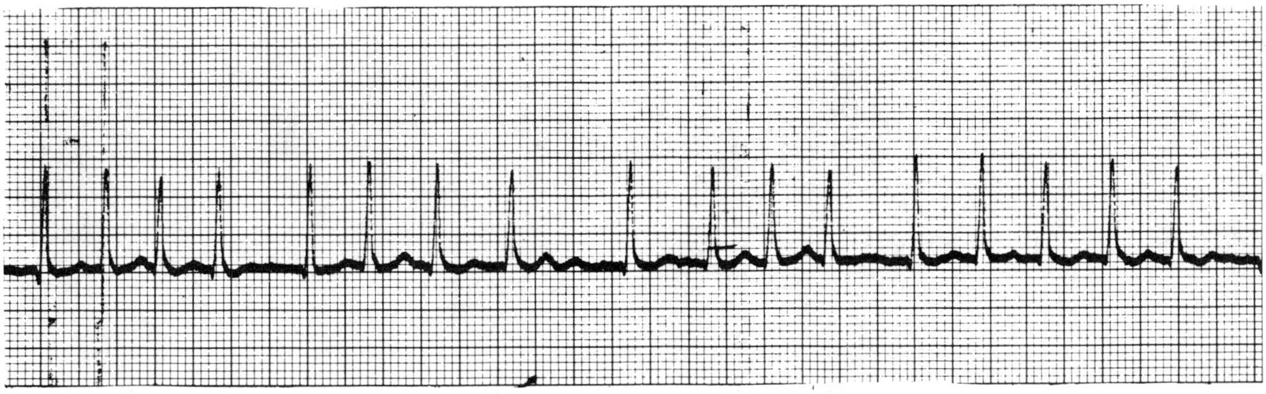

Answer strip 6-17

RHYTHM: *Totally irregular*

RATE: *Ventricular, 160*

P WAVES: *None—fibrillation waves*

PR INTERVAL: *None*

QRS COMPLEX: *0.10 second*

INTERPRETATION: *Uncontrolled atrial fibrillation*

THERAPY: *Digitalis and a Class I agent or verapamil; cardioversion*

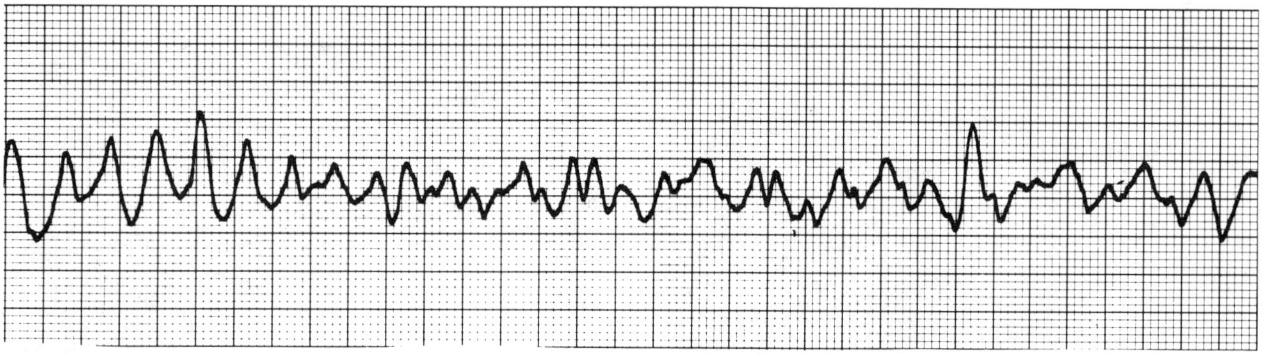

Answer strip 6-18

RHYTHM: *Totally chaotic, irregular*

RATE: —

P WAVES: —

PR INTERVAL: —

QRS COMPLEX: —

INTERPRETATION: *Ventricular fibrillation*

THERAPY: *Defibrillation; CPR; Code Blue*

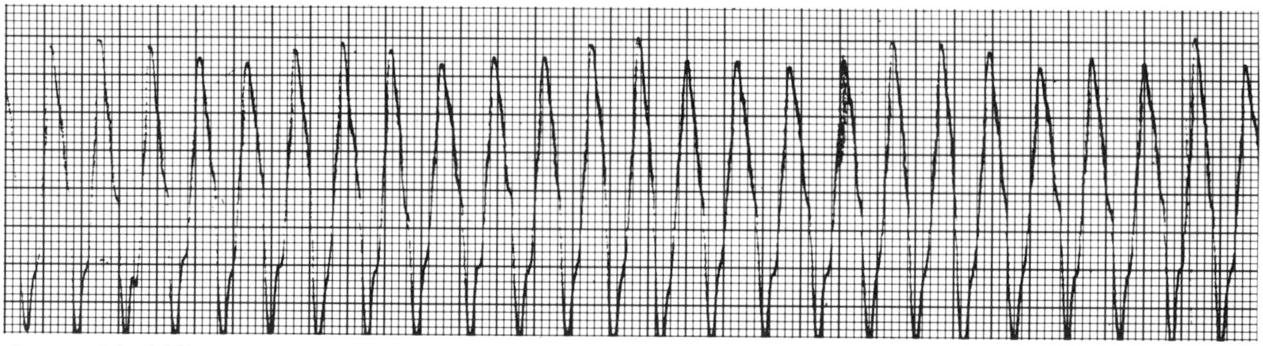

Answer strip 6-19

RHYTHM: *Regular*

RATE: *270*

P WAVES: *None visible*

PR INTERVAL: —

QRS COMPLEX: *Wide, zigzag waveforms*

INTERPRETATION: *Ventricular flutter*

THERAPY: *Code Blue; CPR*

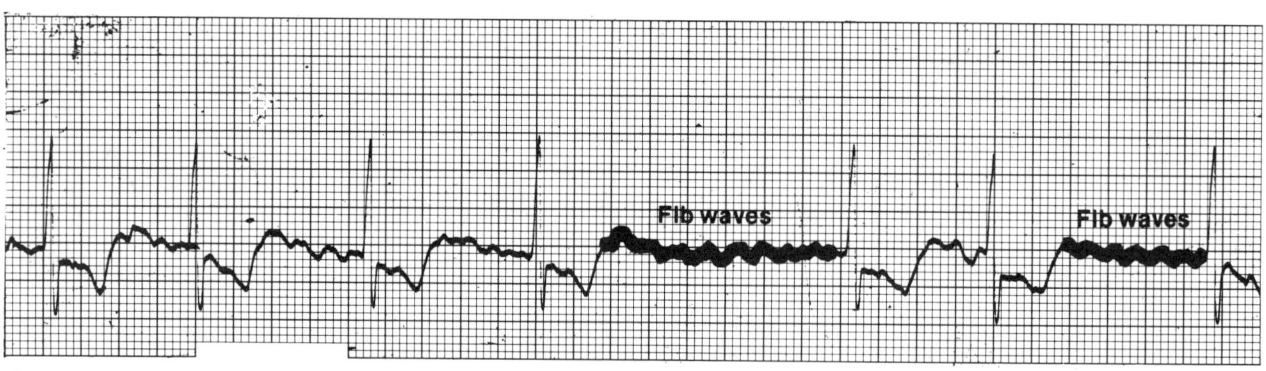

Answer strip 6-20

RHYTHM: *Totally irregular*

RATE: *Ventricular, 60*

P WAVES: *None—fibrillation waves*

PR INTERVAL: —

QRS COMPLEX: *0.10 second*

INTERPRETATION: *Controlled atrial fibrillation*

THERAPY: *Digitalis and a Class I agent, verapamil; cardioversion*

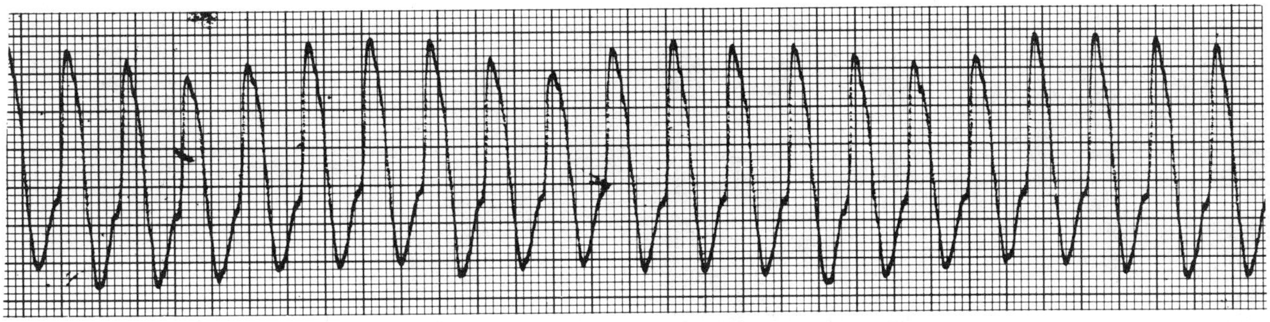

Answer strip 6-21

RHYTHM: *Slightly irregular*

RATE: *210*

P WAVES: *None visible*

PR INTERVAL: *None*

QRS COMPLEX: *Wide and bizarre; changes in configuration from beat to beat*

INTERPRETATION: *Ventricular tachycardia*

THERAPY: *Lidocaine; cardioversion*

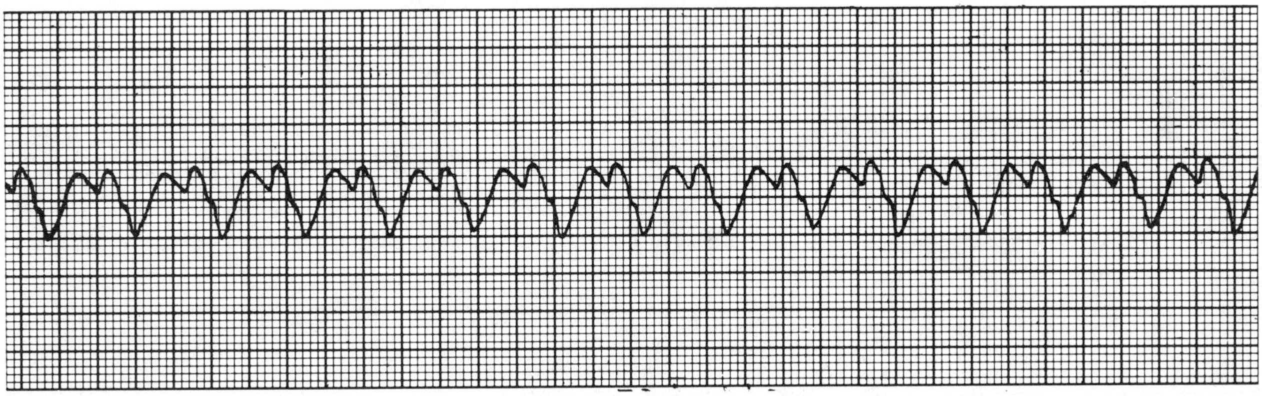

Answer strip 6-22

RHYTHM: *Regular*

RATE: *140*

P WAVES: *Not visible*

PR INTERVAL: —

QRS COMPLEX: *Wide—all beats identical*

INTERPRETATION: *Supraventricular tachycardia with aberrant ventricular conduction*

THERAPY: *Digitalis and a Class I agent, or verapamil; cardioversion*

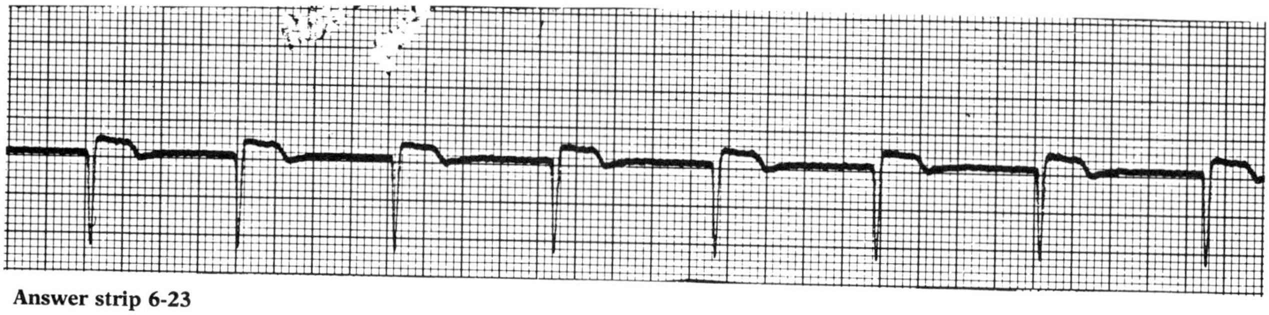

Answer strip 6-23

RHYTHM: *Regular*

RATE: *72*

P WAVES: *None*

PR INTERVAL: —

QRS COMPLEX: *0.06 second*

INTERPRETATION: *Accelerated junctional rhythm*

THERAPY: *Check cause. Suppression—may need atropine if rhythm slows. Irritability—none.*

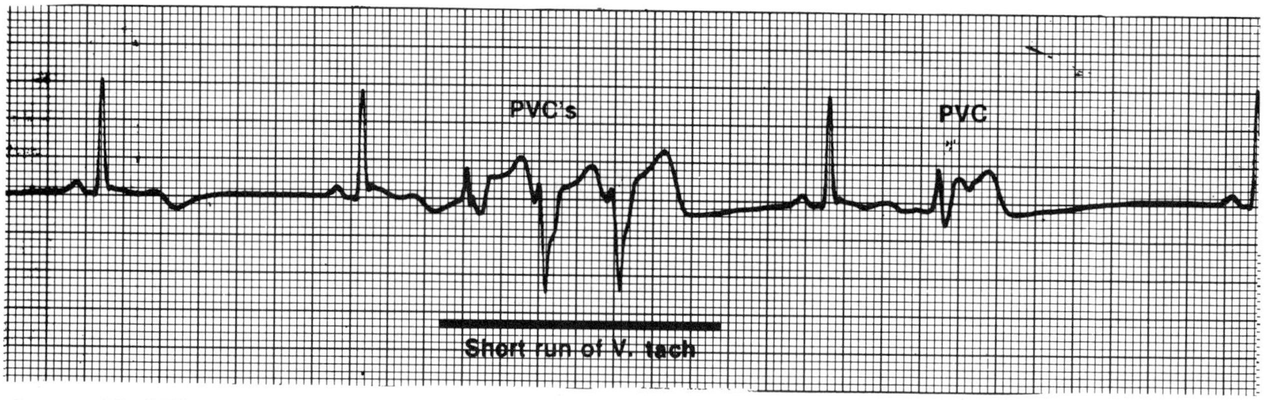

Answer strip 6-24

RHYTHM: *Irregular due to premature beats*

RATE: *Sinus, 48; overall, 70*

P WAVES: *Present—none in premature beats*

PR INTERVAL: *0.16 second*

QRS COMPLEX: *0.08 second; wide and bizarre in premature beats*

INTERPRETATION: *Sinus bradycardia with multifocal PVCs*

THERAPY: *Lidocaine or atropine to ↑ sinus rate to abolish PVCs.*

7

ANTIDYSRHYTHMIC DRUGS

Although we have mentioned the antidysrhythmic drugs commonly used to treat each specific dysrhythmia, a much more detailed discussion of each drug, its dosage and administration, mode of action, and side and toxic effects is needed to cover the pharmacologic therapy completely.

Before beginning the discussion of specific drugs, I think a brief review of the electrophysiology of depolarization and repolarization would be appropriate because these drugs have their effects on the heart and its rhythms by altering different portions of the action potential curve or the spontaneous discharge cycle.

ACTION POTENTIAL CURVE

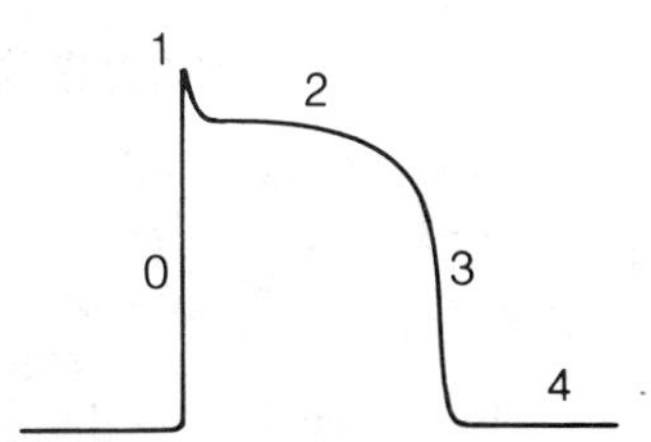

The action potential curve is the electrical activity observed in a cardiac cell that is being activated by a conducted or propagated wave of depolarization.

Phases 0 to 1 are the rapid depolarization stages produced by the rapid ingress of sodium into the cell through the fast channels. The rush of sodium into the cell is allowed because an electrical stimulus hits the cell membrane, opens the gates to the fast channels, and suddenly makes the cell very permeable to sodium. The sodium rushes into the cell, bringing a positive change in with it, and depolarizes the cell.

Phase 2 equates with the absolute refractory period when the cell, if stimulated by another electrical impulse, cannot respond. It is during this plateau in the curve that calcium enters the cell through the slow channels.

Phase 3 is the beginning of repolarization when the potassium leaves the cell, and the cell returns to its electrically balanced state.

During Phase 4, the cell is at its fully repolarized state and has reached its resting potential. The sodium pump is activated in Phase 4 to return the sodium and potassium ions to their repolarized concentrations. Calcium also leaves the cell during Phase 4.

SPONTANEOUS DISCHARGE CYCLE

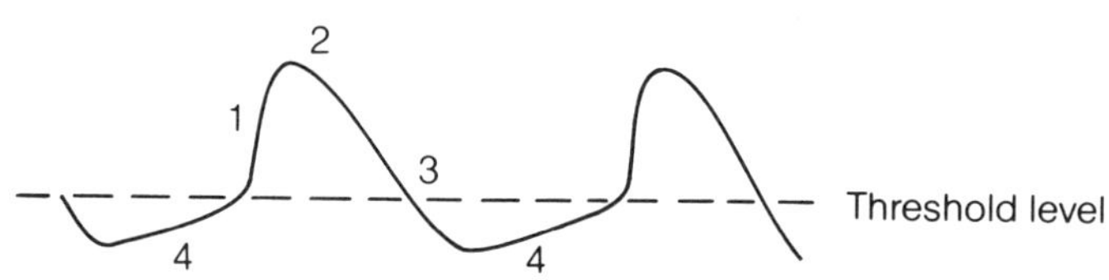

The spontaneous discharge cycle (SDC) is the curve produced by the automatic depolarization of pacing cells. The SDC really begins with Phase 4, when the cell has reached its resting potential. Sodium begins leaking into the cell during this stage of slow diastolic depolarization. As the sodium moves into the cell, the cell becomes more positive inside until the threshold level is reached.

When the threshold level is reached, Phase 1 begins. Sodium rushes into the cell through the fast channels, and the cell rapidly depolarizes.

After depolarization is complete, Phases 2 and 3 occur in the same manner as in the action potential curve repolarizing the cell. As soon as the resting potential is reached, Phase 4 or slow diastolic depolarization begins again, and the SDC repeats.

PHARMACOLOGIC EFFECTS ON ELECTROPHYSIOLOGIC EVENTS

Most of the common antidysrhythmic preparations, particularly those used to treat irritability dysrhythmias, work by producing alterations in either the action potential curve or the SDC.

Some drugs affect the inward current of sodium through the fast channels. These drugs, known as Class I agents, will, of course, have an effect on both spontaneous and propagated depolarization. The Class I preparations have been subdivided further in groups IA, IB, and IC by their electrophysiologic effects on Phase 0 depolarization, conduction, and Phase 3 repolarization.

Class IA preparations include quinidine, procainamide, and disopyramide. These agents slow Phase 0 depolarization markedly, slow conduction moderately, and prolong Phase 3 repolarization.

TABLE 7-1. CLASSIFICATION OF ANTIDYSRHYTHMIC DRUGS

CLASS I	CLASS II	CLASS III	CLASS IV
Group A	Propranolol	Bretylium	Verapamil
Quinidine		Amiodarone	
Procainamide	*Investigational*		*Investigational*
Disopyramide	Metoprolol	*Investigational*	Diltiazem
	Atenolol	Sotalol	Gallopamil
Group B	Acebutolol		Tiapamil
Lidocaine	Nadolol		
Phenytoin	Timolol		
Mexiletine	Oxprenolol		
Tocainide	Alprenolol		
Group C			
Flecainide			
Investigational			
Aprindine			
Lorcainide			
Ethmozin			
Acecainide (NAPA)			
Encainaide			

Class IB agents are lidocaine, phenytoin, tocainide, and mexiletine, and have little effect on Phase 0 depolarization or conduction, and actually shorten repolarization time.

Class IC drugs include encainide and flecainide and also slow Phase 0 depolarization and conduction markedly, but have little effect on repolarization.

Some of these drugs, *e.g.*, quinidine and lidocaine, are old standbys that have been used in the United States for years. Tocainide has just been released for use, and flecainide and mexiletine have been recommended for approval by the Cardio-Renal Advisory Committee of the Food and Drug Administration (FDA). They may soon become available commercially in the United States. Encainide is still classified as an investigational drug. (See the classification of drugs in Table 7-1 for a complete list.)

Other pharmacologic preparations are the Class II agents that act by blocking the effects of sympathetic tone on the heart, thus slowing Phase 4 depolarization. There are many new beta blockers on the market, and it seems that a new one becomes available every so often. However, only one is indicated as an antidysrhythmic—propranolol. The others are used in the treatment of hypertension or angina.

The effects of a third group of drugs widen the whole action potential duration, which very effectively prevents the generation of irritability dysrhythmias. Bretylium tosylate is the only drug in Class III currently approved for use, but amiodarone has received recommendation for approval by the FDA, and may be released in the United States soon.

The calcium antagonists or the slow-channel blockers are the fourth class of drugs. These drugs slow the entry of calcium into the cell. They depress Phase 4 depolarization, and the main antidysrhythmic effect is to prolong AV conduction time. The calcium antagonists currently available in the United States are verapamil, nifedipine, and diltiazem. Of these three, only verapamil is indicated as an antidysrhythmic.

There are two other drugs used to treat suppression rather than irritability—atropine and isoproterenol—that work through sympathetic or parasympathetic mediation.

SUPPRESSIVE DRUGS

Digitalis

ACTIONS Digitalis has two primary actions on the heart—a positive inotropic effect and a negative chronotropic effect. The positive inotropic effect increases the contractility of the myocardium by enhancing the coupling of the electrical activity to the mechanical contraction of the cardiac cell. It will shorten the initial fiber length of cardiac muscle cells so they fall back into the effective contraction range on the Frank-Starling curve. The negative chronotropic effect slows the heart rate by suppressing the automaticity of the SA node and slows conduction through the AV node by prolonging the refractory period. This slowing of SA rate and AV conduction is accomplished by an increase in vagal tone.

USES Because digitalis slows the heart rate and increases contractility of the ventricular muscle, it is most commonly used to treat congestive heart failure. Its use as an antidysrhythmic preparation is mainly to treat supraventricular irritability because it will slow ventricular response to rapid atrial stimuli by blocking down the AV node. However, at higher dosages, digitalis increases both atrial and ventricular irritability and causes many dysrhythmias.

DOSAGE AND ADMINISTRATION The IV administration of digitalis starts with a loading or digitalizing dose of 0.5 to 1.0 mg given in divided doses over a 24-hour period. After that, the maintenance dose is usually 0.125 to 0.5 mg. The usual, daily IV maintenance dose is 0.25 mg, and should be given slowly over a 5-minute time span.

TOXIC AND SIDE EFFECTS Digitalis preparations have many side effects, which cause gastrointestinal (GI) disturbances, central nervous system (CNS) alterations and other problems, but its main problem is digitalis toxicity.

Patients taking any digitalis preparation can become toxic in several ways. First, they can take too much digitalis, bringing their blood levels above the therapeutic range into the toxic range. The blood levels also can be elevated by decreased liver or kidney function, resulting from either organ failure or decreased perfusion of these organs as a result of acute left ventricular failure or cardiogenic shock.

Second, patients can become digitalis toxic with a steady blood level of the drug when their serum potassium levels drop. Frequently, these patients on digitalis are also taking a diuretic. Many diuretics are potassium depleting, and unless careful attention is paid to maintaining the serum level with diets high in potassium or potassium supplements, the patient can become hypokalemic. Hypokalemia sensitizes the myocardium to digitalis and also decreases the positive inotropic effect on contractility.

Taking digitalis in conjunction with other drugs can influence its serum levels. Quinidine, amiodarone, and verapamil cause the blood levels of digitalis to rise, whereas antihistamines, anticonvulsants, barbiturates, and oral hypoglycemic agents may reduce the blood levels.

One of the first signs of digitalis toxicity may be the appearance of dysrhythmias. Digitalis can produce nearly any type of dysrhythmia you might name, because high concentrations increase atrial and ventricular irritability, while slowing conduction through the AV node. Two dysrhythmias very commonly caused by digitalis toxicity are PAT with block and ventricular bigeminy. Other signs and symptoms of digitalis toxicity include GI disturbances such as anorexia, nausea and vomiting, and diarrhea; CNS symptoms such as irritability, headache, vertigo, and generalized muscle weakness; and a curious visual disturbance that causes the patient to see yellow or colored halos around lights.

The treatment for digitalis toxicity is, of course, to stop administering the digitalis until the symptoms of toxicity go away. The serum potassium levels should be checked, and potassium should be replaced if necessary. Phenytoin can be used to suppress digitalis-toxic rhythms.

Quinidine

ACTIONS Quinidine is a Class I agent used to treat irritability dysrhythmias. It is quite easy to remember the actions of quinidine because, very simply, it suppresses everything. As with all Class I agents, it slows the inward flow of sodium into the cell through the fast channels. It lengthens the refractory period, and slows repolarization as well. Quinidine slows the SDC of all pacing foci, but it seems to suppress ectopic pacemakers more than the SA node. It also slows conduction velocity throughout the heart. Quinidine decreases contractility of the myocardium and is also a potent vasodilator, particularly when given IV. Quinidine also has a vagolytic effect.

All of these suppressive actions have definite effects on the ECG, including prolongation of the PR interval, QRS duration, and QT interval. In fact, before the measurement of drug serum levels was readily available, quinidine therapy was monitored by watching the QRS complex widen.

USES Quinidine is used primarily in the treatment of supraventricular irritability dysrhythmias, but is also a second-line drug in the suppression of ventricular irritability. It is used to treat PACs, PVCs, PAT, junctional tachycardia, and atrial flutter and fibrillation.

DOSAGE AND ADMINISTRATION Because quinidine has so many toxic and side effects, a test dose of 200 mg, IM, is recommended. If no untoward effects are produced by the test, then therapy can be instituted. The dosage for IM therapy is 600 mg as an initial dose with repeat doses of

400 mg every two hours, if needed. The IV therapy dose usually is 330 mg or less, but 500 to 750 mg may be needed. The IV solution should be diluted in 50 ml of 5% dextrose in water, and given *slowly* (1 mg/minute). The oral dosage is 200 to 300 mg three to four times a day.

TOXIC AND SIDE EFFECTS Although quinidine's suppressive effects are quite useful in the treatment of irritability dysrhythmias, unfortunately it also suppresses contractility and has a number of very unattractive side effects that make it a difficult and perhaps dangerous drug to use at times.

It has many GI side effects, including nausea and vomiting, abdominal pain, and a rather violent diarrhea that subsides only when the drug is stopped. Many people have an allergic reaction that can be seen as angioedema, asthma, respiratory arrest, and cardiovascular collapse. Its CNS effects are varied and include different visual disturbances, headache, tinnitus, and convulsions.

The suppressive effect quinidine has on myocardial contractility can make this drug impossible to use in a patient with limited cardiac reserve, producing acute left ventricular failure or cardiogenic shock. Its potent vasodilating action can cause extreme hypotensive episodes with IV administration.

Care must be taken when using quinidine to treat atrial flutter. If the AV node is not blocked down with digitalis or some other agent before quinidine is administered, its vagolytic effect may allow 1:1 conduction of the flutter waves as the suppressive effect slows the atrial rate to around 200 beats per minute. Quinidine's effect on conduction velocity can produce or worsen AV block and cause ventricular tachycardia or fibrillation.

Procainamide (Pronestyl)

ACTIONS The actions of procainamide, a Class I agent, are very similar to that of quinidine. It is felt that procainamide has a lesser suppressive effect on contractility than does quinidine.

USES The uses of procainamide are the same as those of quinidine, although some feel that it is less effective in the treatment of atrial dysrhythmias.

DOSAGE AND ADMINISTRATION IV procainamide should be given initially as a boulus of 50 to 100 mg every five minutes, up to a total of 1 g, or until the desired therapeutic effect is achieved. It should be given no faster than 25 to 50 mg per minute. The bolus should be followed by a continuous infusion given at a rate of 2 to 6 mg per minute. When stopping a proçainamide drip, you should taper off the infusion. In reality, procainamide has a half-life of 3 hours, so it tapers itself, but the common practice is to taper the infusion rate to 2 mg per minute and then turn the drip off.

TOXIC AND SIDE EFFECTS These untoward effects are, again, very similar to those produced by quinidine. Procainamide also may cause a lupus-like syndrome with prolonged administration that subsides when therapy is discontinued.

Disopyramide Diphosphate (Norpace)

ACTIONS This drug is another Class I agent similar in action to quinidine and procainamide. It is felt to be better tolerated, having fewer side effects than either of the other two Class I agents discussed.

USES The uses of disopyramide diphosphate are the same as those of quinidine.

DOSAGE AND ADMINISTRATION Disopyramide is only available in the oral form. The dosage is 400 to 800 mg per day in divided doses. The usual dosage is 600 mg per day, given 150 mg every 6 hours or 300 mg of the controlled release form every 12 hours. A loading dose of 300 mg may be given initially, unless the patient has a cardiomyopathy or has marginally compensated contractility. There should be a response to this initial dose within 30 minutes to 3 hours.

TOXIC AND SIDE EFFECTS The toxic and side effects of disopyramide are the same as those of quinidine and procainamide.

Lidocaine

ACTIONS Lidocaine is another Class I agent that is extremely effective in suppressing ventricular irritability dysrhythmias. As with the other Class I agents, it slows entry of sodium through the fast channels, thus decreasing excitability and lengthening the effective refractory period. Lidocaine raises the fibrillation threshold in ischemic myocardium. It also prevents current flow into and out of zones of injury or ischemia produced by MI. It also produces bidirectional block that interrupts the reentry mechanism.

USES The primary use of lidocaine is the suppression of ventricular irritability dysrhythmias—PVCs, ventricular tachycardia, and ventricular fibrillation.

DOSAGE AND ADMINISTRATION Lidocaine is given IV as an initial bolus of 50 to 100 mg (1 mg/kg of body weight), followed by a continuous drip at a rate of 2 mg per minute. Repeat boluses can be given in 50-mg increments every 5 minutes, up to a total of 225 mg. The infusion should be increased by 1 mg per minute with each additional bolus, up to a maximum of 4 mg per minute.

When discontinuing lidocaine therapy, you should taper the drip rate down to 2 mg per minute, but once the rate of administration reaches that level, the drip can be turned off since lidocaine has a half-life of 90 minutes.

TOXIC AND SIDE EFFECTS Lidocaine is a predictable and effective drug with few side effects, and as such, is one of the safest antidysrhythmic preparations. Its adverse effects fall into two categories—allergic and toxic reactions.

Patients with "caine" sensitivities may have an allergic reaction to the initial dose of lidocaine which is manifested by convulsions.

Toxic effects are mainly seen as CNS reactions that include lightheadedness, tinnitus, blurred or double vision, numbness, and respiratory depression or arrest. It also may cause hypotension and cardiovascular collapse.

Phenytoin (Dilantin)

ACTIONS Although it is best known as an anticonvulsant, phenytoin is also a Class I agent with many antidysrhythmic effects similar to those of lidocaine. It decreases automaticity but doesn't slow conduction velocity and, in fact, may even improve conduction. It doesn't seem to decrease contractility as much as other Class I agents.

USES Phenytoin seems to be most effective in suppressing digitalis toxicity-induced dysrhythmias, particularly PAT with block and ventricular bigeminy. Overall, it seems to be best for treating ventricular rather than atrial irritability.

DOSAGE AND ADMINISTRATION The dosage of IV phenytoin is usually 250 mg to 1 g, given IV push, but it must be administered *slowly*, 25 to 50 mg per minute. The higher the dose, the slower the rate of administration must be. If given too rapidly (faster than 50 mg per minute), it can cause vascular collapse, ventricular fibrillation, or AV block.

IV phenytoin is extremely irritating, so you must dilute it with normal saline before using. It is also incompatible with just about everything, so you should flush the IV line before and after administration.

TOXIC AND SIDE EFFECTS There are many side effects, ranging from nausea and vomiting to convulsions, that have been reported following use of phenytoin. IV administration may produce hypotension if the drug is given too rapidly.

Mexiletine (Mexitil)

ACTIONS Mexiletine is a preparation with actions very similar to those of lidocaine, in that it lengthens the effective refractory period by slowing sodium entry through the fast channels but, unlike lidocaine, is well absorbed by the GI tract. It has little effect on blood pressure or heart rate, and only mild negative inotropic effects.

USES Because it can be taken orally and because it has a long half-life of 10 to 26 hours, this drug has a great potential for use in the suppression of chronic ventricular dysrhythmias following acute MI, that put the patient at great risk of sudden death.

DOSAGE AND ADMINISTRATION Mexiletine can be given orally. The daily maintenance dosage runs from 600 to 1000 mg in divided doses given every 8 to 12 hours. The therapeutic plasma level is 1 to 2 μg/ml. An oral loading dose of 600 mg may be required, but an IV loading dose of 150 to 200 mg may be substituted.

TOXIC AND SIDE EFFECTS The side effects are mainly neurologic in nature and include tremors, nystagmus, diplopia, dizziness, and others. Some GI complaints may include nausea and vomiting. Cardiac side effects may include hypotension, bradycardia, and transient AV block seen after IV administration.

Most side effects seem to occur at plasma concentrations greater than 1.5 to 2 μg/ml, and seem to appear most often after the initial administration and disappearing during maintenance therapy.

Tocainide (Tonocard)

ACTIONS Tocainide is a Class IB preparation that has just been released commercially. It is another oral analog of lidocaine similar to mexiletine. It lengthens the absolute refractory period and the action potential duration. It has little or no effect on heart rate or blood pressure, but it does have a mild negative inotropic effect and can increase afterload slightly.

USES This drug is used to suppress ventricular irritability dysrhythmias just as lidocaine does, but it is an oral preparation and can be used to control chronic rhythm problems.

DOSAGE AND ADMINISTRATION The initial dosage recommended by the manufacturer is 400 mg every 8 hours, titrated on the basis of its antidysrhythmic effect. The usual maintenance dosage is 400 to 600 mg, three times a day.

TOXIC AND SIDE EFFECTS The most common side effects include lightheadedness and dizzines, nausea and vomiting, sweating, numbness, and tremor. The GI side effects can be controlled by taking the medication with food. Tremor usually indicates that the blood level is reaching the maximum therapeutic level. The side effects seem to be mild and transient, and dose related. Tocainide should be used cautiously in patients with congestive heart failure or minimal cardiac reserve, particularly if beta blockers also are being given, because of the additive effects. As with any drug that suppresses ventricular irritability, it is contraindicated in patients with AV block unless ventricular pacing is present. Patients also may have allergic reactions as well.

Flecainide (Tambocor)

ACTIONS Flecainide is a member of Class IC agents and as such will slow Phase 0 depolarization and conduction. It seems to have its chief effect on the His-Purkinje and the intraventricular conduction systems. It also shows marked effects on accessory AV pathway and retrograde AV nodal conduction. It has mild negative inotropic properties and it may cause prolongation of sinoatrial node recovery time in patients with preexisting SA dysfunction.

USES Because flecainide works well in the His-Purkinje and intraventricular conduction systems, it is particularly useful for suppressing chronic ventricular dysrhythmias in stable patients. Since it also has been shown to slow conduction through accessory AV pathways and retrograde AV nodal conduction, it is effective in the treatment and prevention of reentrant supraventricular tachycardias such as Wolff-Parkinson-White (WPW) syndrome.

DOSAGE AND ADMINISTRATION Flecainide is easily absorbed from the GI tract. Usually, 100 to 200 mg given orally twice a day seems to provide effective therapy. The effective plasma level ranges from 200 to 1,000 mg/ml, and its elimination half-life is around 20 hours.

TOXIC AND SIDE EFFECTS Because of the mild negative inotropic effect, patients with significantly compromised left ventricular function should use extreme caution when taking this drug.

Other side effects include dizziness and visual disturbances (blurred vision and spots); headache, nausea, dyspnea, and chest pain also have been reported. However, most patients seem to tolerate this drug quite well when taken orally.

Propranolol (Inderal)

ACTIONS Propranolol is the Class II agent or beta blocker currently approved for use as an antidysrhythmic. Many new beta blockers are now on the market for use as antianginal or antihypertensive drugs, but they are not yet indicated for the treatment of dysrhythmias.

Propranolol blocks the effects of catecholamines on the beta receptor sites. Since $beta_1$ sympathetic stimulation increases SA node firing, AV conduction, automaticity, and contractility, beta blockade will slow SA firing and AV conduction and decrease automaticity and contractility. Because it slows rate and decreases contractility, it will decrease myocardial oxygen consumption.

USES Propranolol can be used for both supraventricular and ventricular irritability dysrhythmias; however, its use is not as predictably effective in the ventricles as it is in the atria. Since it slows AV conduction, it can be used to slow ventricular response to rapid atrial stimulation, as seen in atrial flutter or fibrillation, but it has little if any effect on the atrial rate. It also can be used to treat digitalis-toxicity rhythms and suppress PACs, PJCs, and PVCs. It also may control or reduce attacks of paroxysmal supraventricular tachycardia (PSVT) such as PAT, and the Wolff-Parkinson-White or Lown-Ganong-Levine (LGL) syndromes.

DOSAGE AND ADMINISTRATION The oral dosage of propranolol usually is 10 to 30 mg, three to four times a day. This drug can be given IV for life-threatening dysrhythmias, and the IV dose is 1 to 3 mg given at a rate of 1 mg per minute.

TOXIC AND SIDE EFFECTS Propranolol may cause side effects, including GI and CNS problems, similar to many of the other antidysrhythmic drugs. However, the most serious problems arising from its negative inotropic effects on the myocardium, are the decrease in conduction velocity and the $beta_2$ blockade of receptor sites in the lungs.

In a person with limited myocardial reserve, the decrease in contractility produced by propranolol may cause or worsen congestive heart failure. Its effect on conduction velocity can produce or increase AV block. Because it blocks not only the $beta_1$ receptors in the heart but also the $beta_2$ receptors in the lungs, propranolol will cause bronchoconstriction and must be used with caution in patients with asthma or COPD.

Bretylium Tosylate (Bretylol)

ACTIONS Bretylium is the only Class III agent currently approved for use in the United States. Bretylium will lengthen the whole action potential and the effective refractory period. This has the effect of decreasing ventricular irritability and raising the fibrillation threshold. Bretylium is also a positive inotropic drug and will increase contractility.

USES Bretylium is currently used to treat life-threatening, recurrent ventricular tachycardia or fibrillation that has not responded to lidocaine or procainamide. It will suppress ventricular fibrillation within 1 to 2 minutes, but it can take up to 20 minutes to 2 hours to suppress ventricular irritability.

DOSAGE AND ADMINISTRATION The dosage of bretylium to treat intractable ventricular fibrillation is 5 to 10 mg/kg of body weight, given rapidly by IV push. This bolus dose can be repeated at 15- to 30-minute intervals, not to exceed 30 mg/kg.

Treatment of other ventricular irritability dysrhythmias is 5 to 10 mg/kg diluted in 50 ml of normal saline and given over 10 to 30 minutes. This may be repeated in 1 to 2 hours. A continuous drip may be given to maintain the therapeutic blood level at 1 to 2 mg per minute. The half-life of bretylium is 8 to 10 hours, so the blood level also may be maintained by repeating the bolus every 6 to 8 hours.

TOXIC AND SIDE EFFECTS The most common side effects of bretylium is postural hypotension with the initial administration. Patients will develop a tolerance to the hypotension, usually within several days.

Bretylium may produce a transient hypertension with an accompanying increase in the frequency of dysrhythmias. It will also aggravate digitalis toxicity, and may cause nausea and vomiting if given too rapidly IV.

Amiodarone (Cardarone)

ACTIONS Amiodarone is a Class III agent that has just been recommended for approval by the FDA, and may soon be released for use in the United States. It was first introduced as an anti-anginal drug, but it was soon noted to have antidysrhythmic effects as well. As a Class III agent, it prolongs the whole action potential curve, and it has alpha- and beta-blocking effects. It slows the SA node's discharge rate; slows AV node conduction; increases the effective refractory period in AV accessory pathways; and it increases the refractory periods in both the atria and ventricles.

USES Because it slows AV conduction and increases atrial and ventricular refractory periods, amiodarone is effective in suppressing both supraventricular and ventricular irritability dysrhythmias. It works very well in stopping reentrant supraventricular tachycardias such as WPW, but it also can terminate other supraventricular tachycardias as well. It seems to be very effective in converting atrial flutter or atrial fibrillation. It also seems to prevent the tachycardias that are part of sick sinus syndrome without increasing the bradycardia by further suppressing the SA node. Amiodarone also appears to be quite effective in suppressing ventricular irritability, particularly recurrent ventricular tachycardia and ventricular fibrillation.

DOSAGE AND ADMINISTRATION Amiodarone may be given both orally or IV. Usual oral dosage is 600 mg, followed by a maintenance dosage of 200 to 400 mg daily. The IV loading dose is 6 to 10 mg/kg given slowly, followed by an infusion rate of 10 mg/kg per day.

TOXIC AND SIDE EFFECTS After reading all of the wonderful effects, you would tend to think that this drug could be the ideal antidysrhythmic preparation but, unfortunately, it has many side effects, some of which are very distressing. It has produced torsade des pointes (polymorphous ventricular tachycardia) in patients who have had occurrences of this rhythm prior to therapy. It may cause extreme hypotension with rapid I.V. administration. It also has produced a pneumonitis with long-term therapy. Amiodarone also can cause changes in thyroid hormone concentrations. It also has two peculiar side effects seen with long-term therapy—deposits of a yellow-brown pigment in the cornea, and photosensitivity with exposure to the sun that causes a rash or blisters. It also causes a blue-grey pigmentation of the skin, pseudocyanosis (or Smurf Syndrome?), with long-term therapy.

Verapamil (Isoptin, Calan)

ACTIONS Verapamil is the only Class IV agent or slow-channel blocker with an approved antidysrhythmic use. It slows the entry of calcium into the cell. Its antidysrhythmic effect is to slow conduction through the AV node, and it also slows SA firing. Verapamil also decreases contractility of the myocardium.

USES The main antidysrhythmic use of verapamil is to terminate supraventricular tachycardias, particularly those that are paroxysmal reentrant rhythms (PSVT), such as WPW, LGL, or PAT. It is also becoming more widely used to slow the ventricular response to atrial flutter or fibrillation.

DOSAGE AND ADMINISTRATION The initial IV dose of verapamil is 5 to 10 mg/kg of body weight, given as a bolus over 2 minutes. You may give a repeat 10-mg dose in 30 minutes after the initial dose.

The dosage of oral verapamil is 80 to 120 mg given every 8 hours.

TOXIC AND SIDE EFFECTS This drug seems to be well tolerated by most patients. It may produce a transient hypotension and also may cause a rapid ventricular response to atrial stimuli, or extreme bradycardia or asystole. It alters the patient's hemodynamics very slightly, but may produce congestive heart failure. The GI effects are nausea, vomiting, and constipation. CNS effects are headache and dizziness.

Verapamil should be given with extreme caution to patients with hypotension, congestive heart failure, second-degree or third-degree AV block, or sick sinus syndrome. It should not be given to patients taking I.V. beta blockers because of the similarity of their actions and their effects on hemodynamics.

STIMULANT DRUGS

Atropine

ACTIONS Atropine is a vagal blocker. It inhibits parasympathetic tone on the heart, allowing the $beta_1$ effects to predominate in the atria. It therefore increases the rate of SA node firing and speeds conduction velocity through the AV node.

USES Atropine is the first drug of choice in the treatment of symptomatic sinus bradycardia. It also may be used to improve conduction in cases of incomplete AV block.

DOSAGE AND ADMINISTRATION Atropine is given IV as a bolus dose of 0.5 mg that can be repeated every 5 minutes, up to a total of 2 mg. The effects can occur within a few minutes or up to a half hour, and last 4 to 6 hours.

TOXIC AND SIDE EFFECTS The side effects of atropine are mainly anticholinergic and include urinary retention, decreased intestinal motility, dryness of the mouth, enlarged pupils, and confusion. Prolonged administration could exacerbate glaucoma. Atropine has been reported to cause ventricular irritability in the form of ventricular tachycardia or fibrillation.

Care should be taken that the correct dosage is given, since too little of the drug can actually slow the rate more, and too much can cause a tachycardia.

Isoproterenol (Isuprel)

ACTIONS It's easy to remember what isoproterenol does if you know the actions of propranolol. Isoproterenol is a pure beta stimulator whose effect on the heart is exactly opposite that of the beta blockers.

Isoproterenol increases SA node firing and AV conduction. It increases automaticity of ventricular ectopic pacemakers, and greatly increases contractility of the ventricular muscle.

USES Isoproterenol is used to increase heart rate and AV conduction in the presence of second-degree AV block, and in third-degree AV block it may increase the rate of the lower ectopic focus that is pacing the ventricles.

DOSAGE AND ADMINISTRATION Isoproterenol is given IV drip by adding 1 mg of the drug to 250 ml of 5% dextrose in water. The IV drip rate is titrated to achieve a heart rate of 60 to 80 beats per minute. If the drug is given too rapidly, it can produce a tachycardia, and the patient may develop ventricular tachycardia or ventricular fibrillation.

TOXIC AND SIDE EFFECTS Isoproterenol is a dangerous drug with many side effects, and extreme caution should be used when it is being given. Because it increases heart rate and contractility, it greatly increases myocardial oxygen consumption and can provoke angina or even MI. It also increases irritability in the ventricles and can cause PVCs, ventricular tachycardia, or fibrillation. Its use for patients with poor myocardial reserve is contraindicated, since it could put the patient into acute left ventricular failure or cardiogenic shock.

SUMMARY CHART OF DRUG ACTIONS

DRUG	VAGAL TONE	BETA$_1$ TONE	HEART RATE	AV CONDUCTION	CONTRACTILITY	CARDIAC OUTPUT	AUTOMATICITY	CONDUCTIVITY
Digitalis	↑		↓	↓	↑	↑	↓	↓
Quinidine	↓		↓	↓	↓	↓	↓	↓
Procainamide	↓		↓	↓	↓	↓	↓	↓
Disopyramide	↓		↓	↓	↓	↓	↓	↓
Lidocaine							↓	
Phenytoin				↑			↓	↑
Mexiletine					↓		↓	
Tocainide					↓		↓	
Flecainide				↓	↓		↓	↓
Propranolol		↓	↓	↓	↓	↓	↓	↓
Bretylium					↑	↑	↓	↓
Amiodarone		↓	↓	↓			↓	↓
Verapamil			↓	↓	↓	↓	↓	↓
Atropine	↓		↑	↑			↑	↑
Isoproterenol		↑	↑	↑	↑	↑	↑	↑

↑ = increases.
↓ = decreases.

8

THE ELECTRICAL THERAPY OF DYSRHYTHMIAS

In the last chapter we discussed in detail pharmacologic intervention in the therapy of dysrhythmias. Unfortunately, drugs do not always have the desired effects. The patient also may have immediate and disastrous hemodynamic alterations from his particular dysrhythmia that require correction sooner than the usual drug therapy could possibly have effect. At other times, the dysrhythmia becomes a chronic condition, and a long course of drug therapy may not be practical or advisable. In any of these instances, the application of electrical therapy to eliminate or control the dysrhythmia may be the solution to a real problem for the patient.

If the patient is suffering from an irritability dysrhythmia, countershock in the form of cardioversion or defibrillation may be the treatment of choice. If suppression is the problem, a transvenous pacemaker may be used to prevent slow rates and their accompanying hemodynamic alterations.

COUNTERSHOCK

Countershock is simply the delivery of an electrical charge through the abnormally depolarizing heart. This discharge of electrical activity will completely depolarize all of the cells in the entire heart simultaneously. One would hope that countershock will correct any abnormality in the heart's depolarization and allow the SA node to regain control of the rhythm. If the abnormal mechanism producing the tachydysrhythmia is reentry, the shock will break up the reentry circuit and stop the tachycardia. If the mechanism producing the tachycardia is a rapidly firing ectopic focus, the charge should stop this activity. If flutter or fibrillation is the problem, the countershock will depolarize all of the cells and stop the abnormal depolarization, allowing the SA node to regain control.

There are two ways of delivering a countershock, cardioversion and defibrillation, and the method to be used is determined by the dysrhythmia that requires therapy. Defibrillation is used to terminate ventricular fibrillation and everything else should be cardioverted. Defibrillation is achieved by the delivery of an instant electrical charge, but in cardioversion, the delivery of the shock is synchronized with the patient's own cardiac cycle.

Countershocks are delivered with paddles placed on the chest wall. The current is discharged from one paddle through the chest to the other paddle. The paddles usually are placed so that one is just below the clavicle to the right of the sternum, and the other is placed on the left anterior axillary line at the level of the nipple (Fig. 8-1). A variation of paddle placement is the anterior-posterior position where one paddle is placed over the precordium and the other is on the patient's back behind the heart. There is no proof that one method of paddle placement is more effective than the other, and the mechanical convenience of the standard placement is much greater than the anterior-posterior method that requires a special flat posterior paddle and necessitates rolling the patient to position it.

The skin provides resistance to current flow, so a conductive medium such as a gel or special conductive pads must be present between the surface of the paddles and the skin to insure delivery of the optimal amount of electrical energy through the heart, and to prevent burns. In some hospitals, saline-soaked 4-in-square gauze pads are used instead of gel or conductive pads. The gel can be a problem if CPR is being performed because it is very slippery and can cause incorrect hand

Figure 8-1 Paddle placement for countershock.

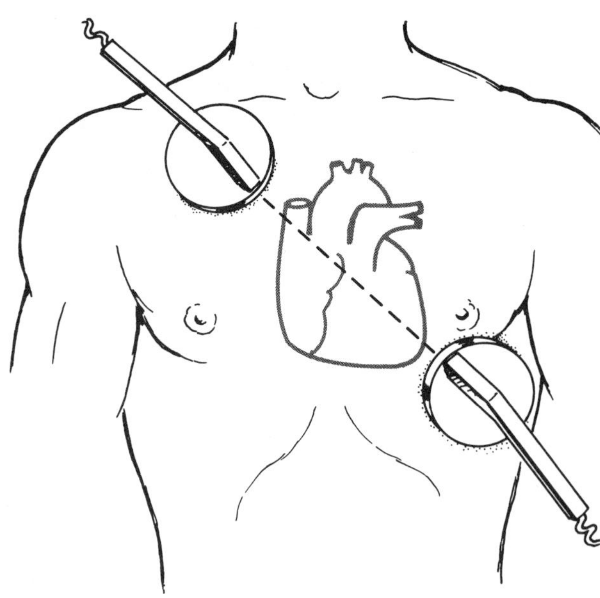

positioning during chest compressions. You must be very careful to keep the gel only under the paddles. If it spreads out over the chest wall, it can dissipate the current and also cause burns. The paddles should be pressed firmly and evenly on the skin, with about 25 pounds of pressure on each paddle to prevent arcing of the current. The fireworks produced by arcing may be impressive, but they are also quite dangerous for you and your patient.

The size of the paddles used on an adult has not really been standardized, but studies appear to show that a 10- to 13-cm diameter surface seems to be most effective. Smaller paddles concentrate the charge in too small an area, which causes greater damage to the myocardium. Obviously, the paddles used on infants and children should be much smaller than those used on an adult.

The amount of electrical energy required to terminate abnormal rhythms is measured in Joules, or watt-seconds, and is determined by the specific dysrhythmia being treated. Another factor to be considered is body size. Some human studies seem to show a correlation, but others seem to point the other way. However, it is obvious that the intensity of the charge should be much less in an infant and child than in an adult.

The amount of energy to be delivered also depends upon the number of previous shocks delivered, because the transthoracic resistance to current flow is reduced with repeated countershocks.

The delivery of a large amount of electrical energy can be a dangerous procedure to the staff if simple safety measures are not observed. Many times the countershock is delivered during a Code Blue with the attendant confusion caused by many persons trying to do different things at the same time. The person controlling the paddles must be very certain no one is touching the patient or the equipment before he delivers the shock. If a member of the code team is touching the patient when the energy is discharged, he or she could receive a shock that might cause muscle cramping, painful burns, convulsions, or even ventricular fibrillation. The person delivering the shock should be certain he or she is not putting himself or herself in danger by careless discharge of the paddles (Fig. 8-2).

The piece of equipment used to deliver countershock may be a defibrillator only, or it also may have the capability of cardioversion as well. In the defibrillation mode, the machine will fire the instant the buttons on the paddles are depressed. However, in the cardioversion mode, the machine will not fire instantaneously. The buttons on the paddles must be depressed and held down until the appropriate time in the patient's cardiac cycle occurs. At this point, namely the down stroke of the R wave, the machine will fire.

Equipment from different manufacturers will vary in the way the energy can be discharged. The safest equipment has two buttons, one on each paddle, that must be depressed simultaneously to fire off the countershock. With this feature, the machine cannot be discharged by anyone other than the code team member in control of the paddles, and he or she can't cause discharge by inadvertently hitting one button.

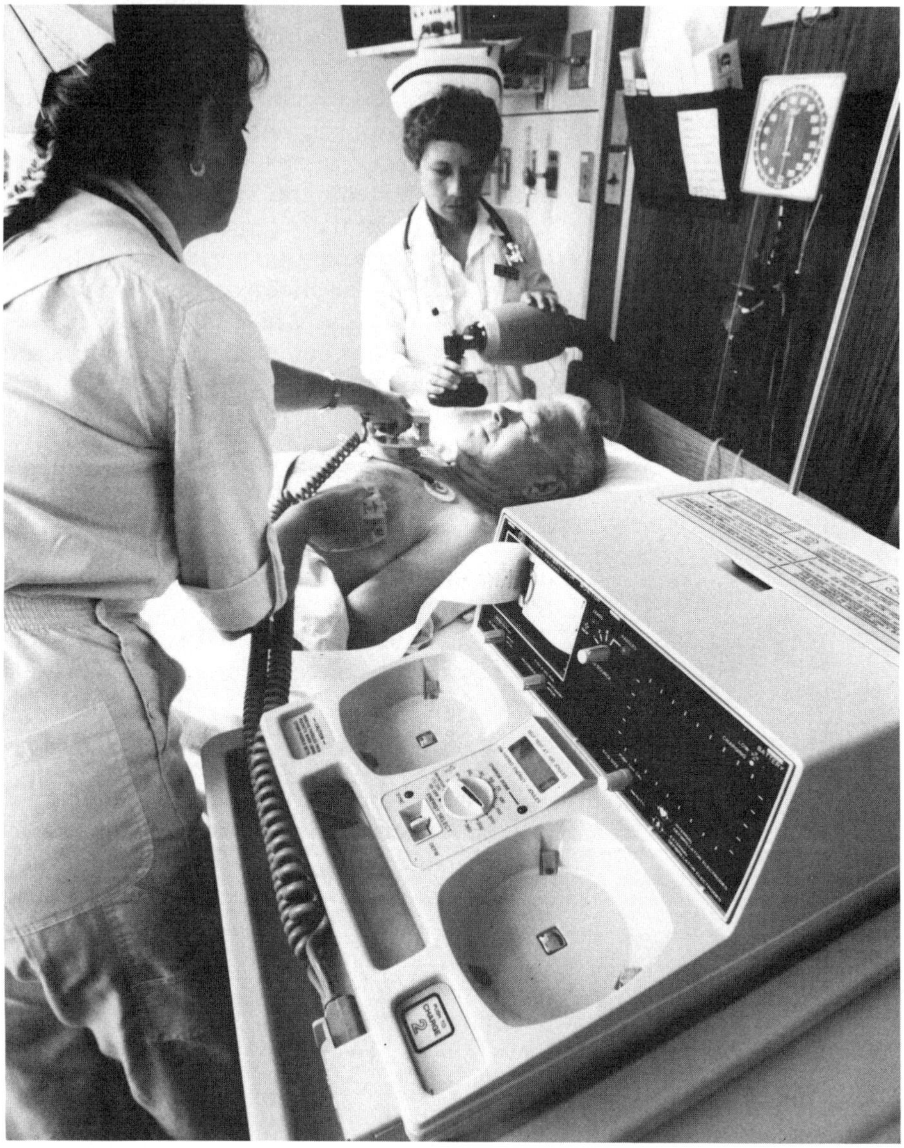

Figure 8-2 Technique for defibrillating patient.

DEFIBRILLATION

Defibrillation is the delivery of an unsynchronized countershock. If set in the defibrillation mode, the machine will fire instantaneously when the buttons are depressed. Defibrillation should be used only when the patient is in ventricular fibrillation. If the patient is experiencing any other tachydysrhythmia requiring countershock, the delivery of an unsynchronized shock could come at that vulnerable period of the cardiac cycle, which occurs on the peak of the T wave, and cause the patient to go into ventricular fibrillation. The only other time defibrillation should be used is for the patient in pulseless ventricular tachycardia when a cardioverter is not immediately available. The reasoning behind this is that pulseless ventricular tachycardia is hemodynamically as disastrous as ventricular fibrillation, and is very likely to rapidly turn into ventricular fibrillation.

The number of watt-seconds to be delivered to successfully defibrillate the patient has not been precisely determined, but the Advanced Cardiac Life Support (ACLS) recommendations are as follows. The initial shock should be between 200 and 300 watt-seconds of delivered energy. If the first shock is not successful, a second shock at the same number of watt-seconds should be given immediately. The watt-seconds delivered in the second shock are not increased because the transthoracic resistance to current flow appears to decrease with each successive countershock. Although precise current requirements for successful defibrillation have not been determined, there appears to be a positive correlation between body size and heart size, and the amount of energy needed to eliminate the abnormal depolarization activity. It is quite apparent that young children with smaller hearts require fewer watt-seconds to terminate ventricular fibrillation.

When the myocardium is anoxic and acidotic, it is less likely to respond to defibrillation. Other factors that will prevent successful defibrillation include electrolyte imbalance or drug toxicity. If any of these situations exist, and the heart does not respond to the first two shocks, ACLS protocol recommends that CPR be initiated to reperfuse the myocardium with oxygenated blood to correct the anoxia, and sodium bicarbonate be given to reduce the acidosis. It also has been shown that fine ventricular fibrillation is more refractory to countershock than a coarser fibrillation wave. Epinephrine will turn fine fibrillation into coarse fibrillation, which is much more likely to respond to countershock.

Care must be taken when defibrillating a patient that the machine is in the defibrillation mode. If the synchronizer circuit inadvertently is turned on, the machine will wait for an R wave to fire, and there are no R waves in ventricular fibrillation. With the synchronizer on, the machine won't fire and the patient continues to fibrillate.

CARDIOVERSION

Cardioversion differs from defibrillation in that the delivery of the shock is synchronized with the patient's own rhythm. The cardioverter is designed to deliver the countershock at the safest time in the cardiac cycle which occurs on the downstroke of the R wave. Administering the energy at this predetermined interval reduces the amount of watt-seconds needed to achieve successful termination of the dysrhythmia and prevents the R-on-T wave phenomenon possible with unsynchronized countershock that could precipate ventricular fibrillation.

Cardioversion is the electrical therapy for all tachydysrhythmias, both supraventricular and ventricular in origin. Cardioversion is indicated when conventional drug therapy has been unsuccessful, or when the patient is suffering decreased hemodynamic function because of the fast rate or the loss of atrial kick that can occur with these rhythms.

Cardioversion may be an elective procedure when the patient needs the tachycardia terminated but is in no immediate danger. It also may be an emergency procedure when the patient's hemodynamic situation is deteriorating rapidly.

Certain precautions must be observed during cardioversion. The synchronizer circuit must be activated on the machine to insure the proper timing of the countershock to prevent the production of ventricular fibrillation. Most cardioverters also have the defibrillation mode, and because of safety regulations, the synchronizer circuit turns off after each time the machine is fired. Once the synchronizer is off, the machine is a defibrillator and will deliver an unsynchronized instantaneous shock the next time it is fired unless the synchronizer is reactivated.

When the countershock is to be given, the buttons on the paddles must be pushed and held until the energy is delivered. Some machines sense the first R wave that comes along after the buttons are pushed, but don't fire until the second R wave. In any case, there will be a delay from the time the buttons are depressed until the energy is discharged, unlike defibrillation which has an instantaneous discharge. In the synchronized mode, if the buttons are pushed and released, the machine may never fire.

When setting the patient up for cardioversion, the ECG lead being used must have an R wave of sufficient voltage to be sensed by the synchronizer circuit. If the R-wave height is too small, the machine won't sense the complex and won't fire. If the T wave has a greater amplitude than the R wave, the machine will fire on the T wave. Most cardioverters will put an indicator mark resembling a pacemaker spike on the monitor at the point in the patient's cardiac cycle when the synchronized shock will be delivered. Some machines also have a blinking light that indicates synchronization as well.

The amount of current to be delivered in cardioversion varies, and some dysrhythmias may be converted with as little as 10 watt-seconds. ACLS standards recommend an initial countershock of 200 watt-seconds if the situation is an emergency cardioversion.

PACEMAKERS

The electrical therapy for slow-rate dysrhythmias is pacemaking. There are many different types of pacemakers, both external and implanted, and many modes or ways of pacing the heart. To cover everything about pacing in a complete manner would require a book in itself, so this discussion will be limited to temporary transvenous pacing.

As early as the 1800s, scientists knew that the myocardial tissue of animals would contract if stimulated by an artificial electrical charge. But it wasn't until the 1950s that physicians applied this knowledge to the human myocardium. It was the space program with its resulting advances in electronic technology and miniaturization that provided dependable equipment that made pacemakers one of the major methods of treating bradydysrhythmias and AV blocks.

INDICATIONS FOR PACING

Pacemakers are inserted for many reasons, the main one being dysrhythmias that cause slow ventricular rates that have not responded to drug therapy or are compromising the patient's hemodynamic status. Pacemakers also may be inserted prophyllactically in patients with known problems before they undergo elective surgical procedures or coronary angiography. During a cardiac catheterization, radio-opaque dye is injected into the coronary arteries. The blood is replaced with the contrast material, and many times the heart rate slows drastically. Some cardiologists insert a pacer before the ciné angiograms are taken to prevent the drop in rate, and then remove the pacing wire at the end of the procedure.

Pacers also may be inserted to over-drive tachydysrhythmias. This may be accomplished in two ways. First, the patients with a brady-tachy syndrome may have premature beats and breakthrough tachycardias simply because the sinus rate is so slow. The tachycardia can't break out when the patient's underlying rate is accelerated, so a pacemaker is inserted to keep the ventricular rate up. Second, a patient with a tachycardia that has not responded to drugs or countershock sometimes can be converted by a special pacer which starts capturing at a rate faster than the tachycardia. One hopes that pacer capture will terminate the tachycardia at which time the pacemaker rate is turned down until the SA node regains control.

Some specific dysrhythmias that may require pacemaker therapy include sinus bradycardia; second-degree, type II, high-grade, or third-degree AV blocks; sick sinus syndrome; and bi- and trifasicular blocks. These rhythms may be caused by acute processes such as MI or cardiac trauma, but they also may be produced by long-term coronary insufficiency with chronic ischemia and the resulting fibrosis. Congenital anomalies such as ventricular septal defects may cause a permanent complete heart block.

Pacing after acute MI may be temporary in nature because the dysrhythmia probably will subside as the acute process heals. However, at times, the dysrhythmia becomes a chronic rhythm and the temporary pacer then must be replaced by a permanent one.

PACING EQUIPMENT

A temporary transvenous pacemaker consists of two parts—the pulse generator and a bipolar electrode pacing catheter.

The Pacing Catheter

The pacing catheter, made of radio-opaque material, is inserted into a vein and passed through the venous system to the right side of the heart, where it is wedged either in the right atrium or behind the trabeculae at the apex of the right ventricle. The internal end of the pacing catheter has two electrodes: the tip or distal electrode, and the ring or proximal electrode. The tip electrode is the negative pole of the circuit that delivers the electrical stimulus to the myocardium. The ring electrode is the positive pole of the circuit. The electrical activity of the myocardium is sensed between the positive and negative electrodes. The external end of the catheter has two terminals that attach to the pulse generator. The proximal electrode terminal should connect to the positive pole on the pulse generator, the distal electrode to the negative (Fig. 8-3).

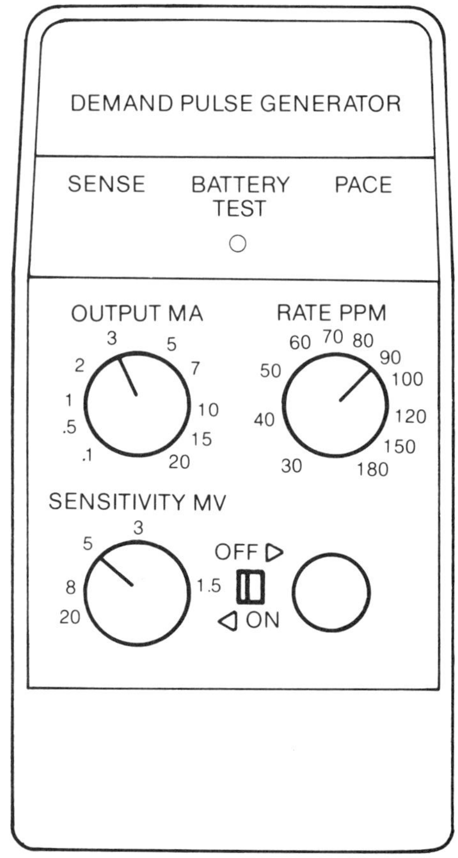

Figure 8-3 Pulse generator.

There are many pacing catheters available from different manufacturers, but there are three general types. The first is made of a semirigid material that is easily inserted and directed. It can be advanced by pushing, and directed by rotating the hub of the catheter. The second is called a semi-floating catheter which is made of a lighter, more flexible material. It can be pushed to advance it, and the lightweight construction lets it float with the returning blood flow to the right side of the heart. The third is a floating catheter that has a balloon at the tip between the two electrodes. It is extremely lightweight. After insertion into a large vein the balloon is inflated, which then pulls the catheter to the right heart with the venous return, not unlike a Swan-Ganz catheter. There is one other pacing device that is used only in extreme emergency situations. This is a transthoracic pacing stylet that is placed in the right ventricle through an intracardiac needle.

The Pulse Generator

The pulse generator is a battery-powered device that controls and generates pacing activity. There are several different brands of temporary transvenous pulse generators available. They differ in design, but all have similar controls.

The on-off switch usually is a sliding button that is easily moved to the on position. This switch has a built-in safety device to prevent the possibility of inadvertently turning the pacemaker off.

The rate control dial sets the lower rate limit for the pacemaker. If, for example, you set the rate dial at 75 beats per minute, the pacemaker's firing will be inhibited as long as the patient's own rate stays above 75. However, if the patient's own rate drops below 75 beats per minute, the pacemaker will begin to fire, and it will fire at a rate of 75.

The output dial controls the amount of electrical activity delivered to the myocardium with each pacing stimulus. The energy is measured in milliamperes (mA). The setting on the output dial must be above the patient's electrical threshold level for the pacing stimulus to cause depolarization of the myocardium. The threshold level measurement is part of the insertion procedure. After the threshold level is determined, the output dial usually is set at two to three times the threshold measurement. The higher setting compensates for any change in the patient's threshold level during the period of pacemaker therapy.

The sensitivity dial controls the demand mechanism that allows the pulse generator to sense the patient's own electrical activity. If the sensitivity control is in the off position, it turns the pulse generator into a set-rate pacemaker with no sensing capability, which fires regularly with no regard for the patient's own underlying rhythm. The sensitivity dial should be kept in the full demand position. As you turn the sensitivity down, a larger amount of the patient's own electrical activity is required in order to be seen by the pacemaker. This control is analogous to the gain control on a cardiac monitor. If the gain is turned down, the QRS complexes on the oscilloscope become too small to be sensed by the rate meter and the alarm system.

Most pulse generators have indicator dials or lights that tell you whether the QRS complex is being initiated by the pacemaker or the patient. There is usually a battery test indicator that tells if the battery is functional. Battery life is usually about a month, but this depends entirely on the amount of firing that is occurring. The sensing function takes less energy than firing, so if the patient's own ventricular rate is such that the pulse generator is only firing occasionally, the battery will last longer.

PACEMAKER INSERTION PROCEDURE

The insertion of a temporary transvenous pacemaker is a sterile procedure performed by the physician. The method of insertion and the site used is determined by the individual physician's preference. Two methods are commonly used for insertion: the percutaneous puncture or the cut-down approach.

In the percutaneous puncture approach, a special needle with an external dilator sheath and an internal stylet is inserted into a vein. The vein is dilated, and the pacing catheter is introduced. With the cut-down approach, a venesection is performed, and the pacing catheter is inserted directly into the small incision in the vein.

The sites for pacemaker insertion also are determined by the individual physician's preference. Veins generally used are the femoral,

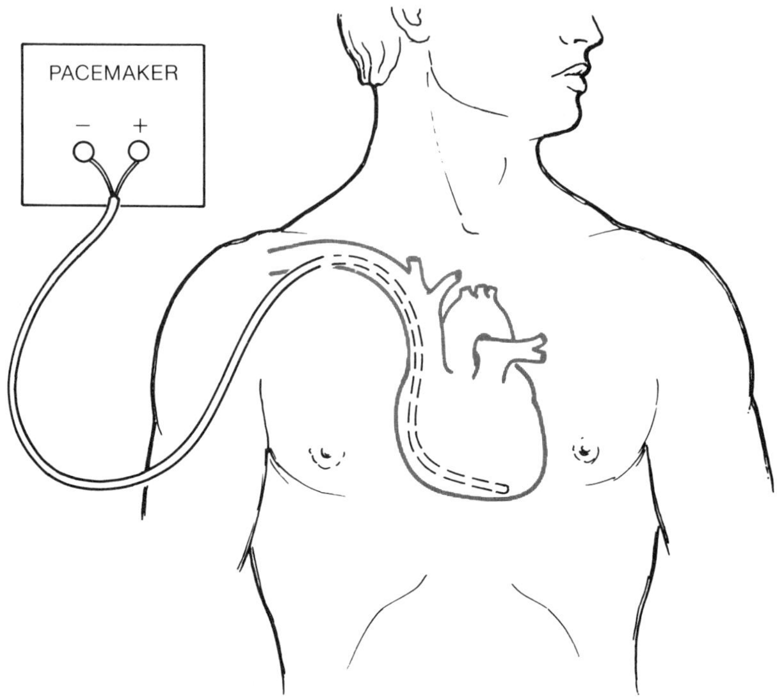

Figure 8-4 Placement of catheter for cardiac pacing.

subclavian, medial cephalic, basilic, or jugular. If the femoral or subclavian vein is selected, the percutaneous approach is used. If a smaller vein is selected, a cut-down is usually performed (Fig. 8-4).

After the site is selected, the skin must be meticulously cleansed with a povidone-iodine preparation. If the insertion site has a significant hair growth, it should be carefully shaved. The skin is then anesthesized, and the vein is cannulated, either by puncture or cut-down. The pacing catheter is inserted and advanced to the right heart. The catheter usually is advanced visually, using fluoroscopy, but if necessary, an ECG trace can be employed, using the tip of the pacing catheter as the exploring electrode. As the catheter advances through the venous system and into the heart, typical wave configurations are reflected on the ECG that locate the position of the catheter tip. The catheter tip is wedged in the right heart, and the proximal and distal lead connectors are attached to the pulse generator. The pulse generator is turned on and the rate is set at the level determined by the physician. The threshold level of the patient's myocardium is determined by turning the output control to its lowest setting, and then slowly increasing the milliamperes until capture is confirmed on the ECG monitor. The lowest level at which capture occurs is the threshold level. The output control is usually set at two to three times the threshold level. The sensing function is tested. Then the catheter is sutured to the skin, and an antibacterial ointment is applied to the insertion site. A sterile dressing is put in place with caution taken not to put too much pressure on the site that could occlude venous return.

Nursing responsibilities after insertion of a pacemaker include daily dressing changes, with careful inspection of the site for signs of infection or inflammation of the vein. Another nursing responsibility is the frequent observation of the ECG monitor to determine if the pacemaker is continuing to function normally. Patient instruction, both before and after insertion, is also an important nursing function.

Electrical Safety

Anytime a patient has a line into the circulatory system, such as an IV, Swan-Ganz, or arterial lines, they are much more susceptible to electrical accidents. Extremely small currents caused by something as simple as static electricity building up in the nurse's uniform could put the patient in ventricular fibrillation if the current is discharged at the vulnerable period in the cardiac cycle. A patient with a pacing catheter in place is at the very greatest risk, since he or she has a low-resistance pathway for current to flow directly to the ventricular myocardium. A nurse caring for a patient with a temporary transvenous pacemaker in place must be very careful to protect the patient from an electrical accident.

A little common sense tells you that you shouldn't touch the exposed ends of the catheter terminals without wearing rubber gloves. These terminals should always be protected with finger cots or some other insulator if they are not attached to the pulse generator. The newer pulse generators are designed as a closed circuit where the distal and proximal terminals of the pacing wire are completely enclosed at the positive and negative connection sites. However, some of the older models had screw type connectors that left the terminal ends exposed. We hope that none of these unsafe pieces of equipment are still in use, but if they are, they should be completely enclosed in a rubber glove to prevent dangerous current flow to the patient's heart.

PACEMAKER FUNCTIONS

The usual purpose of a pacemaker is to prevent the patient's rate from dropping below a predetermined minimal point. As you are well aware, at very slow ventricular rates the cardiac output will drop, causing the blood pressure to fall, which produces a decrease in tissue perfusion. The patient will become hypotensive and exhibit signs and symptoms that show inadequate tissue perfusion of different organ systems, such as mental confusion, lethargy, loss of consciousness, decreased urinary output, and cool clammy skin. When a pacemaker is inserted, the patient's ventricular rate can never drop below the rate set on the pulse generator, preventing the hemodynamic alterations.

A pacemaker has three main functions: firing, capturing, and sensing.

Firing

Firing is the delivery of a preset amount of electrical energy to the myocardium. The number of milliamperes to be delivered is determined by the output dial, and how fast these stimuli are delivered is set on the rate dial of the pulse generator. Firing is seen on the ECG as a pacemaker spike (see ECG at top of p. 252).

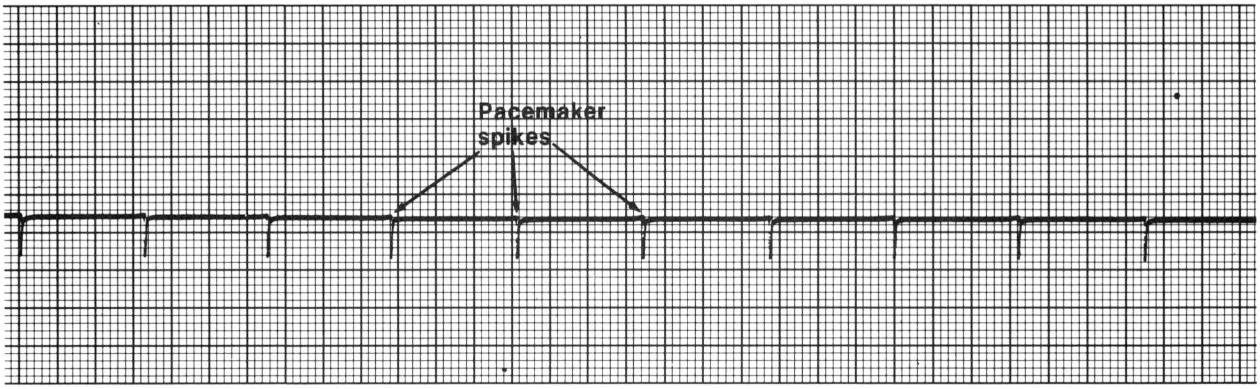

Capture

Capture occurs when the pacing stimulus is of great enough amplitude to cause depolarization of the myocardium. This simply means that the milliamperes delivered were above the patient's electrical threshold level. Ventricular capture is seen on an ECG as a wide, bizarre QRS complex that immediately follows the pacemaker spike. These QRS

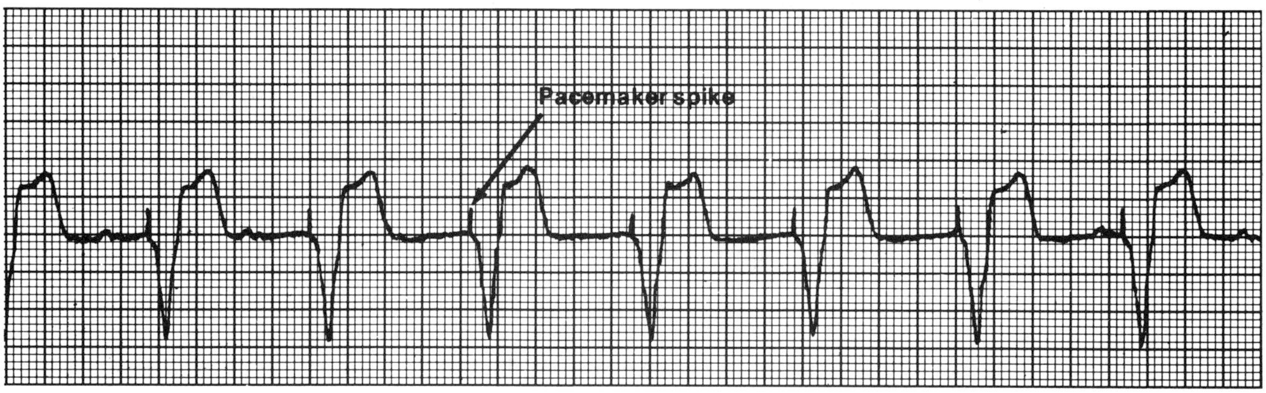

complexes will have the same footprints as any ventricular beat because they are, after all, an artificial idioventricular rhythm. Atrial capture would be seen on an ECG (below) as an abnormal P wave immediately following the pacemaker spike.

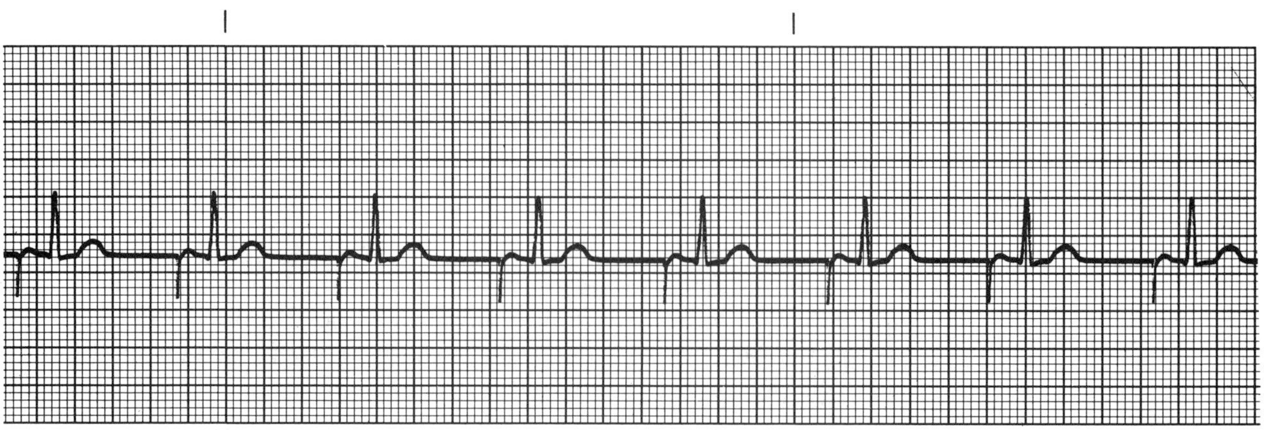

Sensing

Sensing is the capability that allows the pulse generator to "see" the patient's own complexes and to fire only on demand when the patient's natural rhythm slows or fails. As long as the patient's own rate stays above the rate set on the pulse generator, the firing mechanism is turned off. If however, the rate drops below that set on the pacemaker, the pulse generator turns on the firing mechanism and begins to pace at the preset rate (below).

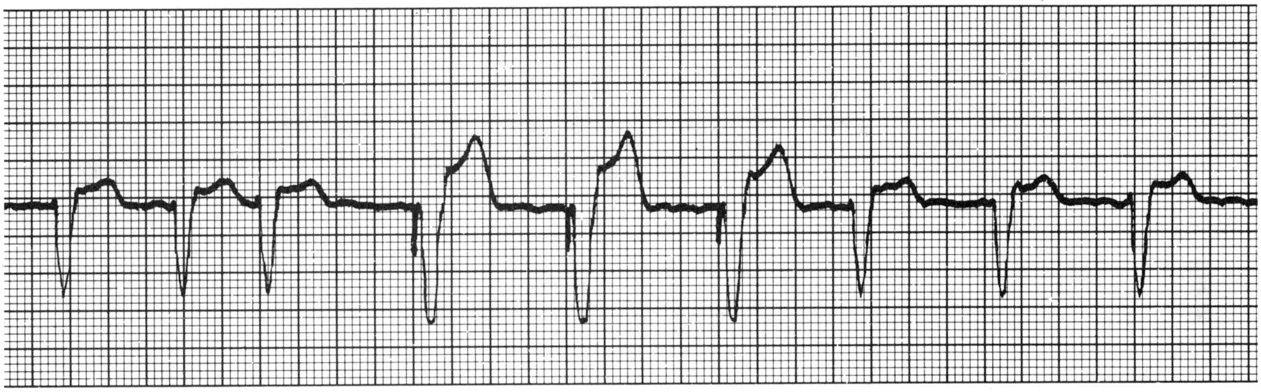

Automatic and Escape Intervals

There are two intervals programmed into the pulse generator that affect the pacing function: the automatic interval and the escape interval. The automatic interval is the amount of time, in milliseconds, occurring between paced beats when the pulse generator is firing continuously.

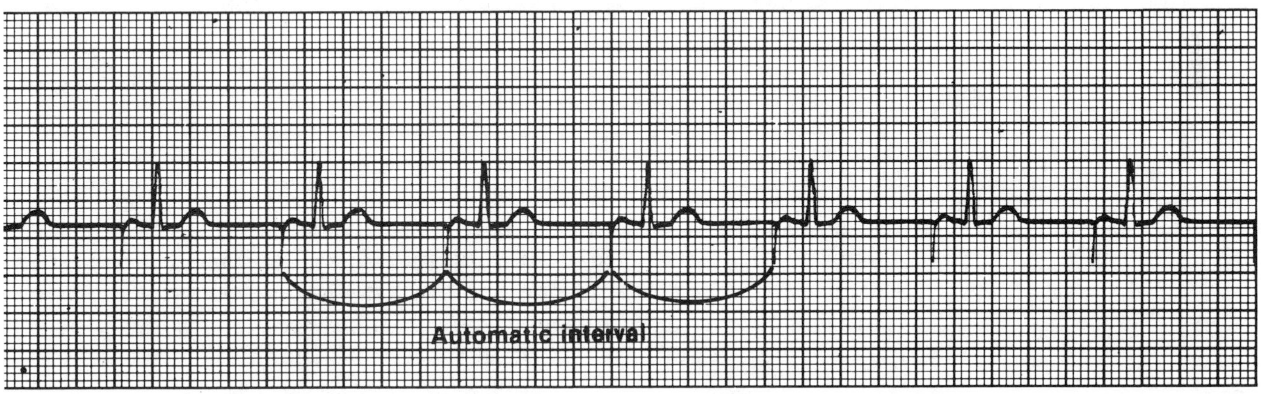

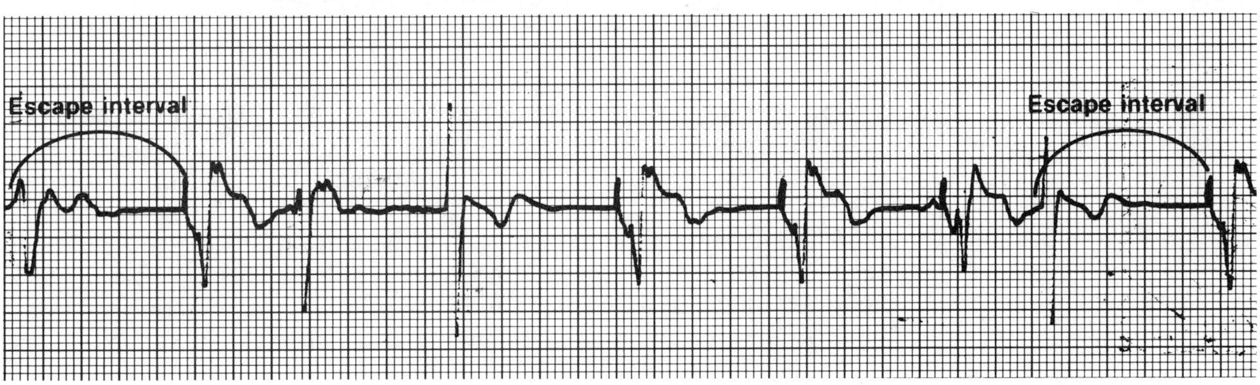

The escape interval is the amount of time the pacemaker waits, after the patient's own beat, before firing.

In most temporary, external pulse generators both the escape interval and the automatic interval are programmed by setting the rate dial, and they are the same in duration. However, in some permanent pacemakers the escape interval is longer in duration than the automatic

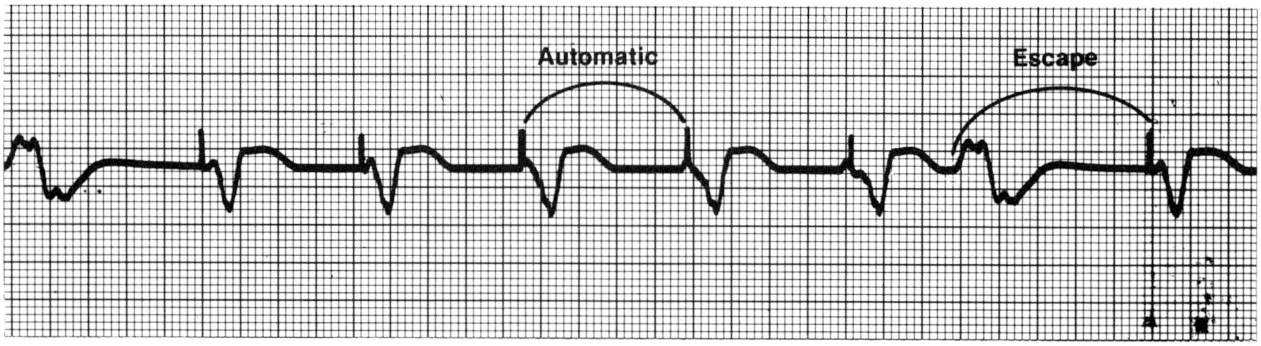

interval. This is known as pacemaker hysteresis. Hysteresis is advantageous because it allows the patient more time to get in another beat of his own before the pacemaker has to fire again. This can be beneficial for the patient in two ways. First, the patient's own beats may have a P wave in front of the QRS complex that will provide atrial kick, a situation that is usually better hemodynamically. Ventricular paced beats may not have atrial kick, and in patients with limited cardiac reserve, the loss of atrial kick can result in congestive heart failure. Second, the more patient beats that occur, the less the pacemaker has to fire, thus prolonging battery life.

PACING MODALITIES

There are many different pacing modalities available, and each pacemaker, particularly permanent implanted ones, has varied capabilities. A three-letter pacemaker code has been devised to identify the capabilities of each type of pulse generator. This three-letter code identifies the chamber sensed, the chamber paced, and the mode of pacing.

Chamber Paced	*Chamber Sensed*	*Mode of Pacing*
A—Atrium	A—Atrium	I—Inhibit
V—Ventricle	V—Ventricle	T—Triggered
D—Atrium and ventricle	D—Atrium and ventricle	D—Inhibit and triggered
O—Not applicable	O—Not applicable	O—Not applicable

The letter in the first position of the code indicates the chamber paced. The letter in the second position indicates the chamber sensed. The letter in the third position indicates the pacing mode of response. The term "inhibited" means the pacemaker's firing is turned off by the patient's own beats. "Triggered" means the patient's beat causes the pacemaker to fire during the absolute refractory period on the downstroke of the R wave.

Thus, a ventricular demand pacemaker that fires and senses in the ventricle and has its firing inhibited by the patient's own beats would be coded VVI. An atrial demand pacemaker that works the same as a ventricular demand pacemaker would be coded AAI. AV sequential pacemakers that pace in both the atrium and ventricle, but sense only in the ventricle, are coded DVI.

Obviously, there are many different pacing modalities, but since we are limiting this discussion to temporary transvenous pacing, we will cover only those modes commonly used. These are VVI, AAI, and DVI.

Ventricular Demand

Ventricular demand, or VVI, pacing is the most commonly used, temporary pacing modality. The bipolar electrode catheter is located at the apex of the right ventricle, wedged behind the trabeculae to hold it in place. It senses the patient's own QRS complexes and is inhibited from firing by them. When the patient's QRS complexes slow down or stop, the pacemaker fires on demand and causes the ventricles to depolarize.

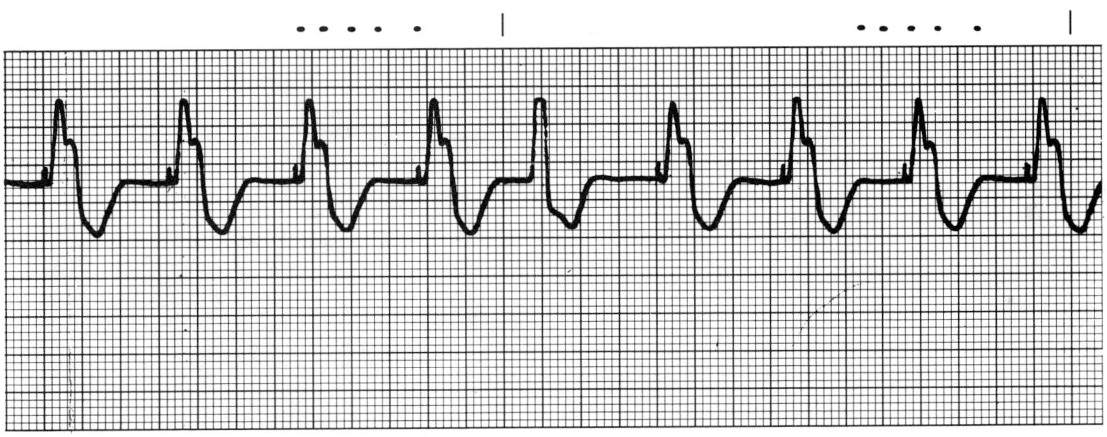

Atrial Demand

Atrial demand, or AAI, pacing is just like VVI pacing, but the pacing catheter is anchored in the right atrium. Because the catheter is in the atrium, it does not sense QRS complexes, it senses P waves. The patient's own atrial activity inhibits pacer fire, and when the patient's P waves slow or stop, the pacemaker will fire and depolarize the atria. On the ECG, you will see a pacemaker spike immediately followed by a funny looking P wave (see ECG for atrial capture, p. 252). The PR interval and QRS complex following the paced P wave should be normal, since this pacing modality cannot be used if the patient has AV block or bundle branch block. The conduction system from the AV node on down must be intact. Atrial pacing is reserved for patients with sick sinus syndrome or sinus bradycardia that has not responded to conventional drug therapy. AAI pacing is better hemodynamically than VVI because there is atrial kick with each paced beat.

AV Sequential Pacing

AV sequential, or DVI, pacing differs from VVI or AAI in that there are two pacing catheters in the heart. One is anchored in the right atrial appendage and the other is at the right ventricular apex. DVI pacemakers pace both the atrium and ventricle, but can sense only in the ventricle. DVI pacing is most beneficial in patients who need AV synchrony. In some patients, the loss of atrial kick seen in VVI pacing decreases contractility of the ventricles enough to put the patient into congestive heart failure. Other patients need AV synchrony to prevent the start of reentry tachycardias.

There are two intervals that have to be programmed into the pulse generator for AV sequential pacing, the VV interval and the AV interval. A third interval, the VA interval, is determined by the other two settings.

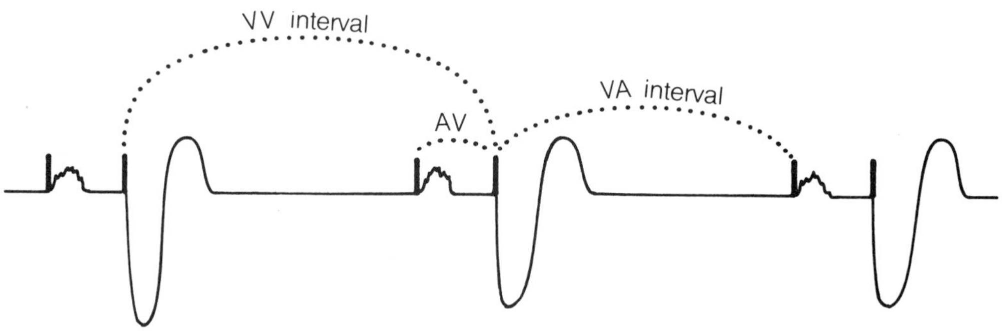

The VV interval is the ventricular demand rate. The pulse generator will pace the atrium and the ventricle if no patient QRS complexes occur. The AV interval is the same as the PR interval of a normal beat, and is the factor that provides AV synchrony. The VA interval is the escape interval. If no ventricular event occurs before the end of the VA interval, the pulse generator will deliver an atrial stimulus. If a patient QRS complex does occur before the end of the VA interval, the pulse generator is inhibited from firing, and the pacing cycle is reset.

You can see how this can get very confusing, and you almost have to know what the interval settings are in order to determine pacemaker function or malfunction. In general, the following is a description of the different ways an AV sequential pacemaker functions.

If the patient's ventricular rate is slower than the programmed rate, then the AV sequential pacemaker will pace both atria and ventricles.

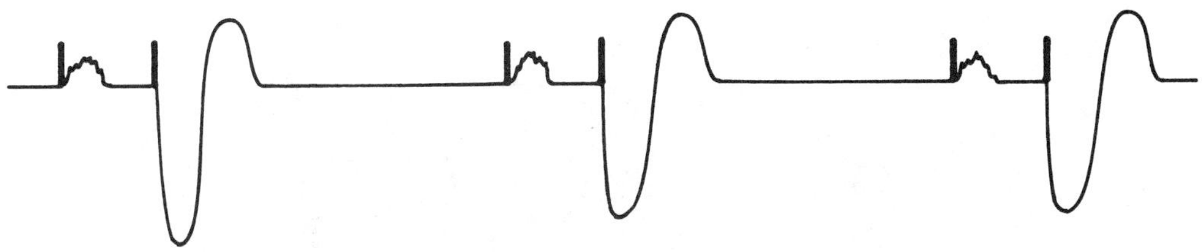

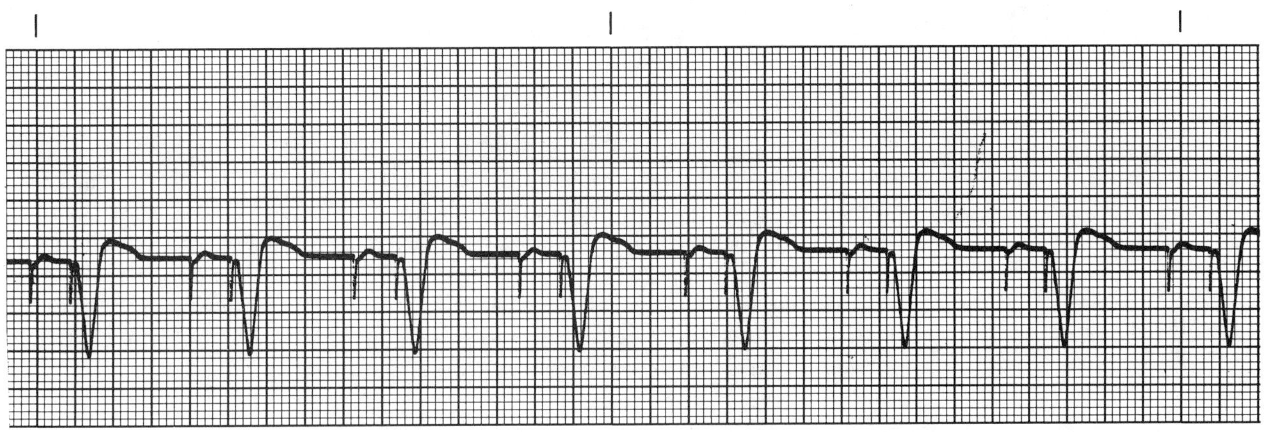

Because there is sensing in the ventricle, if the atrial pacing stimulus is conducted normally to the ventricle before the end of the AV interval, then the ventricular pacing activity is inhibited.

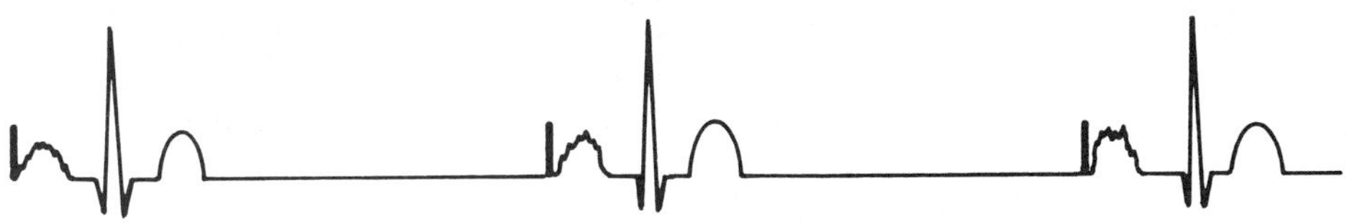

If a patient's own ventricular activity occurs before the end of the VA interval, then both the atrial and ventricular pacing activities are inhibited. This could occur if the patient's own rate is greater than the VV interval rate, in which case you would see only the patient's own rhythm.

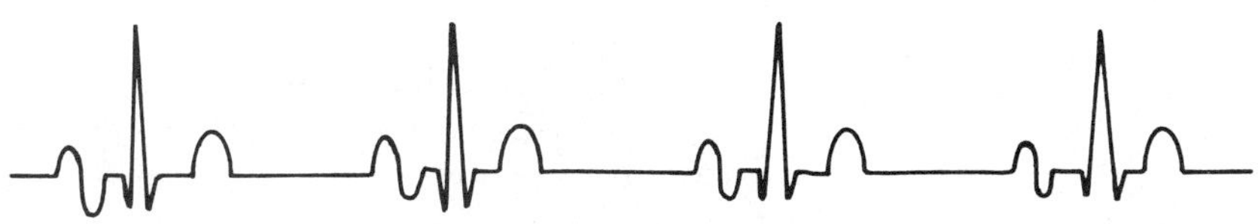

If the patient has an early beat such as a PVC, or a normal beat that occurs within the VA interval, then both atrial and ventricular pacing are inhibited, and the timing of the pulse generator is reset.

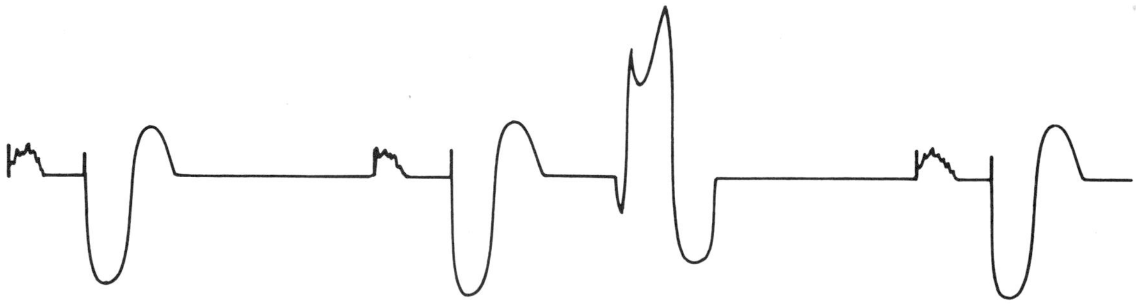

There is one possible problem with AV sequential pacing, which occurs because there isn't any sensing mechanism in the atria. The atrial pacing spike can compete with the SA node. The atrial spike also can fall on the peak of the T_p wave (the atrial T wave) and cause atrial fibrillation. This usually can be avoided by carefully setting the AV and VV intervals. A universal or DDD pacemaker that paces and senses in both atria and ventricles will soon be available. DDD pacing is still in clinical trials, but it nevertheless looks promising.

PACEMAKER COMPLICATIONS

Infection

Infection at the insertion side is one complication with the use of a pacemaker. If meticulous sterile technique is used during insertion, and if the continuing care of the insertion site on a daily basis includes sterile dressing changes, application of an appropriate ointment, and careful inspection by the nurse, the incidence of infection should be minimized. Generally, infection does not directly influence the function of the pacemaker. The longer the pacer wire is in place, the greater is the incidence of infection.

Displacement

The most common complication of pacemaker insertion is displacement of the tip of the pacing catheter. The tip may be free-floating in the right ventricle, or it may have moved into the pulmonary artery or the right atrium.

Another less common event is perforation of the ventricular wall by the tip of the catheter. This may cause pericardial tamponade, or the pacemaker could start capturing the diaphragm, in which case, the patient would have hiccups at what ever rate the pacemaker was set.

Displacement can very well interfere with pacer function, and cause loss of sensing or loss of capture.

PACEMAKER MALFUNCTIONS

Lastly, we will discuss the three types of pacemaker malfunction—loss of firing, loss of capture, and loss of sensing—their causes, and necessary nursing intervention.

Loss of Firing

Loss of firing occurs because of malfunction of the pulse generator or the wire connections. The pulse generator will stop firing if the battery is low, or if a mechanical malfunction in the circuitry is present. Loss of firing also can occur if a terminal becomes disconnected from the pacing catheter, or if there is a wire fracture inside the pacing catheter.

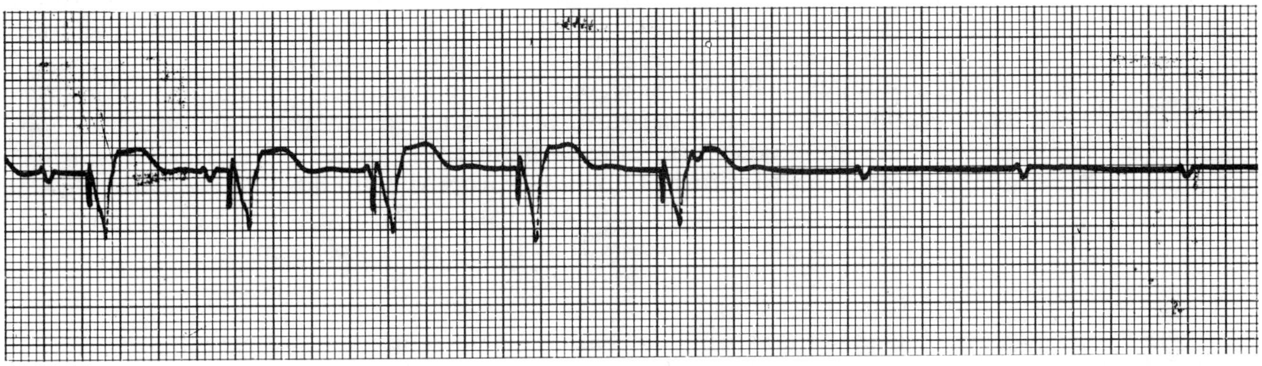

Loss of firing is detected by the disappearance of the pacing spike on the ECG monitor, despite the fact that the patient's own ventricular rate is lower than the escape rate set on the pulse generator.

Nursing intervention should include (1) Check the patient for symptoms that indicate a drop in cardiac output. (2) Check the pulse generator. Is it on? Is the battery dead? (3) Check the wire connections to be certain that they are intact. The physician should be notified immediately, and if the patient is symptomatic because of a very slow ventricular rate, supportive therapy may be needed until the pacemaker rhythm is restored.

Loss of Capture

Loss of capture is most commonly caused by displacement of the pacing catheter tip, but it also can occur because of increased ischemia that raises the electrical threshold level of the myocardium.

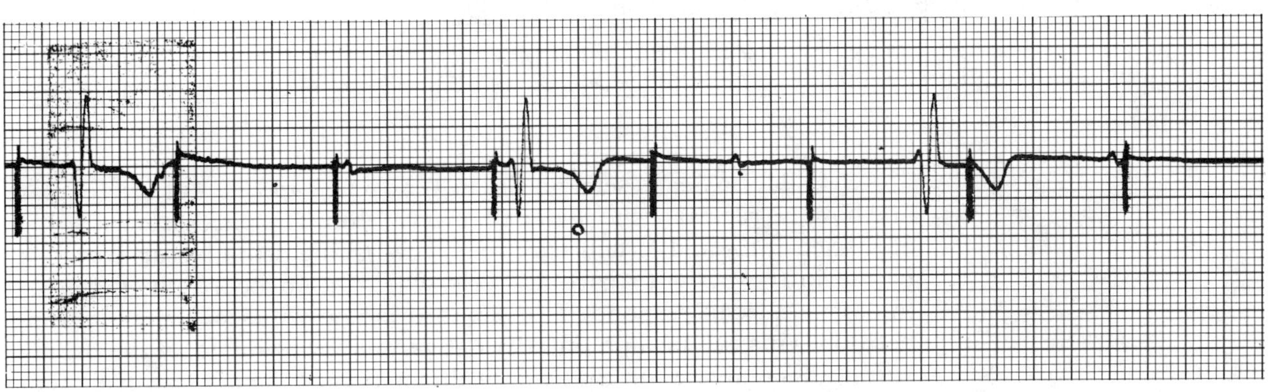

Loss of capture is determined on the ECG by the presence of pacer spikes that have no QRS complex following them. Occasionally, when the tip of the catheter is free-floating in the right ventricle, the loss of capture will be intermittent; if the catheter is against the wall of the ventricle when firing occurs, capture may follow.

Nursing Intervention. To regain capture, the pacing catheter must be repositioned by the physician, but there are some things that the nurse can do which may increase the number of capture beats until the doctor arrives. The first thing to do is to check the patient for symptoms caused by a decrease in cardiac output. The nurse can turn the patient onto his or her left side, or put the patient back into the position he or she was in when capture was last noted. This is done with the hope that gravity will pull the catheter tip against the ventricular wall and capture will return. If loss of capture is caused by an increased threshold level of the myocardium, turning up the MAs on the output control of the pulse generator will facilitate return of capture.

Loss of Sensing

Loss of the sensing mechanism may result from several different causes. If the pacer tip is displaced, sensing may or may not be lost, or it may be intermittent. Other causes of loss of sensing could be malfunction of the circuitry of the pulse generator, wire fracture, or terminal disconnection. The most common cause of loss of sensing is poor positioning of the pacing catheter. In this case, the ring electrode is situated near a portion of the ventricular myocardium that, as a result of injury, ischemia, or fibrosis, is not generating adequate electrical potentials for the pacemaker to sense.

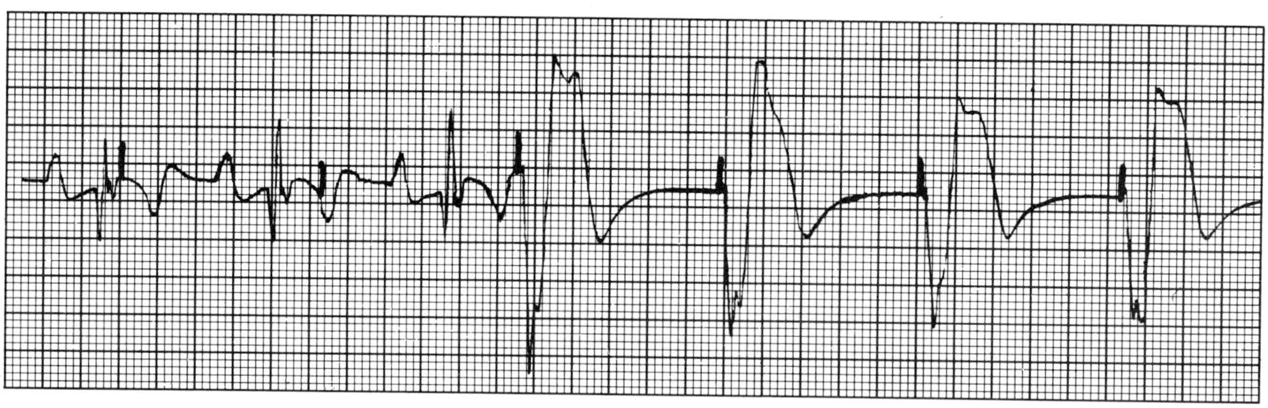

Loss of sensing is seen on the ECG as pacer spikes that are regular and have no regard of the patient's own rhythm. The pacemaker is firing at a fixed rate, and it will capture if the pacing stimulus arrives at a period in the patient's cardiac cycle when the myocardium is nonrefractory and can respond. This rhythm is known as pacemaker competition. This can be a potentially dangerous situation, for if the pacing stimulus is delivered in that vulnerable period of the cardiac cycle that corresponds with the peak of the T wave, ventricular tachycardia or ventricular fibrillation may result.

Nursing intervention in this case first involves determining the patient's underlying rate, and if the patient's rate is satisfactory, the pacemaker should be turned off and the physician notified immediately. If the patient's own rate is very slow, it may not be feasible to turn the pacemaker off. However, with a very slow underlying rate, the chance of a pacing stimulus being delivered during the vulnerable period of the cycle is much less than at a faster underlying rate.

Repositioning the pacing catheter in an area of the right ventricle that is generating greater electrical potentials will allow the pulse generator to regain the sensing mechanism. Another solution to the problem of loss of sensing is to unipolarize the pacemaker. This is accomplished by disconnecting the proximal lead connector of the pacing catheter from the positive terminal of the pulse generator, and capping the lead connector. A regular monitoring electrode is placed on the patient's chest in a position that is picking up adequate R wave potentials. The chest electrode is connected to the positive terminal of the pulse generator.

BIBLIOGRAPHY

BOOKS

American Heart Association: Textbook of Advanced Cardiac Life Support. Dallas, American Heart Association, 1983

Andreoli KG: Comprehensive Cardiac Care. St Louis, CV Mosby, 1983

Baker CE (publisher): Physicians' Desk Reference. Oradell, Medical Economics, 1983

Best CH: The Physiologic Basis of Medical Practice. Baltimore, Williams & Wilkins, 1966

Dubin D: Rapid Interpretation of EKGs. Tampa, COVER Publishing, 1982

Friedburg CK: Diseases of the Heart. Philadelphia, WB Saunders, 1969

Goldman MJ: Principles of Clinical Electrocardiography. Los Altos, Lange Medical Publishers, 1970

Mangiola S: Cardiac Arrhythmias. Philadelphia, JB Lippincott, 1974

Marriott HJL: Workshop in Electrocardiography. Oldsmar, FL, Tampa Tracings, 1972

Marriott HJL: Practical Electrocardiography. Baltimore, Waverly Press, 1977

Meltzer LE: Intensive Coronary Care, a Manual for Nurses. Bowie, MD, Robert J. Brady, 1983

Netter FH: The CIBA Collection of Medical Illustrations, volume 5, The Heart. Summit, NJ, CIBA, 1969

Phillips RN: The Cardiac Rhythms. Philadelphia, WB Saunders, 1980

Ritota MC: Diagnostic Electrocardiography. Philadelphia, JB Lippincott, 1969

ARTICLES

Arnsdorf MF: Electrophysiologic properties of antidysrhythmic drugs as a rational basis for therapy. Med Clin North Am 60:213–231, 1976

Bigger JT (ed): Symposium on flecainide acetate. Am J Cardiol 53:1B–122B, 1984

Braunwald E: Introduction to calcium channel blockers. Am J Cardiol 46:1045–1046, 1980

Gibson DG: Pharmacodynamic properties of beta adrenergic receptor blocking drugs in man. Drugs 7:8–38, 1974

Henry PD: Comparative pharmacology of calcium antagonists. Am J Cardiol 46:1047–1055, 1980

Katz AM: Ion channels in membranes. Circulation 65(Supp I): I-2–I-10, 1982

Mehta J: Mexiletine. Am J Cardiol 49:455–460, 1982

Morganroth J, Panidis I, Lee G: Flecainide vs. quinidine for treatment of chronic ventricular arrhythmias. Circulation 67(5):1117–1123, 1983

Nademanee K: Advances in antiarrhythmic therapy. JAMA 247:217–222, 1982

Sloskey G: Amiodarone: A unique antiarrhythmic agent. Clin Pharm 2:330–340, 1983

Snyder DW: Clinical uses of calcium antagonist agents. Hosp Form 18:541–548, 1983

Winkle RA: Beta blockers in the treatment of acute arrhythmias. Heart Lung 6:62–67, 1977

Zipes DP: New antiarrhythmic agents. Am J Cardiol 41:1005–1019, 1978

APPENDIX: EXERCISES ON ECG INTERPRETATION

PRACTICE STRIPS

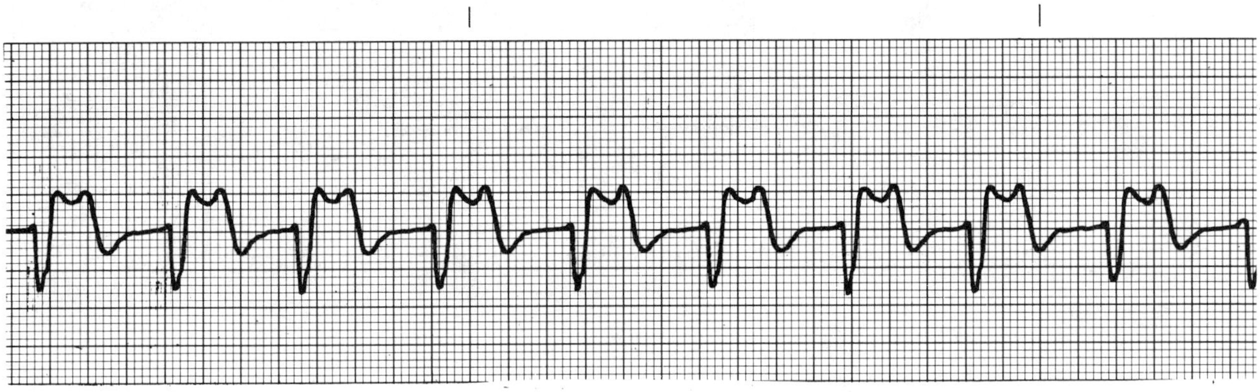

Practice strip A-1

RHYTHM:
RATE:
P WAVES:
PR INTERVAL:
QRS COMPLEX:
INTERPRETATION:
THERAPY:

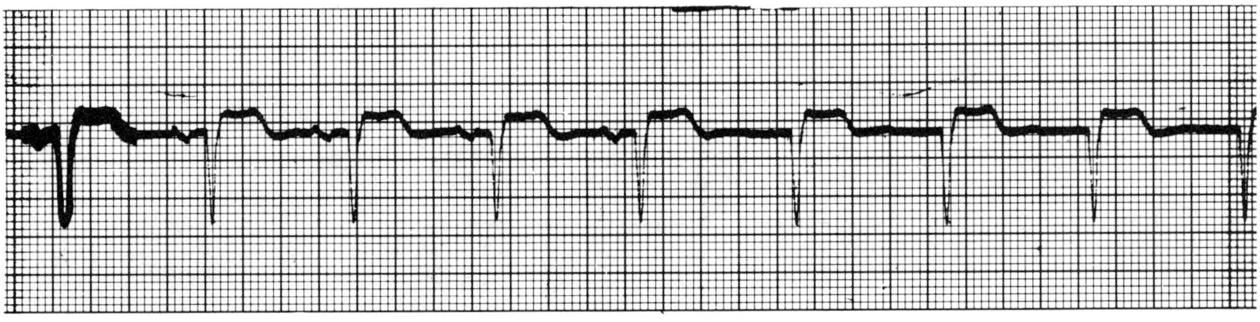

Practice strip A-2

RHYTHM:
RATE:
P WAVES:
PR INTERVAL:
QRS COMPLEX:
INTERPRETATION:
THERAPY:

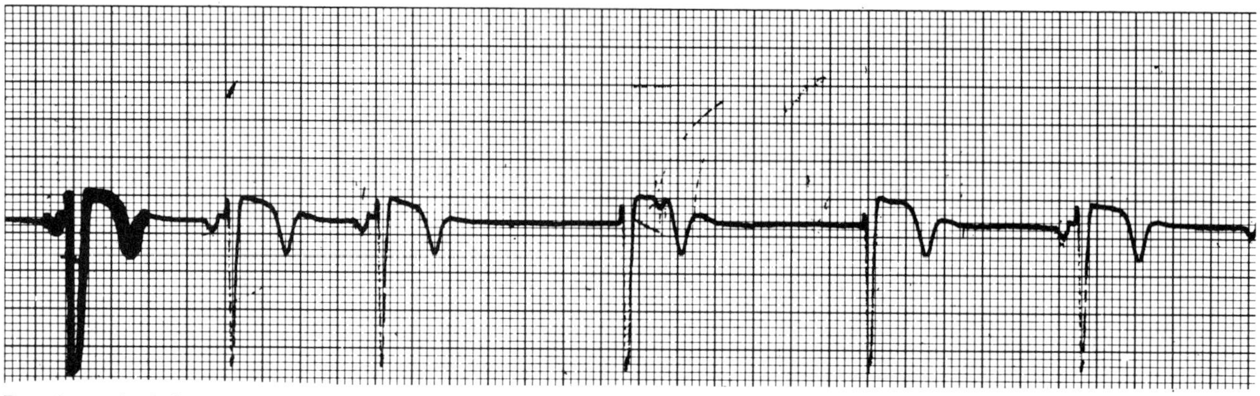

Practice strip A-3

RHYTHM:

RATE:

P WAVES:

PR INTERVAL:

QRS COMPLEX:

INTERPRETATION:

THERAPY:

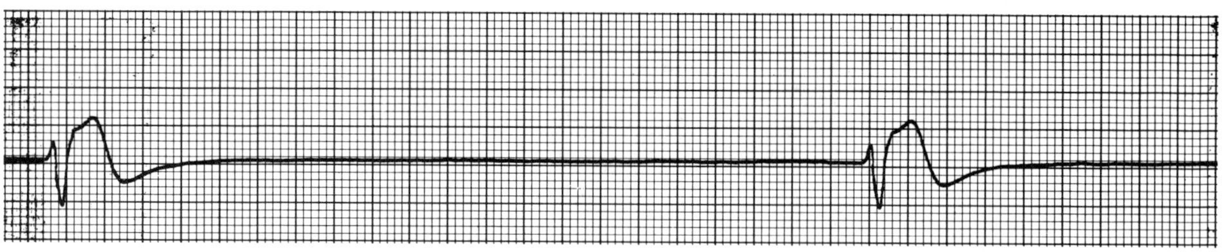

Practice strip A-4

RHYTHM:

RATE:

P WAVES:

PR INTERVAL:

QRS COMPLEX:

INTERPRETATION:

THERAPY:

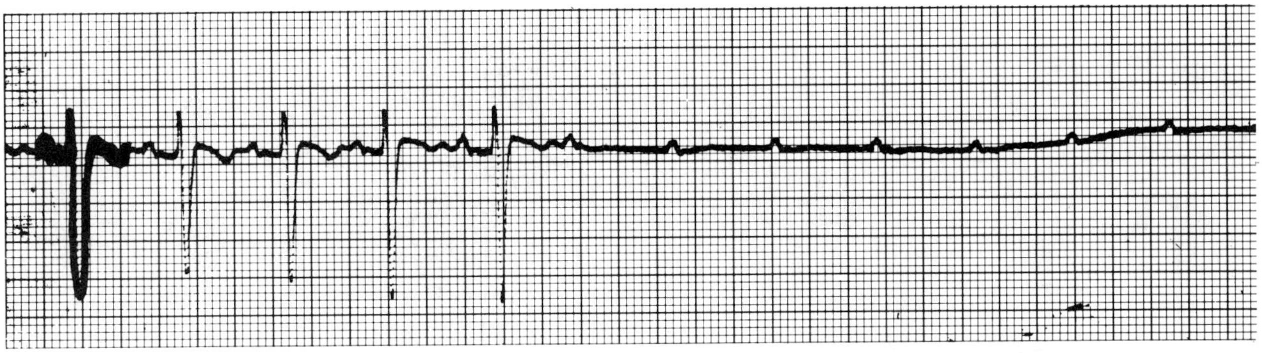

Practice strip A-5

RHYTHM:

RATE:

P WAVES:

PR INTERVAL:

QRS COMPLEX:

INTERPRETATION:

THERAPY:

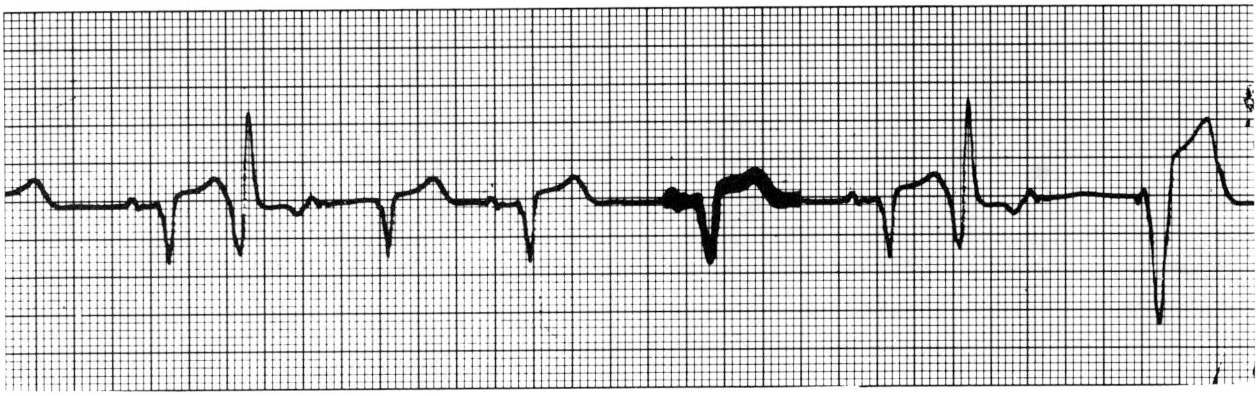

Practice strip A-6

RHYTHM:

RATE:

P WAVES:

PR INTERVAL:

QRS COMPLEX:

INTERPRETATION:

THERAPY:

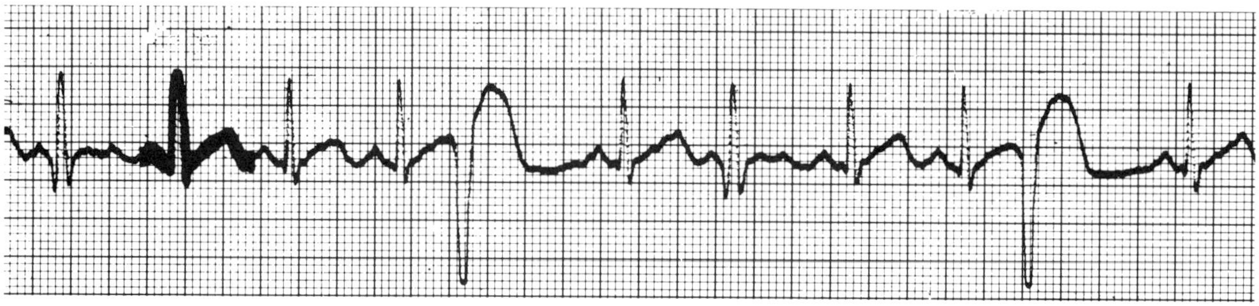

Practice strip A-7

RHYTHM:

RATE:

P WAVES:

PR INTERVAL:

QRS COMPLEX:

INTERPRETATION:

THERAPY:

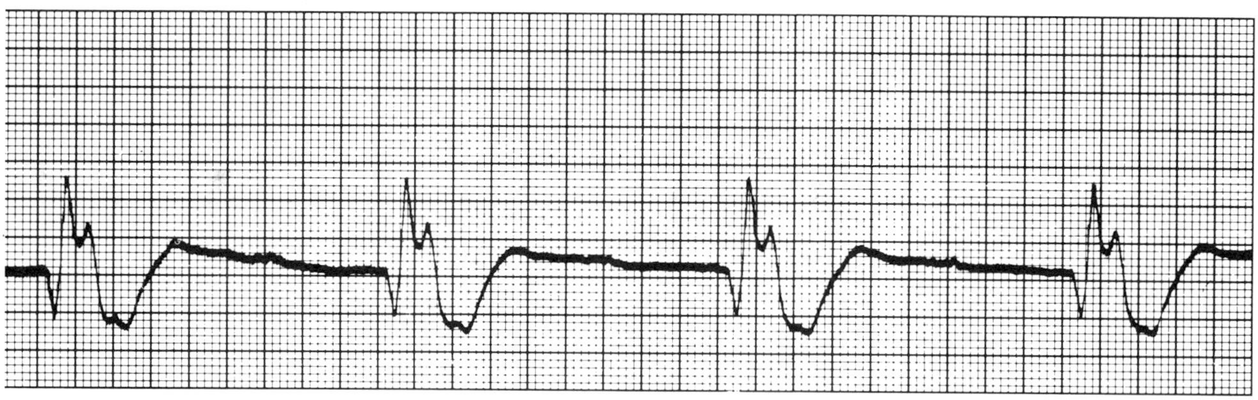

Practice strip A-8

RHYTHM:

RATE:

P WAVES:

PR INTERVAL:

QRS COMPLEX:

INTERPRETATION:

THERAPY:

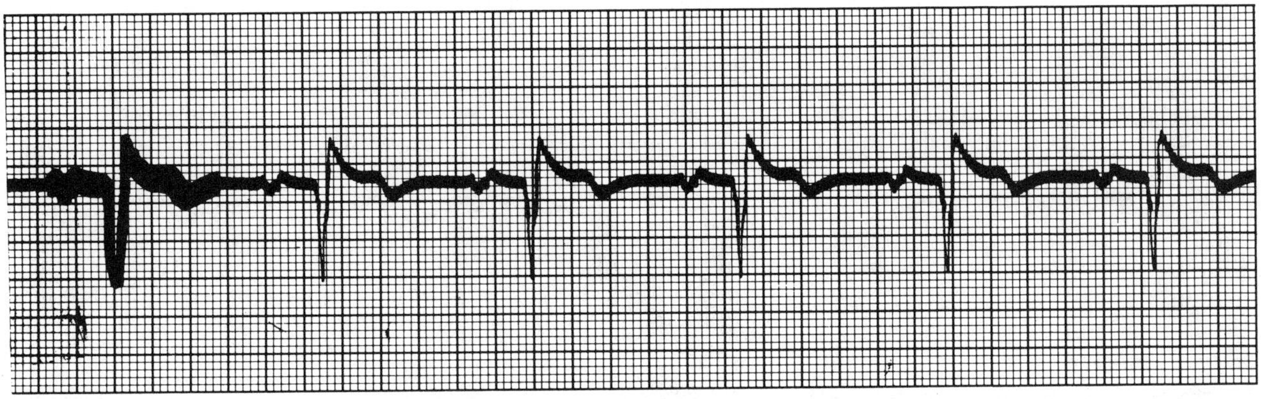

Practice strip A-9

RHYTHM:

RATE:

P WAVES:

PR INTERVAL:

QRS COMPLEX:

INTERPRETATION:

THERAPY:

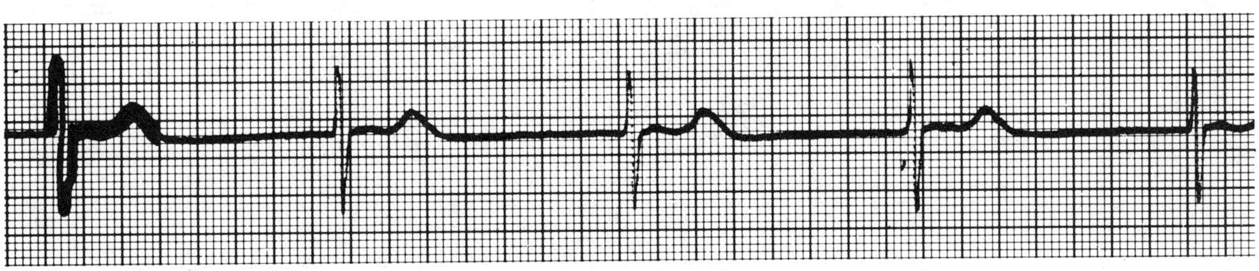

Practice strip A-10

RHYTHM:

RATE:

P WAVES:

PR INTERVAL:

QRS COMPLEX:

INTERPRETATION:

THERAPY:

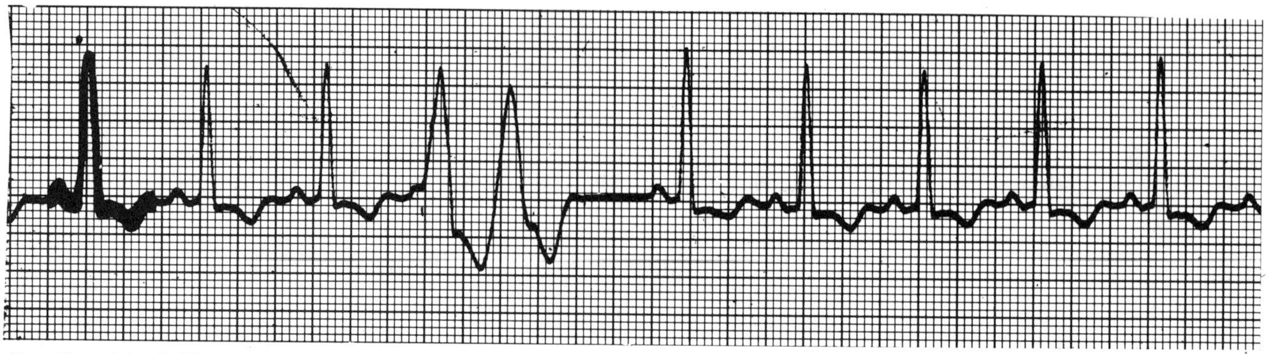

Practice strip A-11

RHYTHM:

RATE:

P WAVES:

PR INTERVAL:

QRS COMPLEX:

INTERPRETATION:

THERAPY:

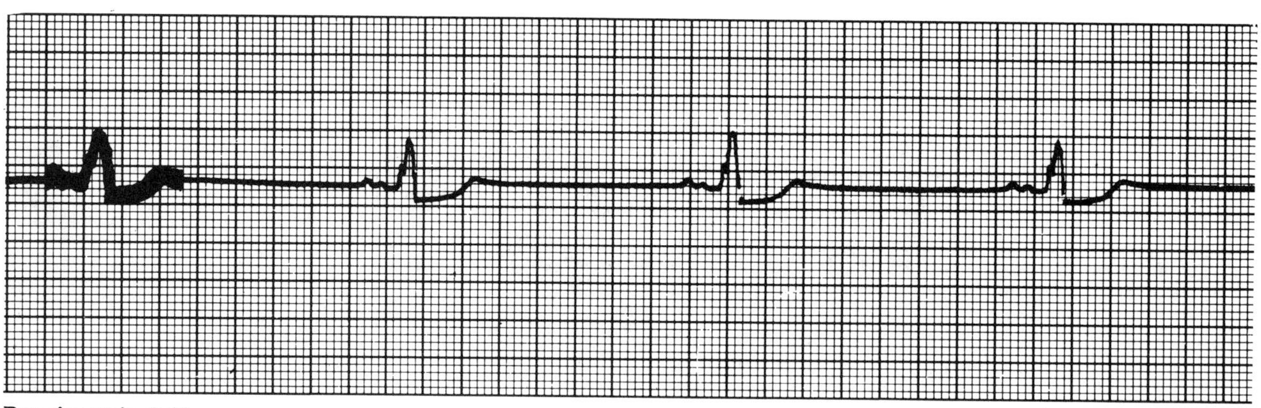

Practice strip A-12

RHYTHM:

RATE:

P WAVES:

PR INTERVAL:

QRS COMPLEX:

INTERPRETATION:

THERAPY:

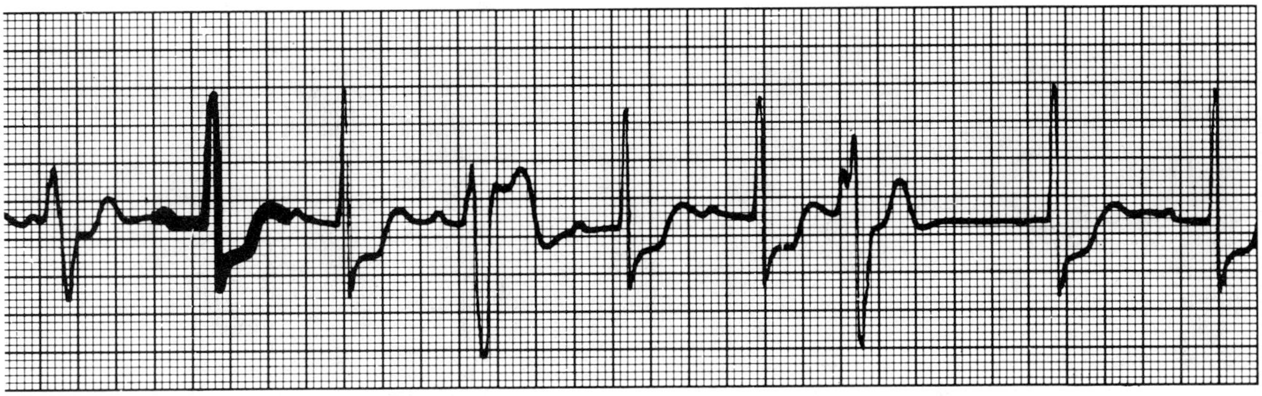

Practice strip A-13

RHYTHM:
RATE:
P WAVES:
PR INTERVAL:
QRS COMPLEX:
INTERPRETATION:
THERAPY:

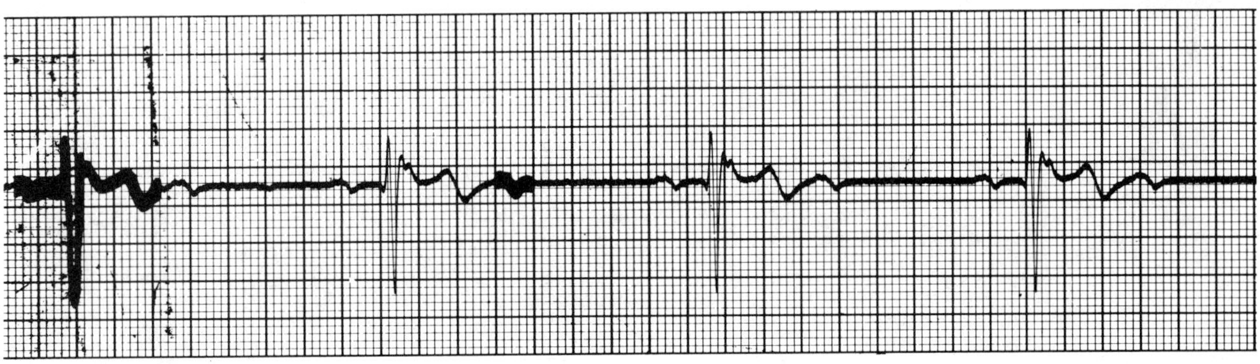

Practice strip A-14

RHYTHM:
RATE:
P WAVES:
PR INTERVAL:
QRS COMPLEX:
INTERPRETATION:
THERAPY:

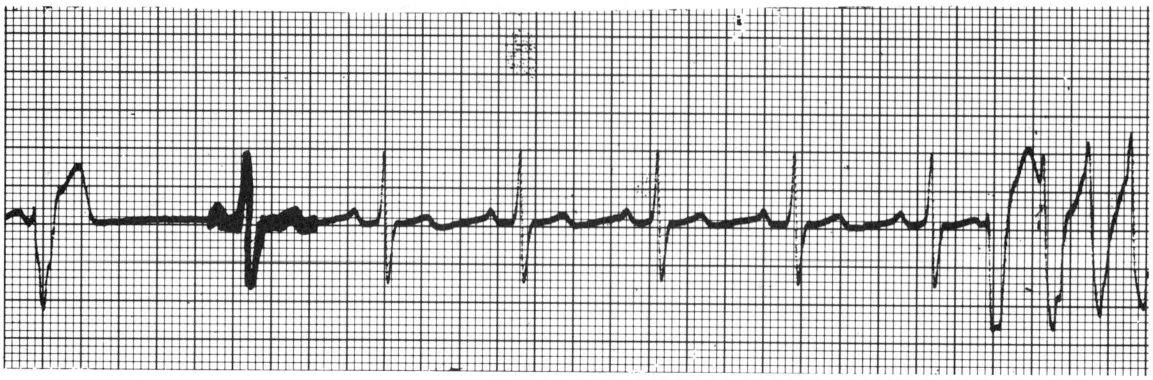

Practice strip A-15

RHYTHM:

RATE:

P WAVES:

PR INTERVAL:

QRS COMPLEX:

INTERPRETATION:

THERAPY:

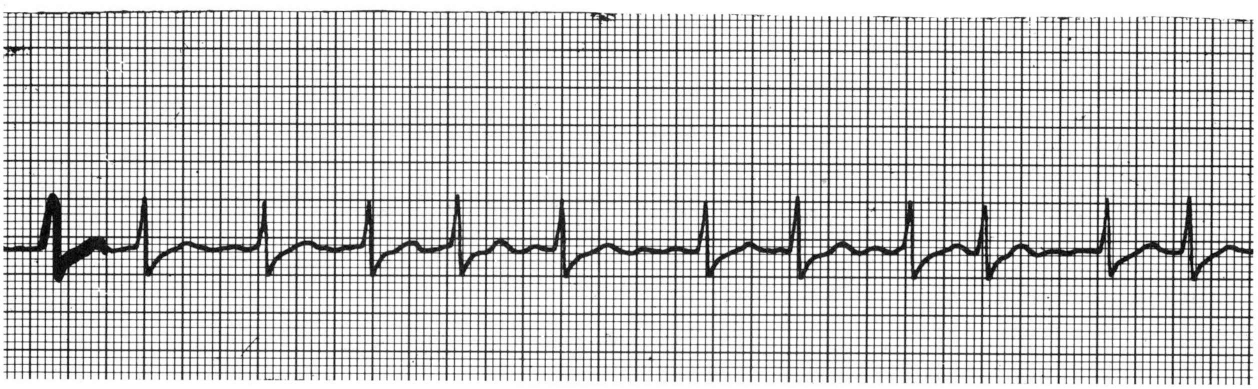

Practice strip A-16

RHYTHM:

RATE:

P WAVES:

PR INTERVAL:

QRS COMPLEX:

INTERPRETATION:

THERAPY:

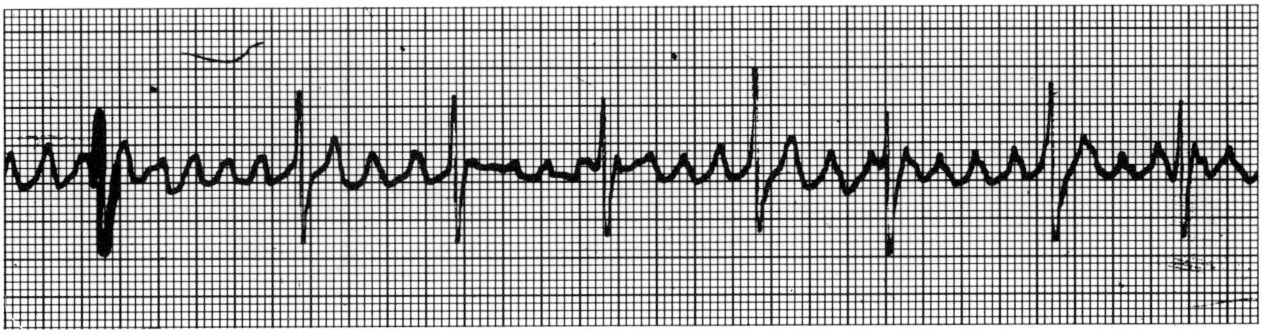

Practice strip A-17

RHYTHM:

RATE:

P WAVES:

PR INTERVAL:

QRS COMPLEX:

INTERPRETATION:

THERAPY:

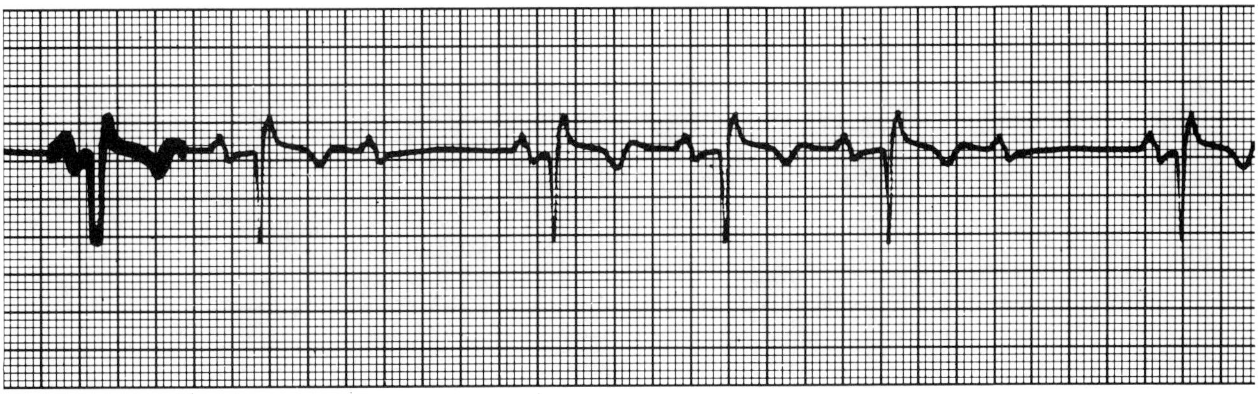

Practice strip A-18

RHYTHM:

RATE:

P WAVES:

PR INTERVAL:

QRS COMPLEX:

INTERPRETATION:

THERAPY:

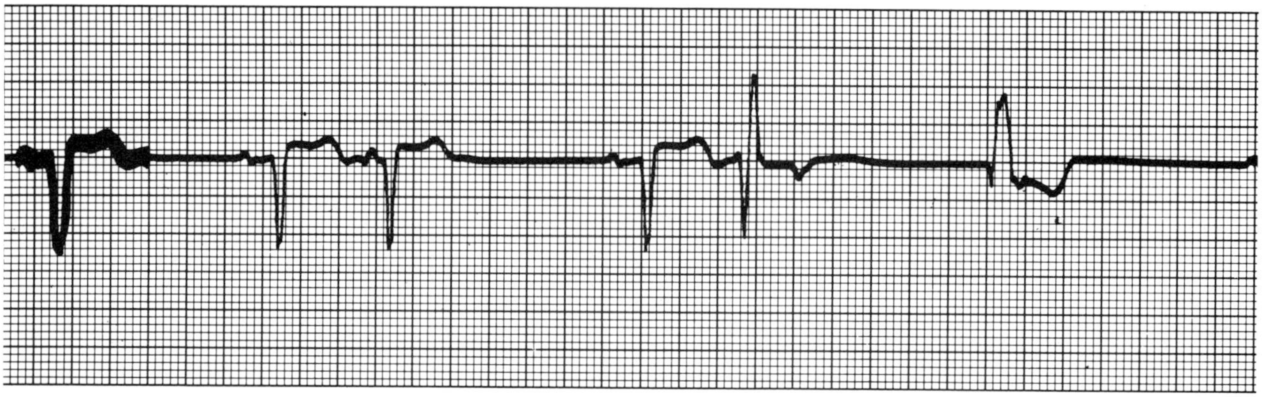

Practice strip A-19

RHYTHM:

RATE:

P WAVES:

PR INTERVAL:

QRS COMPLEX:

INTERPRETATION:

THERAPY:

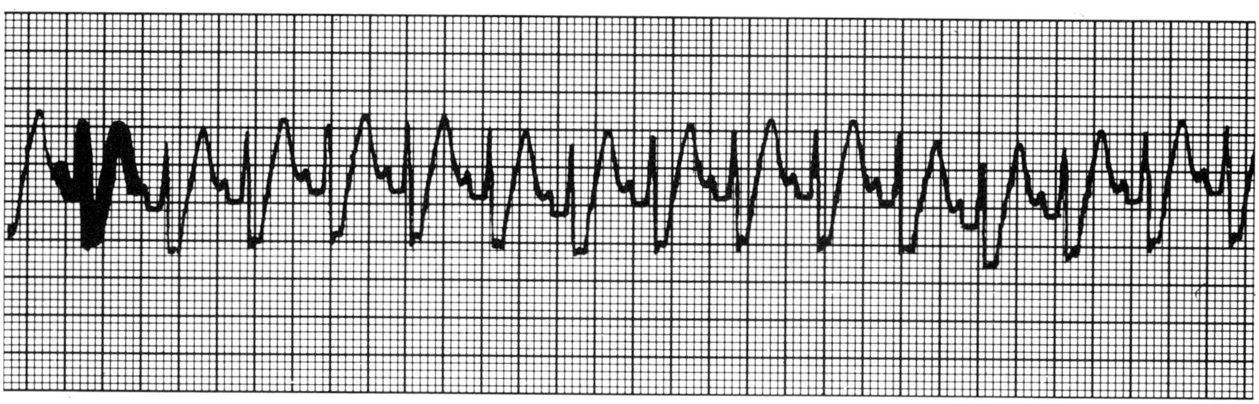

Practice strip A-20

RHYTHM:

RATE:

P WAVES:

PR INTERVAL:

QRS COMPLEX:

INTERPRETATION:

THERAPY:

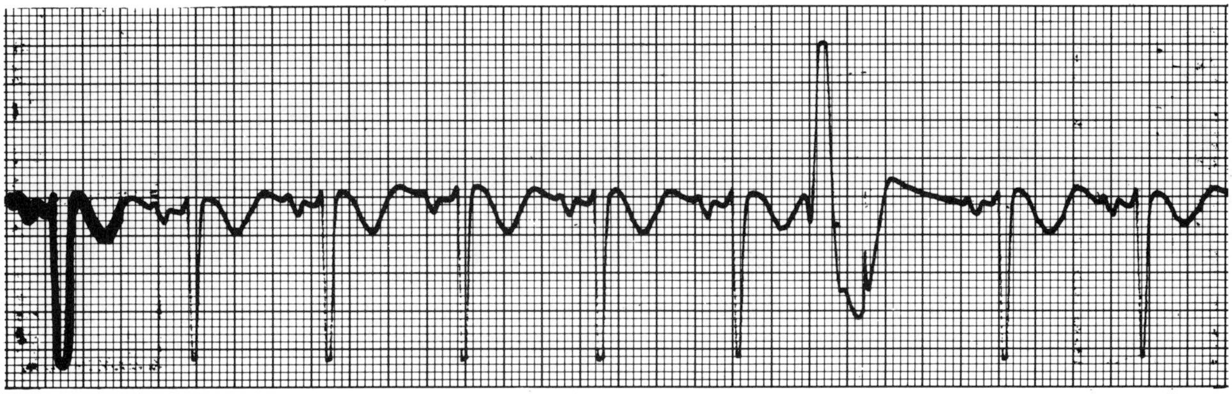

Practice strip A-21

RHYTHM:
RATE:
P WAVES:
PR INTERVAL:
QRS COMPLEX:
INTERPRETATION:
THERAPY:

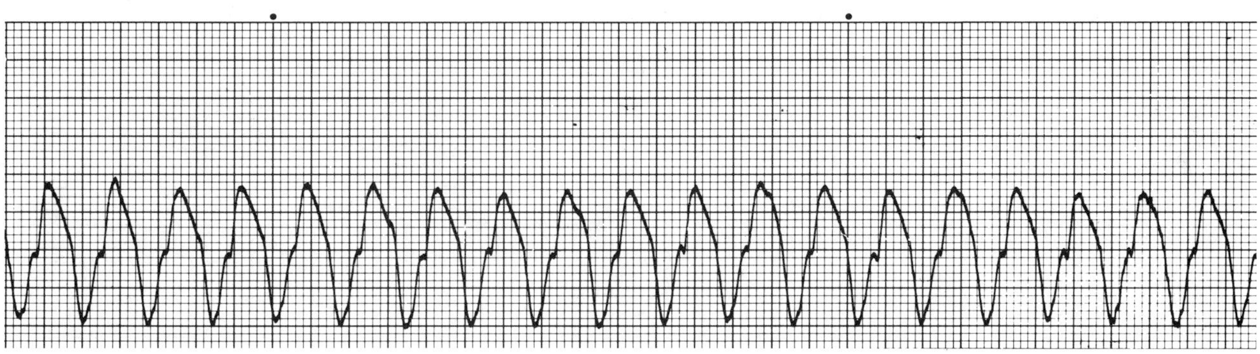

Practice strip A-22

RHYTHM:
RATE:
P WAVES:
PR INTERVAL:
QRS COMPLEX:
INTERPRETATION:
THERAPY:

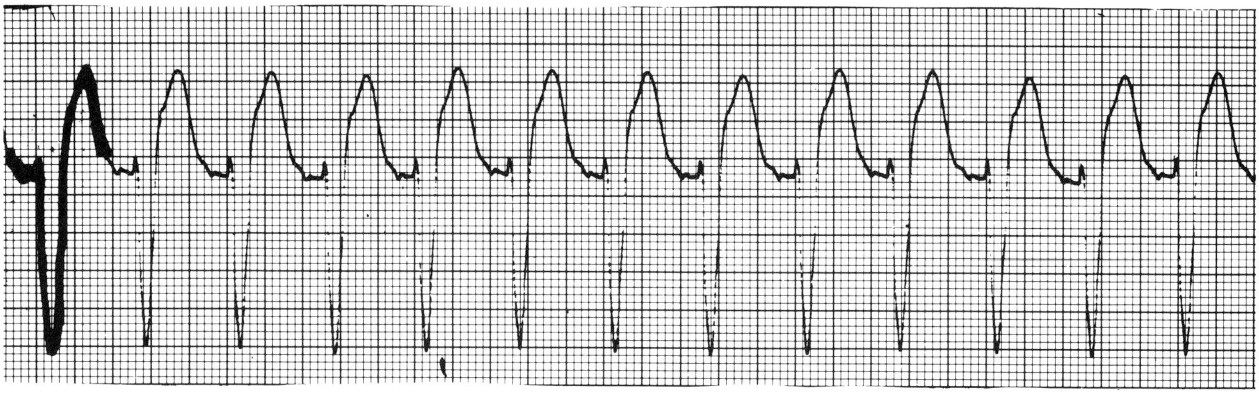

Practice strip A-23

RHYTHM:

RATE:

P WAVES:

PR INTERVAL:

QRS COMPLEX:

INTERPRETATION:

THERAPY:

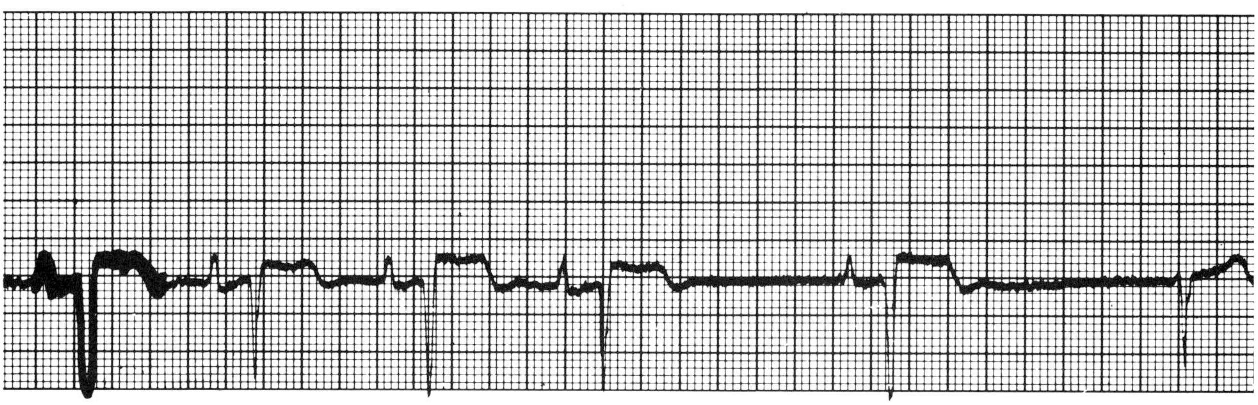

Practice strip A-24

RHYTHM:

RATE:

P WAVES:

PR INTERVAL:

QRS COMPLEX:

INTERPRETATION:

THERAPY:

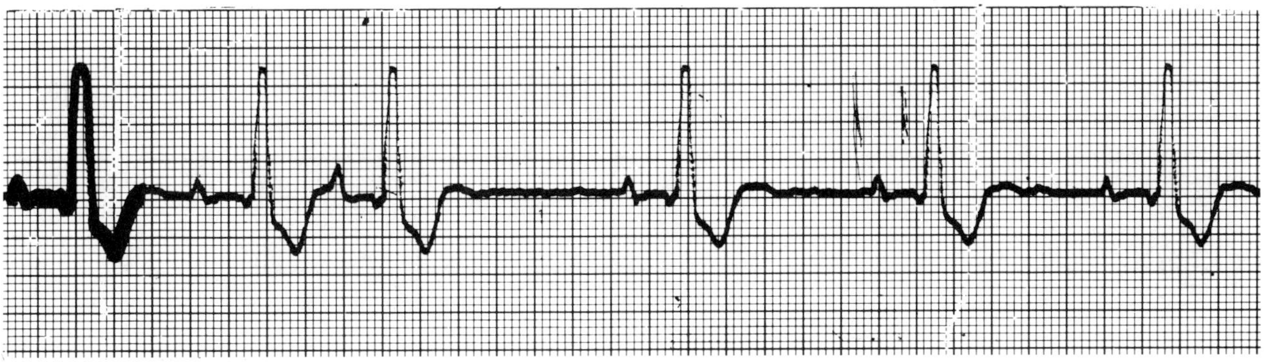

Practice strip A-25

RHYTHM:
RATE:
P WAVES:
PR INTERVAL:
QRS COMPLEX:
INTERPRETATION:
THERAPY:

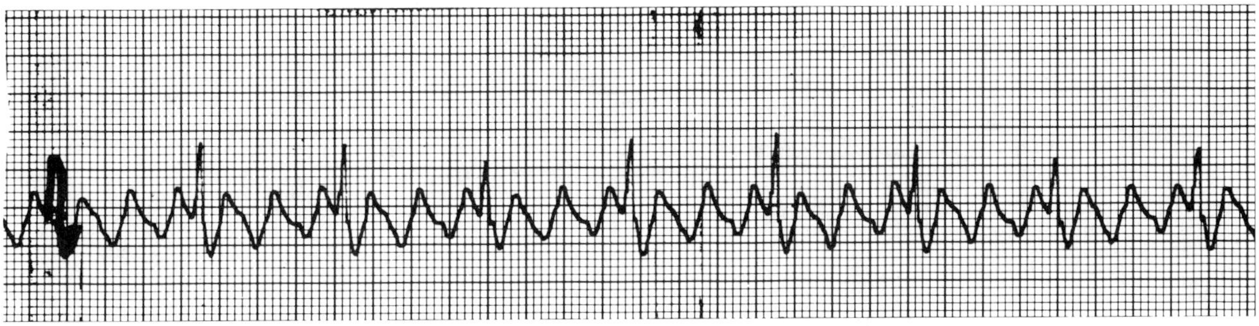

Practice strip A-26

RHYTHM:
RATE:
P WAVES:
PR INTERVAL:
QRS COMPLEX:
INTERPRETATION:
THERAPY:

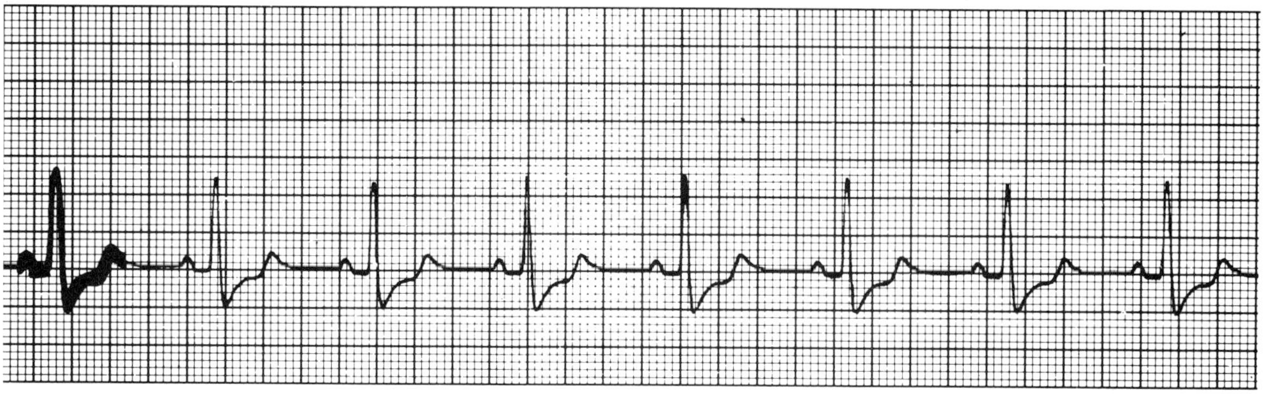

Practice strip A-27

RHYTHM:

RATE:

P WAVES:

PR INTERVAL:

QRS COMPLEX:

INTERPRETATION:

THERAPY:

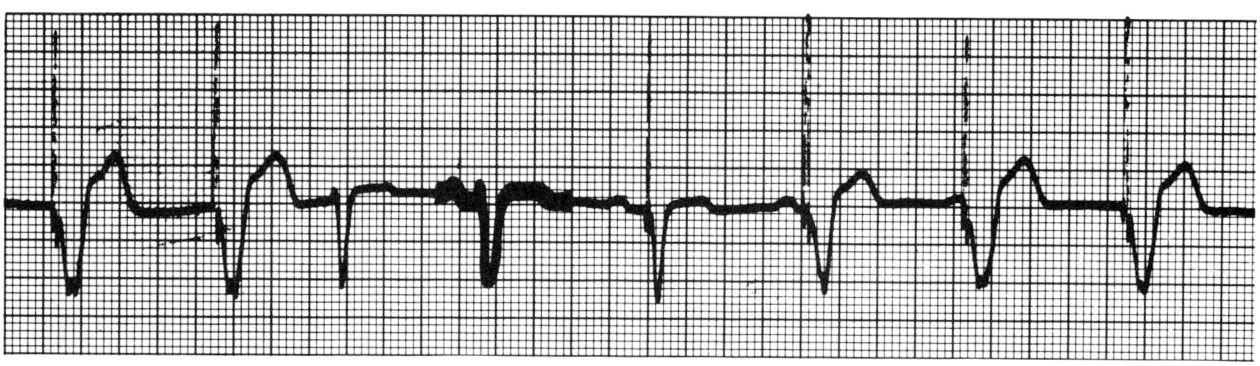

Practice strip A-28

RHYTHM:

RATE:

P WAVES:

PR INTERVAL:

QRS COMPLEX:

INTERPRETATION:

THERAPY:

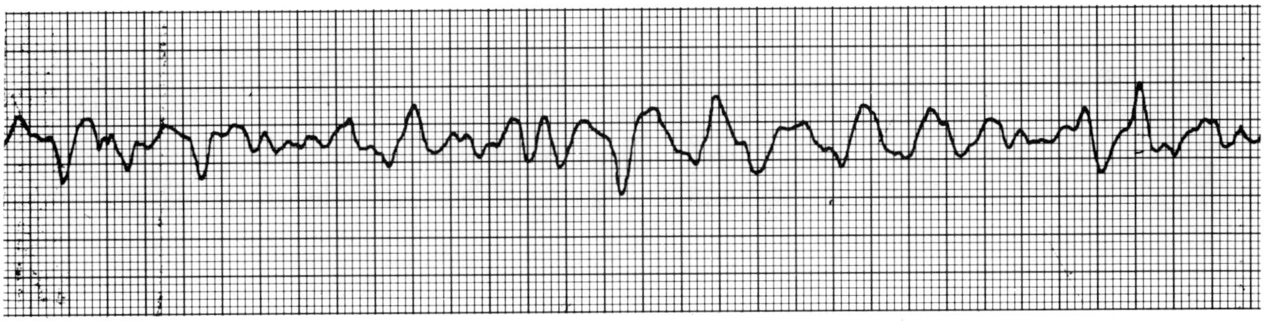

Practice strip A-29

RHYTHM:

RATE:

P WAVES:

PR INTERVAL:

QRS COMPLEX:

INTERPRETATION:

THERAPY:

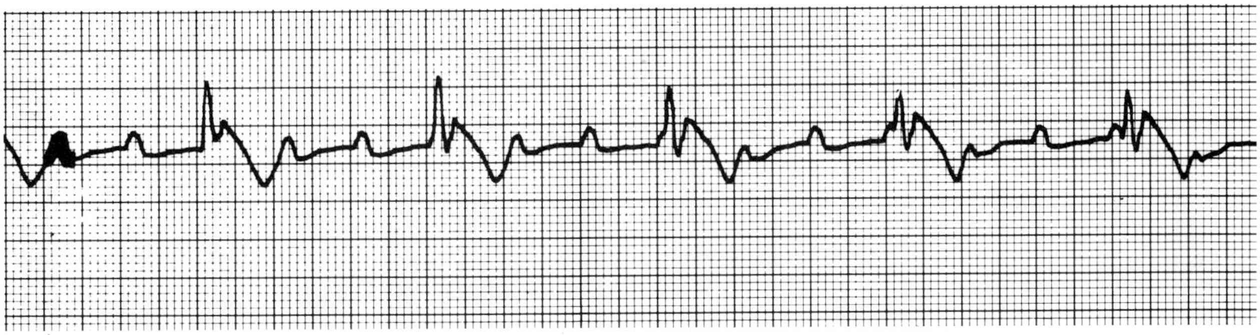

Practice strip A-30

RHYTHM:

RATE:

P WAVES:

PR INTERVAL:

QRS COMPLEX:

INTERPRETATION:

THERAPY:

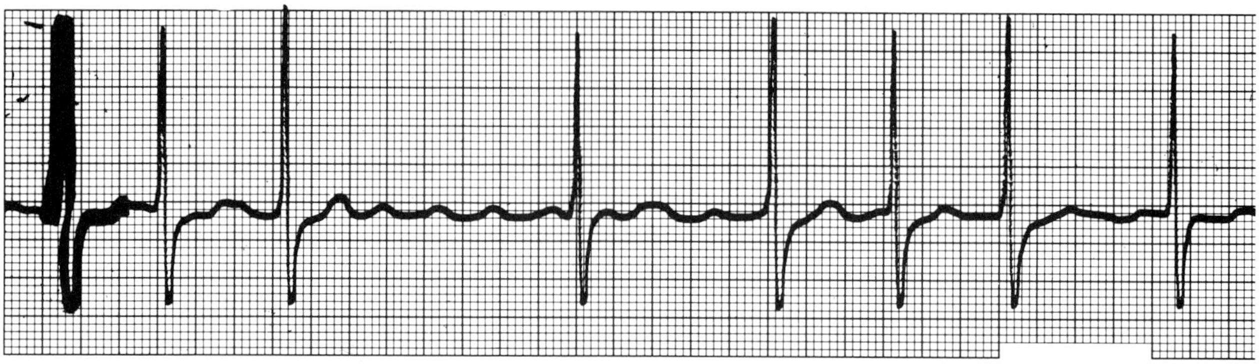

Practice strip A-31

RHYTHM:

RATE:

P WAVES:

PR INTERVAL:

QRS COMPLEX:

INTERPRETATION:

THERAPY:

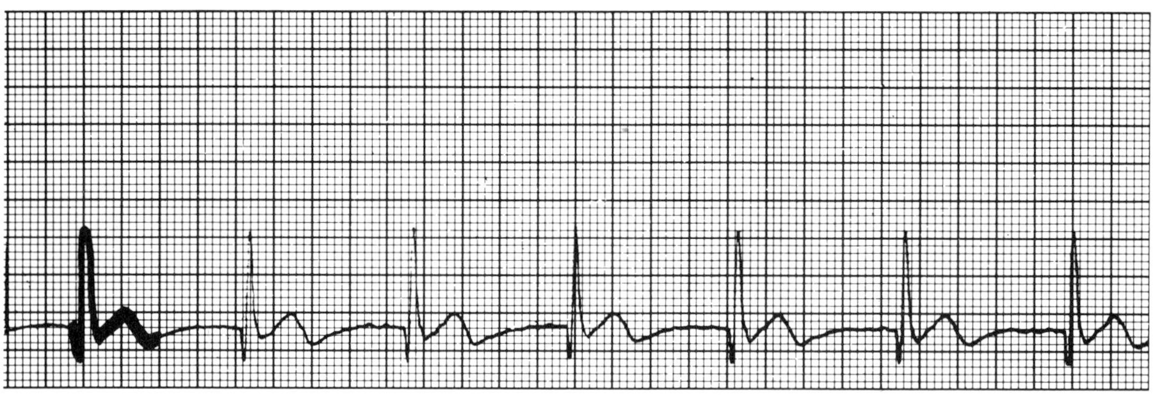

Practice strip A-32

RHYTHM:

RATE:

P WAVES:

PR INTERVAL:

QRS COMPLEX:

INTERPRETATION:

THERAPY:

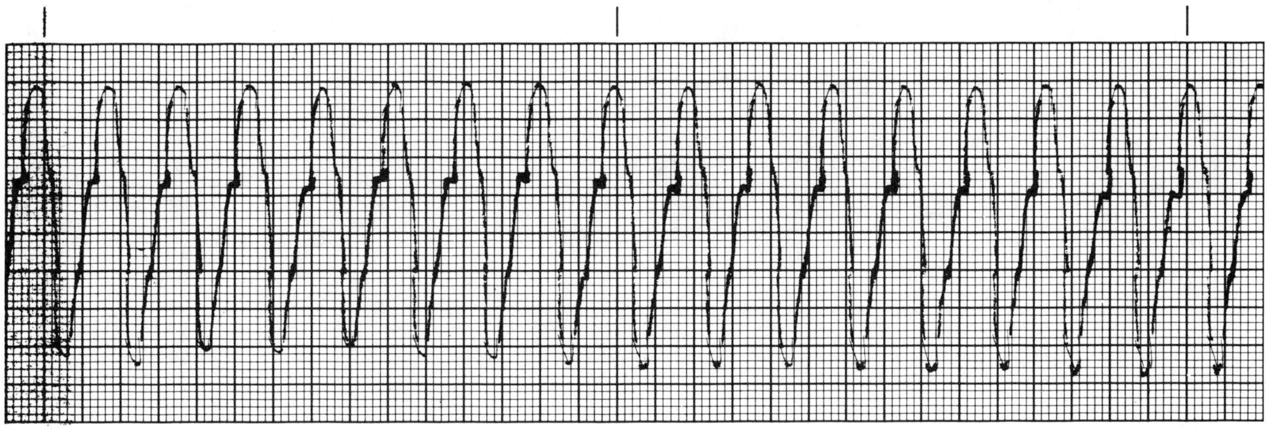

Practice strip A-33

RHYTHM:
RATE:
P WAVES:
PR INTERVAL:
QRS COMPLEX:
INTERPRETATION:
THERAPY:

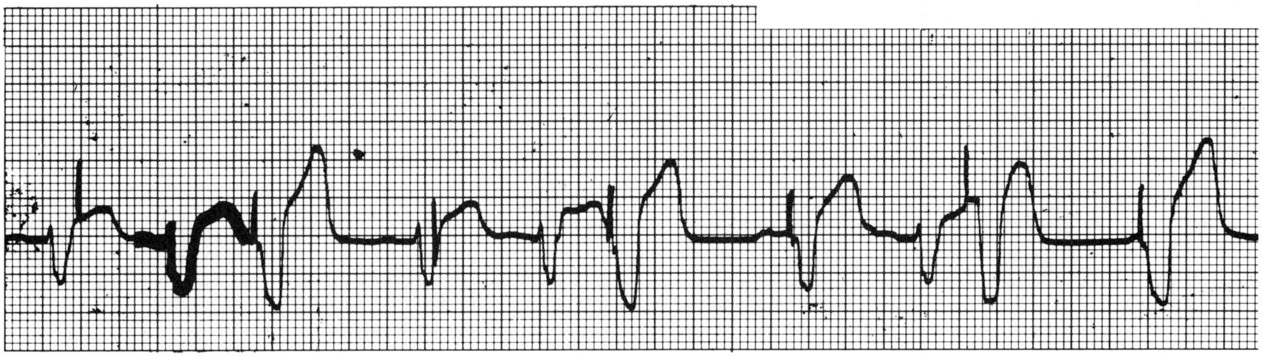

Practice strip A-34

RHYTHM:
RATE:
P WAVES:
PR INTERVAL:
QRS COMPLEX:
INTERPRETATION:
THERAPY:

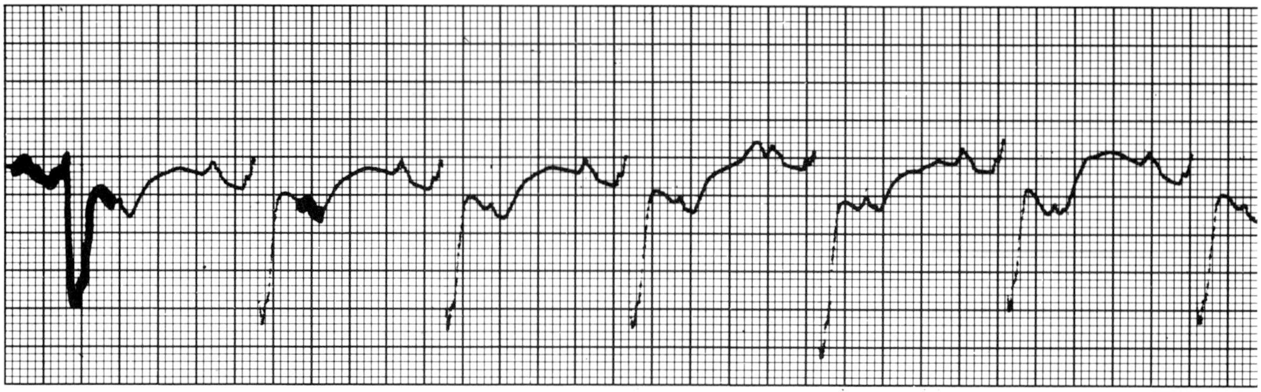

Practice strip A-35

RHYTHM:

RATE:

P WAVES:

PR INTERVAL:

QRS COMPLEX:

INTERPRETATION:

THERAPY:

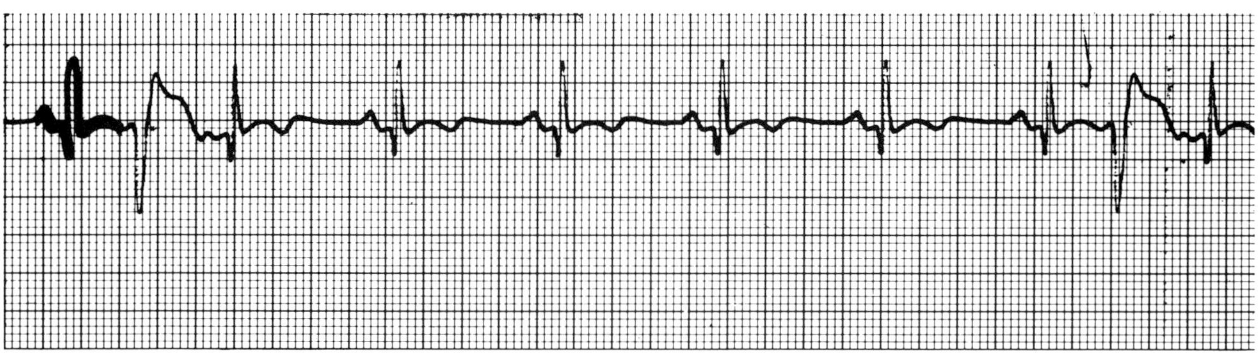

Practice strip A-36

RHYTHM:

RATE:

P WAVES:

PR INTERVAL:

QRS COMPLEX:

INTERPRETATION:

THERAPY:

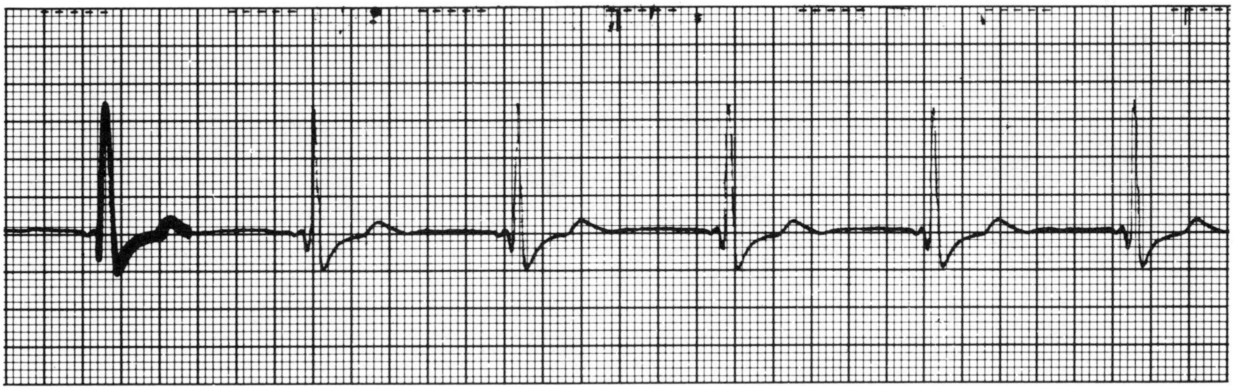

Practice strip A-37

RHYTHM:

RATE:

P WAVES:

PR INTERVAL:

QRS COMPLEX:

INTERPRETATION:

THERAPY:

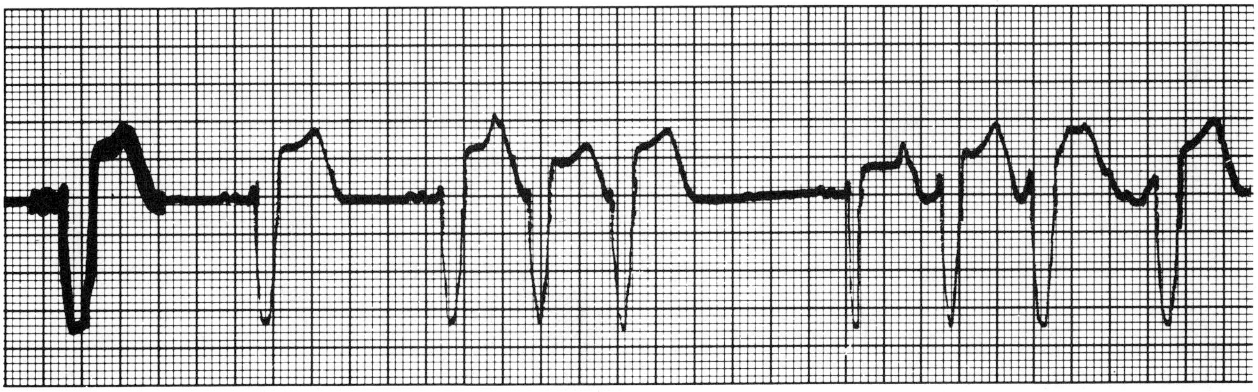

Practice strip A-38

RHYTHM:

RATE:

P WAVES:

PR INTERVAL:

QRS COMPLEX:

INTERPRETATION:

THERAPY:

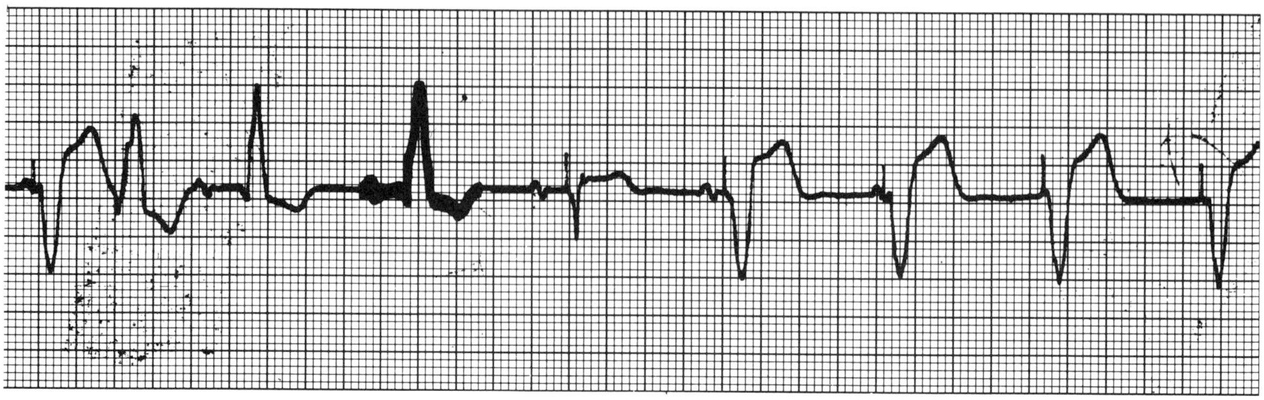

Practice strip A-39

RHYTHM:

RATE:

P WAVES:

PR INTERVAL:

QRS COMPLEX:

INTERPRETATION:

THERAPY:

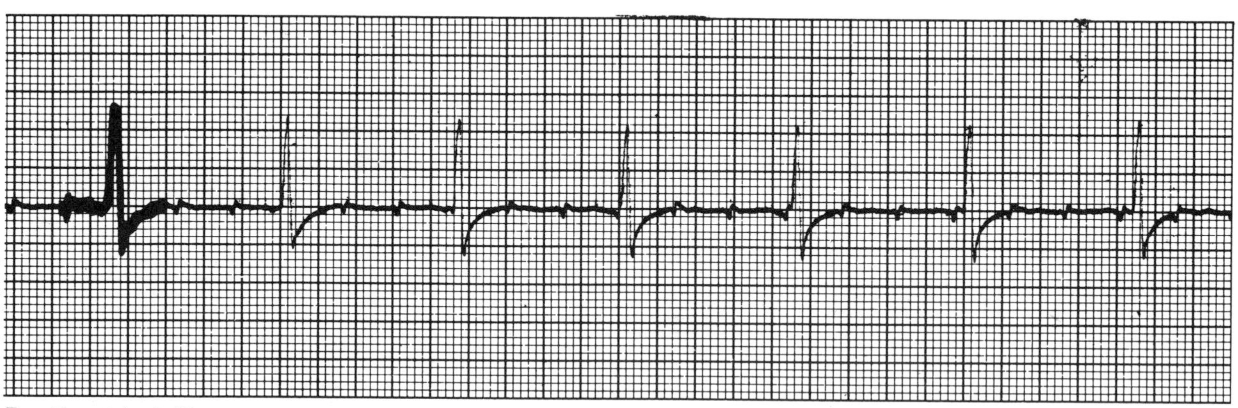

Practice strip A-40

RHYTHM:

RATE:

P WAVES:

PR INTERVAL:

QRS COMPLEX:

INTERPRETATION:

THERAPY:

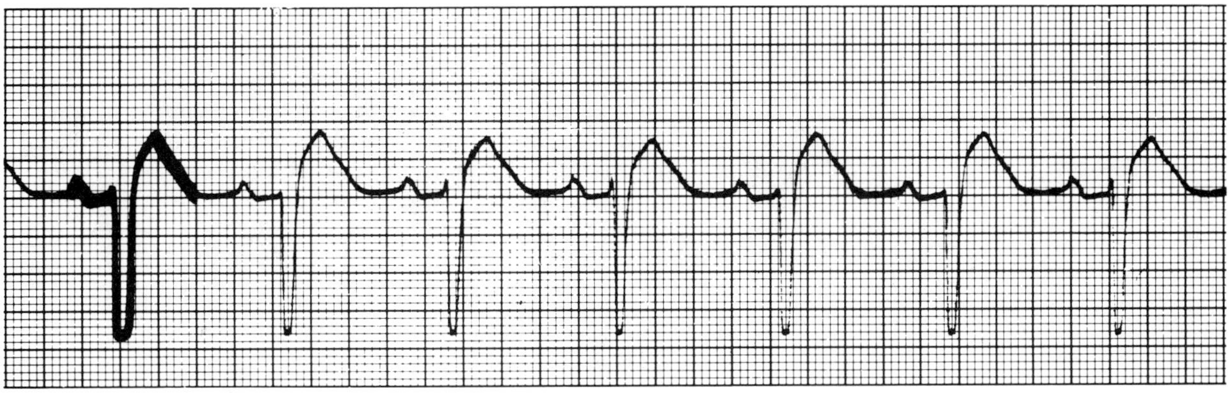

Practice strip A-41

RHYTHM:
RATE:
P WAVES:
PR INTERVAL:
QRS COMPLEX:
INTERPRETATION:
THERAPY:

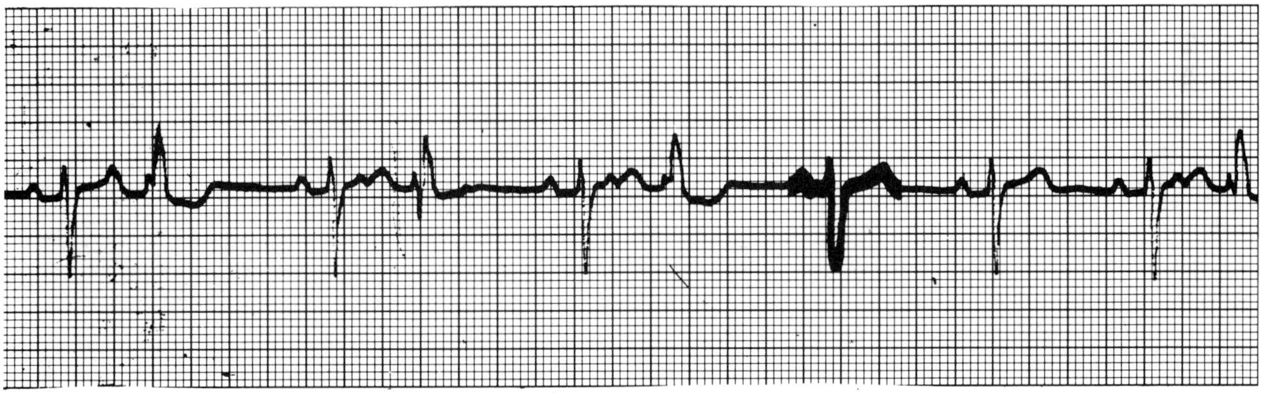

Practice strip A-42

RHYTHM:
RATE:
P WAVES:
PR INTERVAL:
QRS COMPLEX:
INTERPRETATION:
THERAPY:

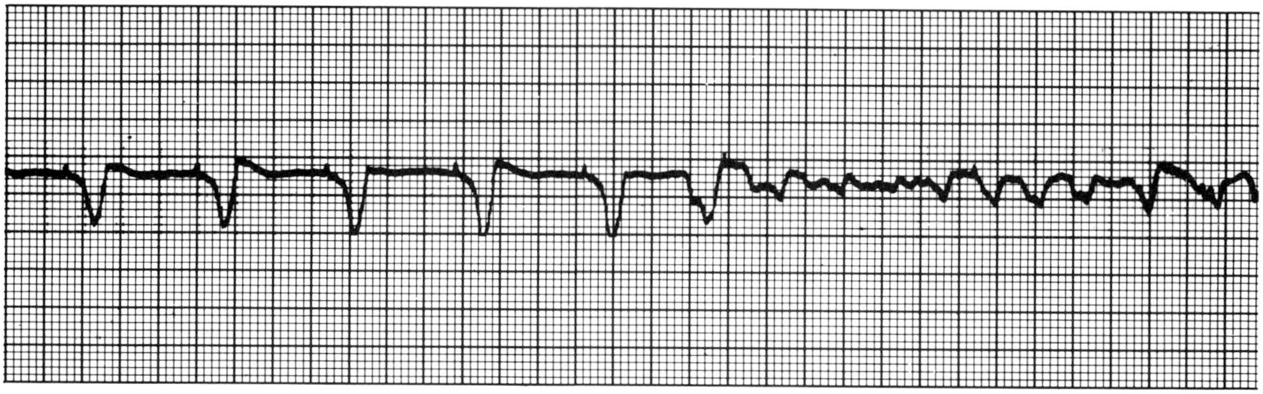

Practice strip A-43

RHYTHM:

RATE:

P WAVES:

PR INTERVAL:

QRS COMPLEX:

INTERPRETATION:

THERAPY:

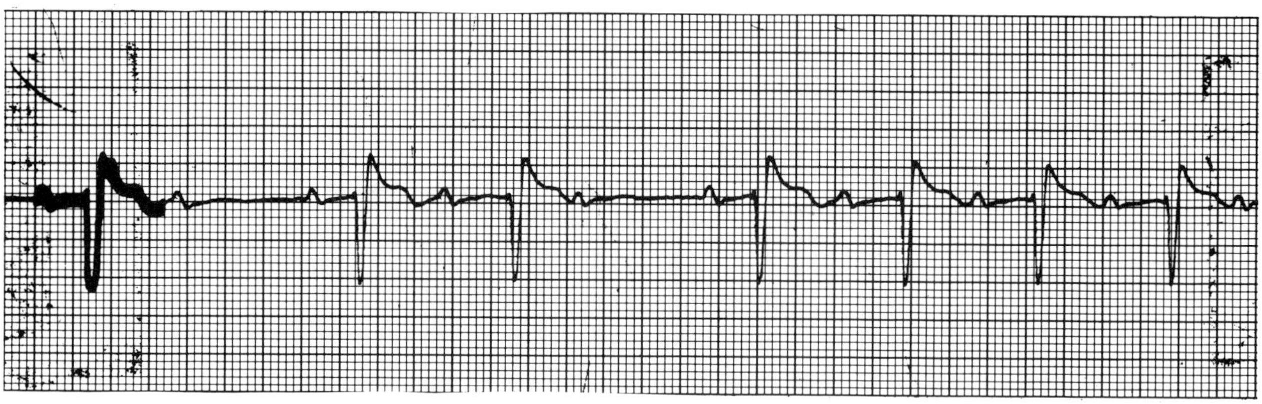

Practice strip A-44

RHYTHM:

RATE:

P WAVES:

PR INTERVAL:

QRS COMPLEX:

INTERPRETATION:

THERAPY:

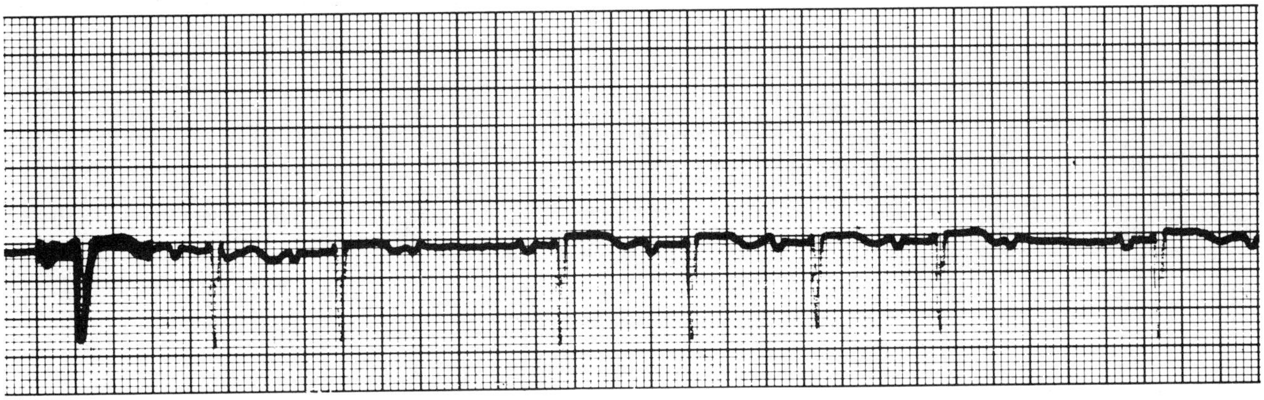

Practice strip A-45

RHYTHM:
RATE:
P WAVES:
PR INTERVAL:
QRS COMPLEX:
INTERPRETATION:
THERAPY:

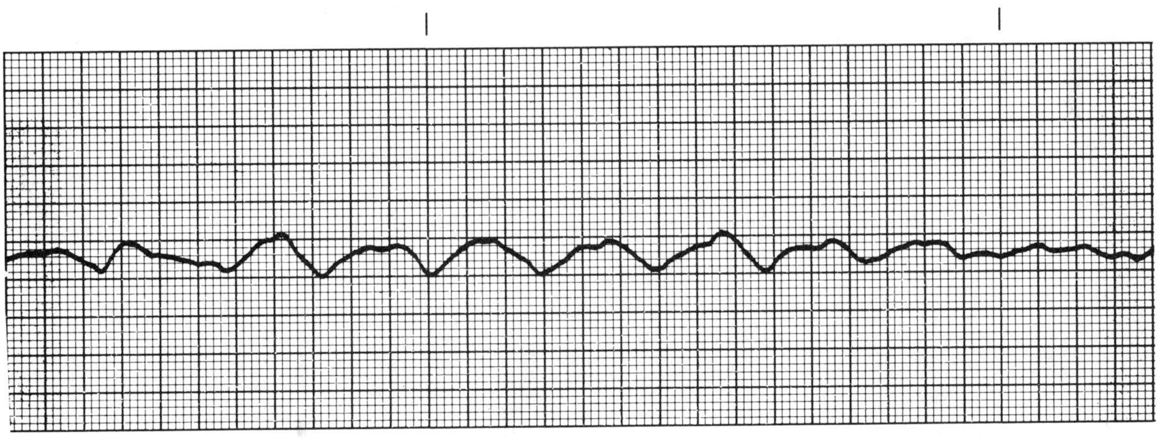

Practice strip A-46

RHYTHM:
RATE:
P WAVES:
PR INTERVAL:
QRS COMPLEX:
INTERPRETATION:
THERAPY:

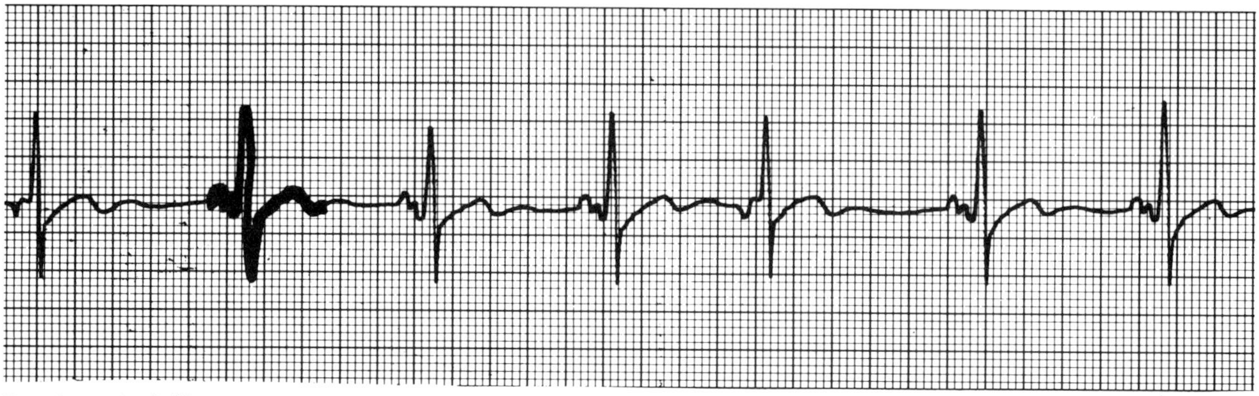

Practice strip A-47

RHYTHM:

RATE:

P WAVES:

PR INTERVAL:

QRS COMPLEX:

INTERPRETATION:

THERAPY:

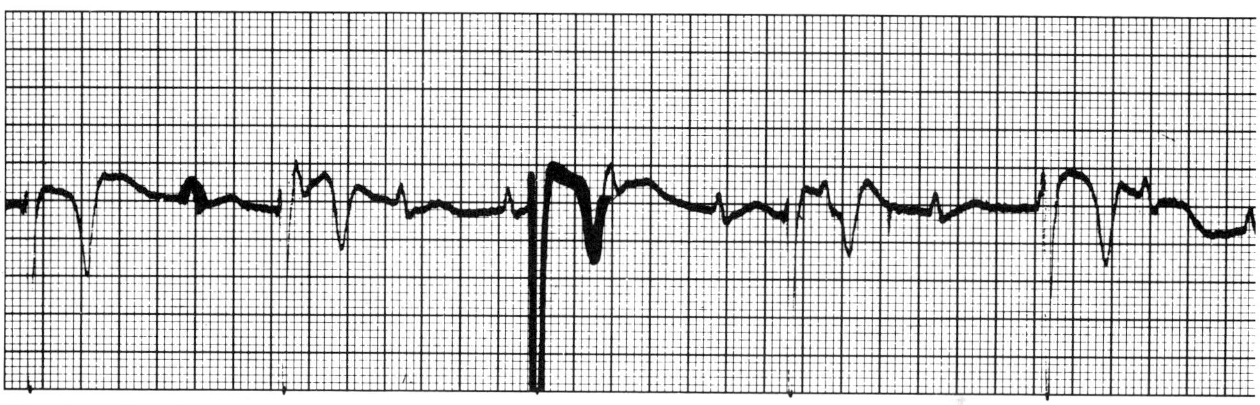

Practice strip A-48

RHYTHM:

RATE:

P WAVES:

PR INTERVAL:

QRS COMPLEX:

INTERPRETATION:

THERAPY:

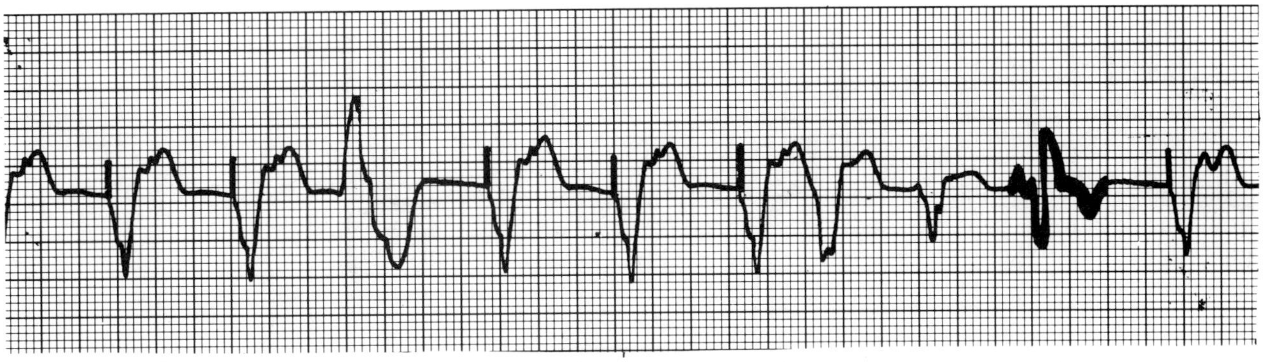

Practice strip A-49

RHYTHM:

RATE:

P WAVES:

PR INTERVAL:

QRS COMPLEX:

INTERPRETATION:

THERAPY:

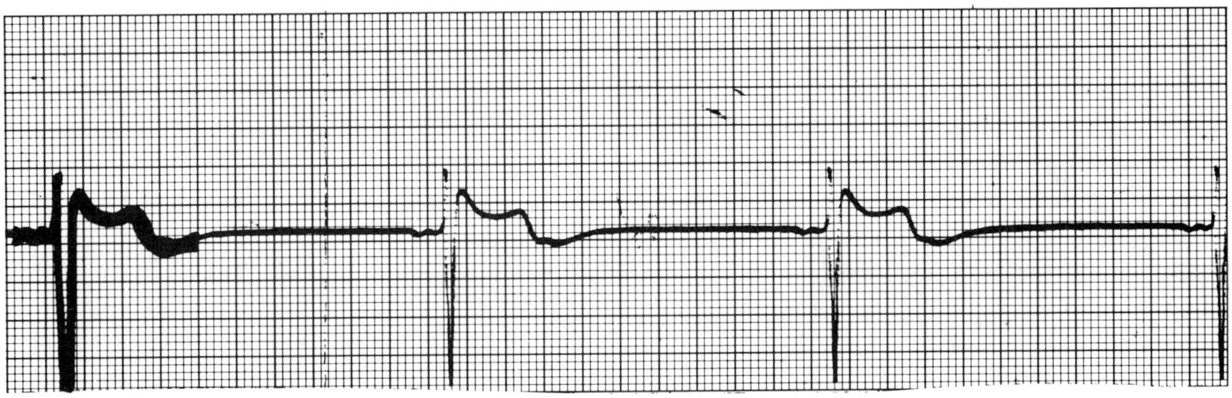

Practice strip A-50

RHYTHM:

RATE:

P WAVES:

PR INTERVAL:

QRS COMPLEX:

INTERPRETATION:

THERAPY:

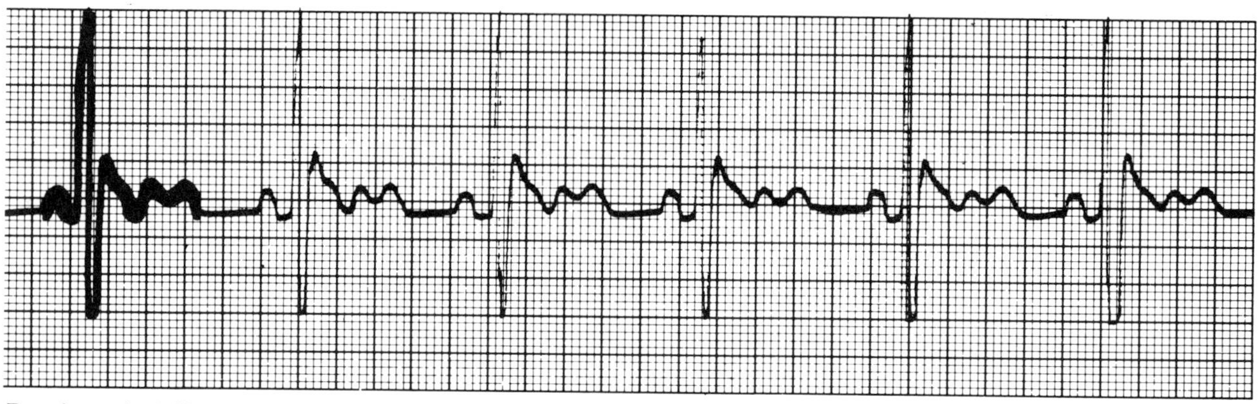

Practice strip A-51

RHYTHM:

RATE:

P WAVES:

PR INTERVAL:

QRS COMPLEX:

INTERPRETATION:

THERAPY:

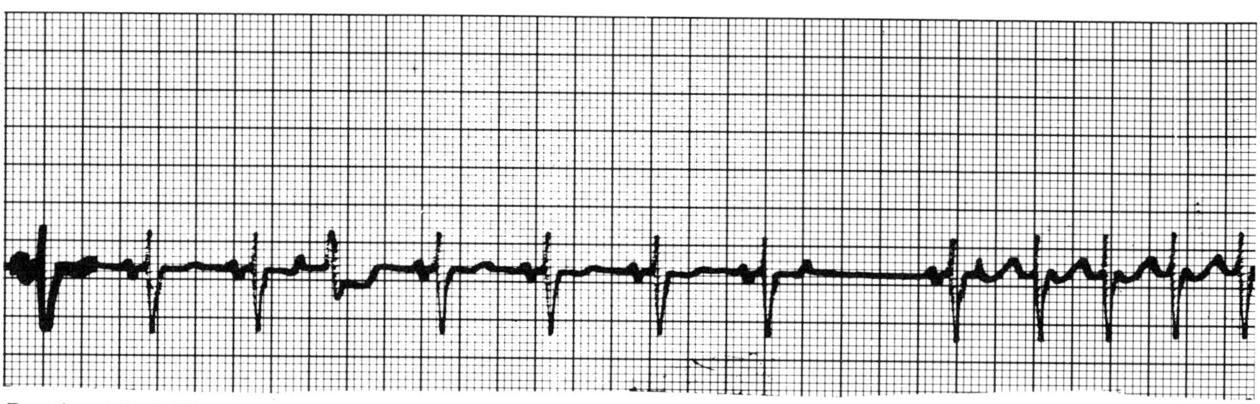

Practice strip A-52

RHYTHM:

RATE:

P WAVES:

PR INTERVAL:

QRS COMPLEX:

INTERPRETATION:

THERAPY:

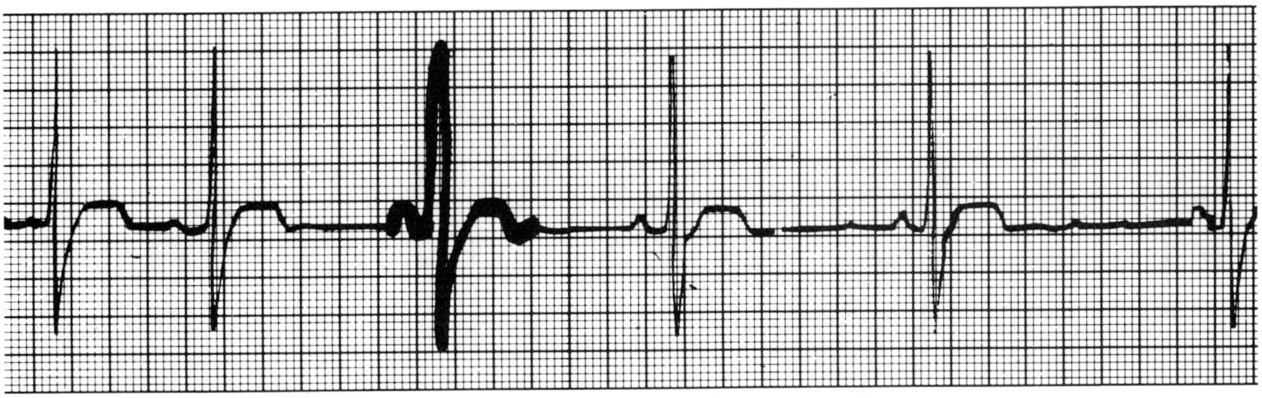

Practice strip A-53

RHYTHM:

RATE:

P WAVES:

PR INTERVAL:

QRS COMPLEX:

INTERPRETATION:

THERAPY:

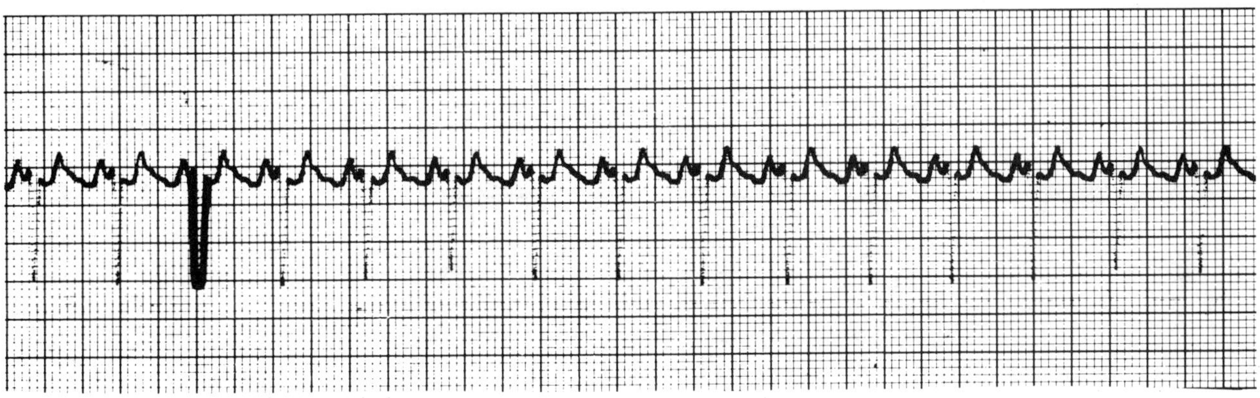

Practice strip A-54

RHYTHM:

RATE:

P WAVES:

PR INTERVAL:

QRS COMPLEX:

INTERPRETATION:

THERAPY:

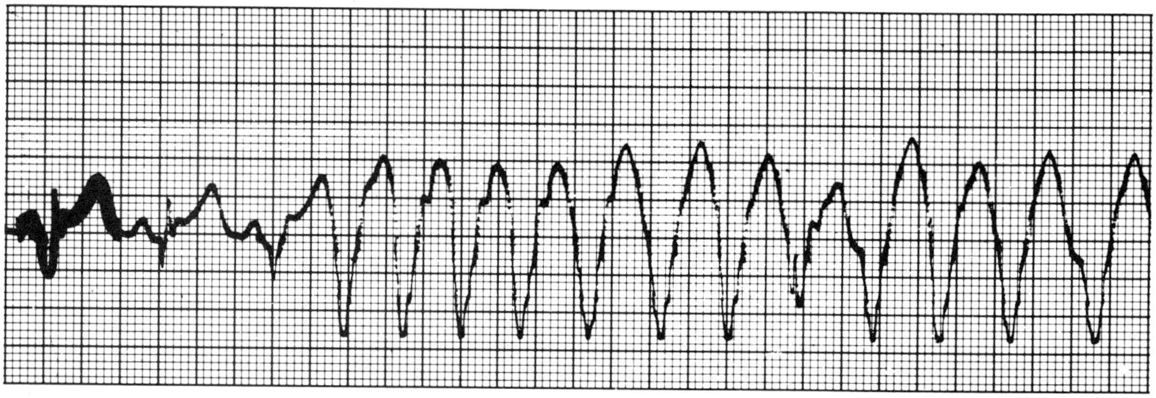

Practice strip A-55

RHYTHM:
RATE:
P WAVES:
PR INTERVAL:
QRS COMPLEX:
INTERPRETATION:
THERAPY:

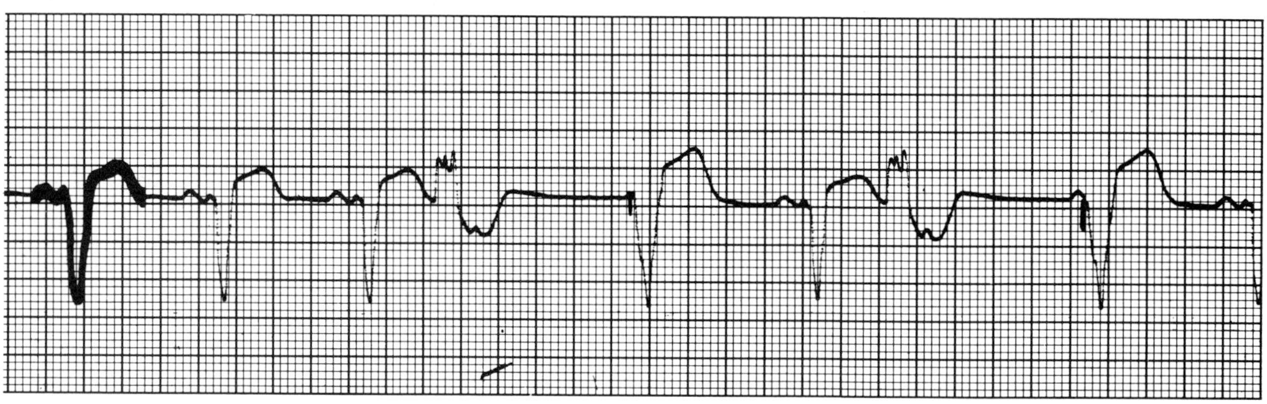

Practice strip A-56

RHYTHM:
RATE:
P WAVES:
PR INTERVAL:
QRS COMPLEX:
INTERPRETATION:
THERAPY:

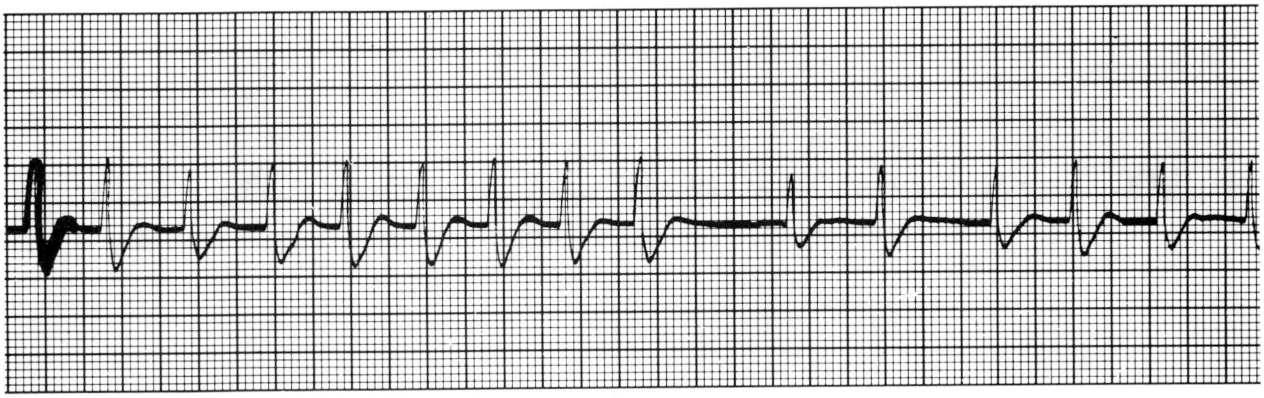

Practice strip A-57

RHYTHM:
RATE:
P WAVES:
PR INTERVAL:
QRS COMPLEX:
INTERPRETATION:
THERAPY:

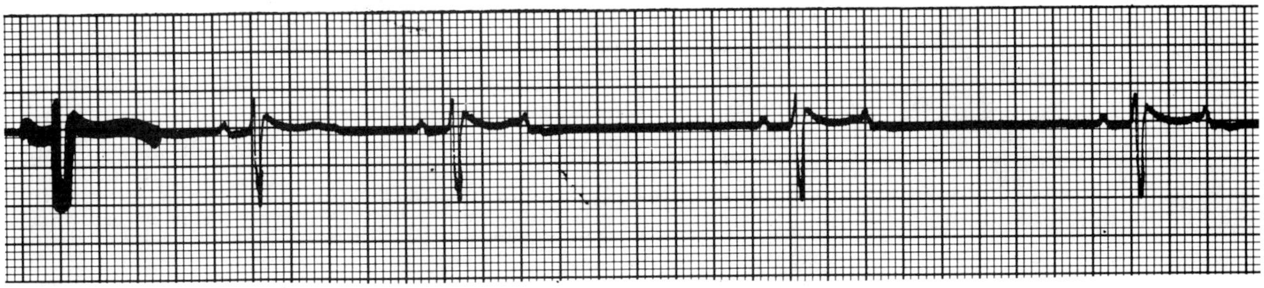

Practice strip A-58

RHYTHM:
RATE:
P WAVES:
PR INTERVAL:
QRS COMPLEX:
INTERPRETATION:
THERAPY:

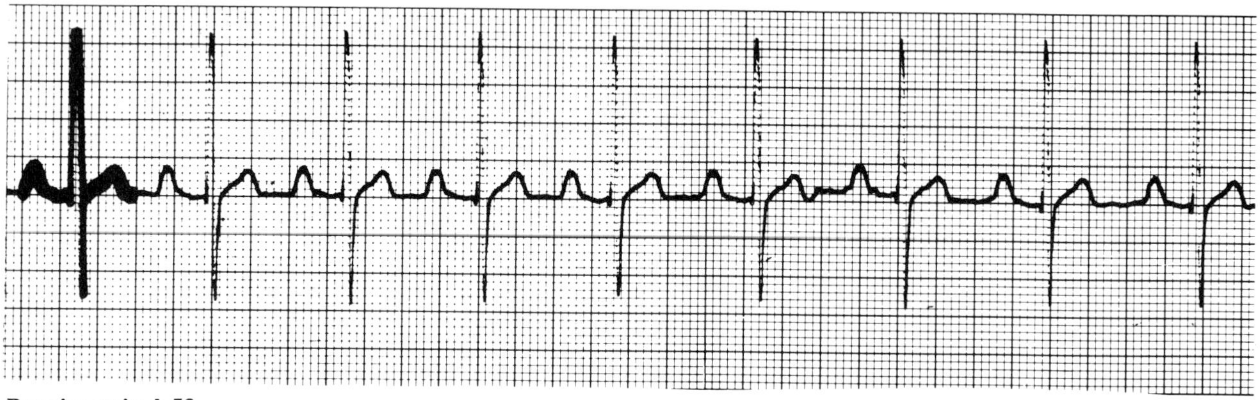

Practice strip A-59

RHYTHM:

RATE:

P WAVES:

PR INTERVAL:

QRS COMPLEX:

INTERPRETATION:

THERAPY:

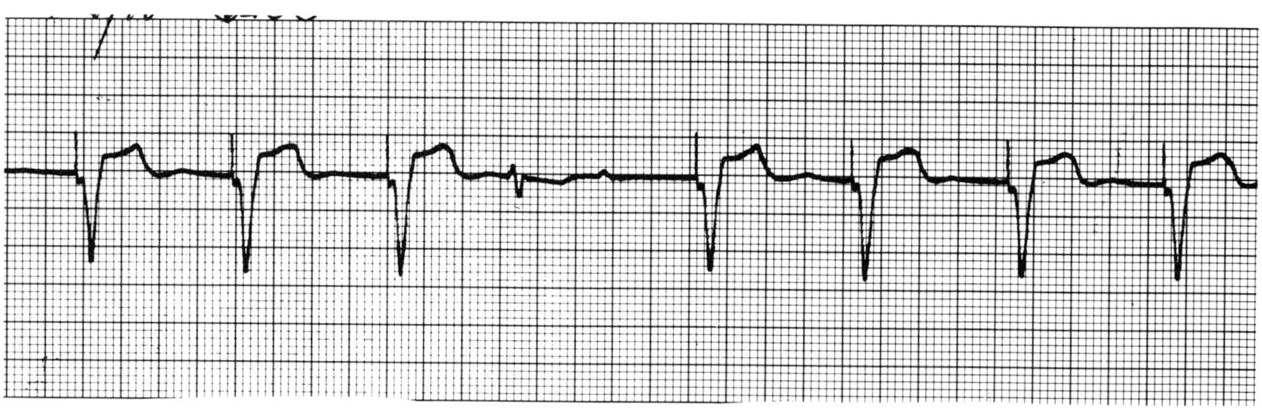

Practice strip A-60

RHYTHM:

RATE:

P WAVES:

PR INTERVAL:

QRS COMPLEX:

INTERPRETATION:

THERAPY:

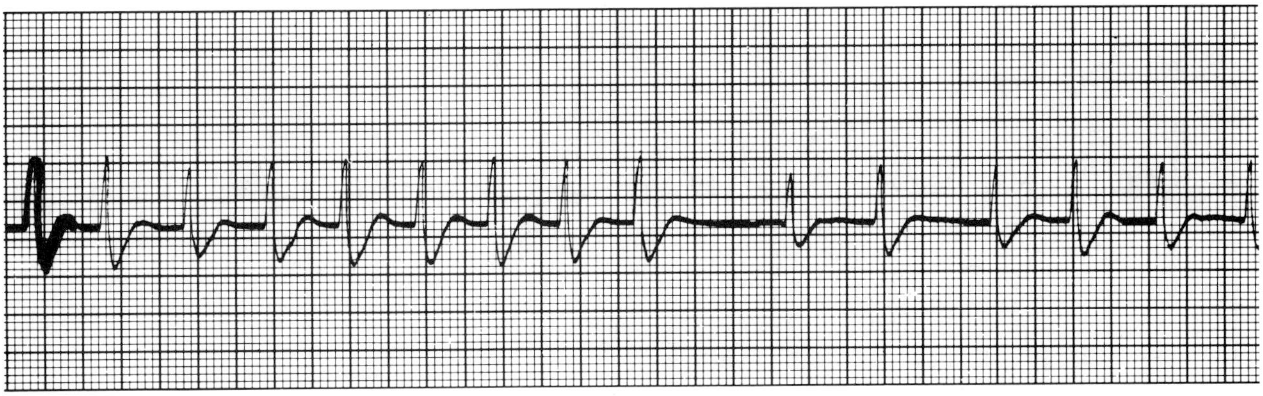

Practice strip A-57

RHYTHM:

RATE:

P WAVES:

PR INTERVAL:

QRS COMPLEX:

INTERPRETATION:

THERAPY:

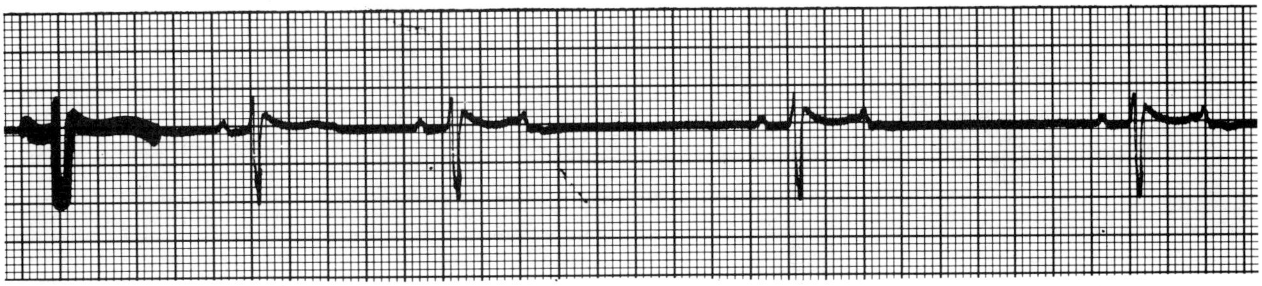

Practice strip A-58

RHYTHM:

RATE:

P WAVES:

PR INTERVAL:

QRS COMPLEX:

INTERPRETATION:

THERAPY:

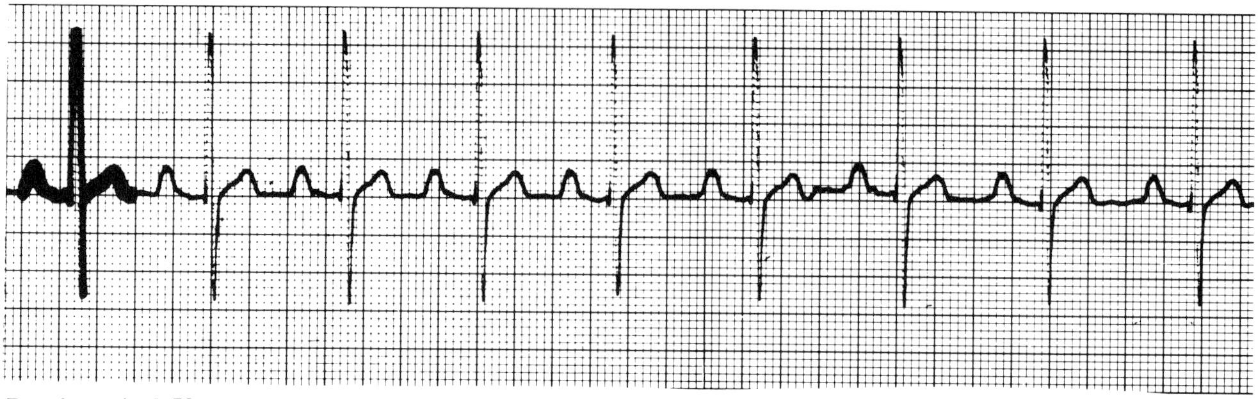

Practice strip A-59

RHYTHM:

RATE:

P WAVES:

PR INTERVAL:

QRS COMPLEX:

INTERPRETATION:

THERAPY:

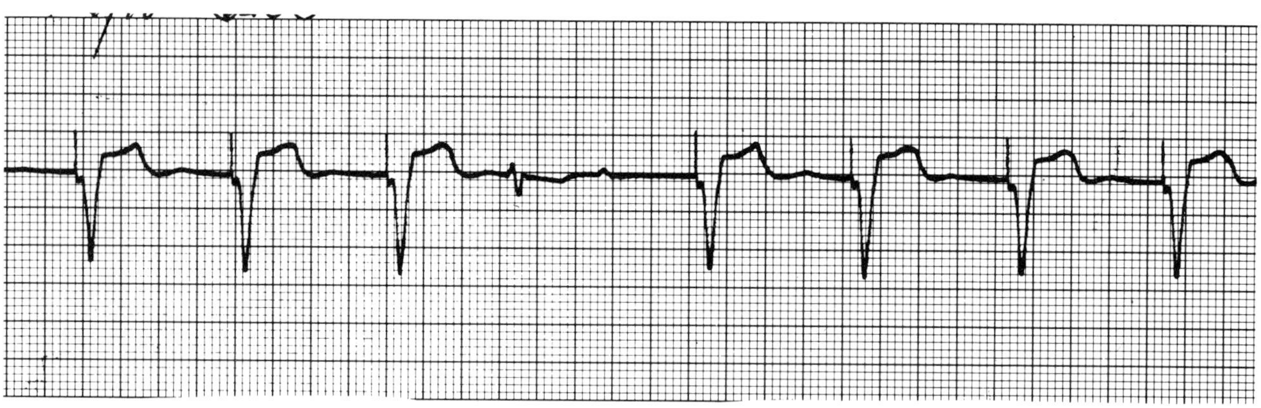

Practice strip A-60

RHYTHM:

RATE:

P WAVES:

PR INTERVAL:

QRS COMPLEX:

INTERPRETATION:

THERAPY:

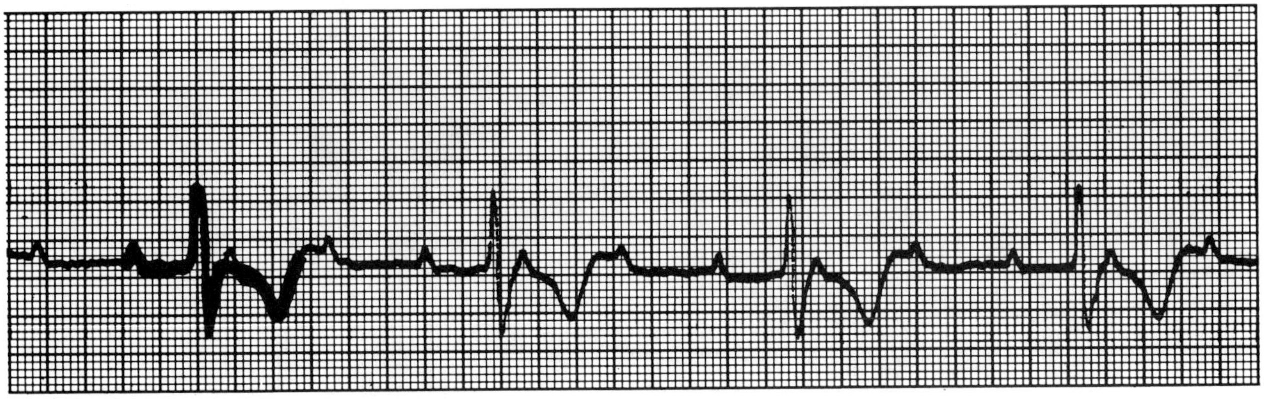

Practice strip A-61

RHYTHM:

RATE:

P WAVES:

PR INTERVAL:

QRS COMPLEX:

INTERPRETATION:

THERAPY:

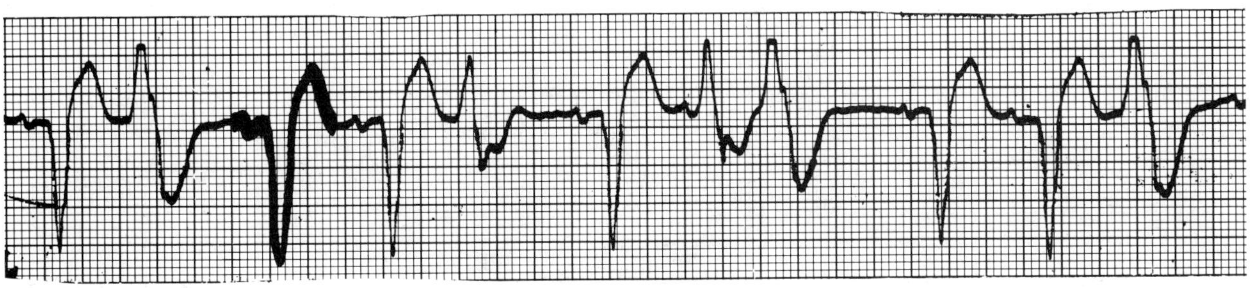

Practice strip A-62

RHYTHM:

RATE:

P WAVES:

PR INTERVAL:

QRS COMPLEX:

INTERPRETATION:

THERAPY:

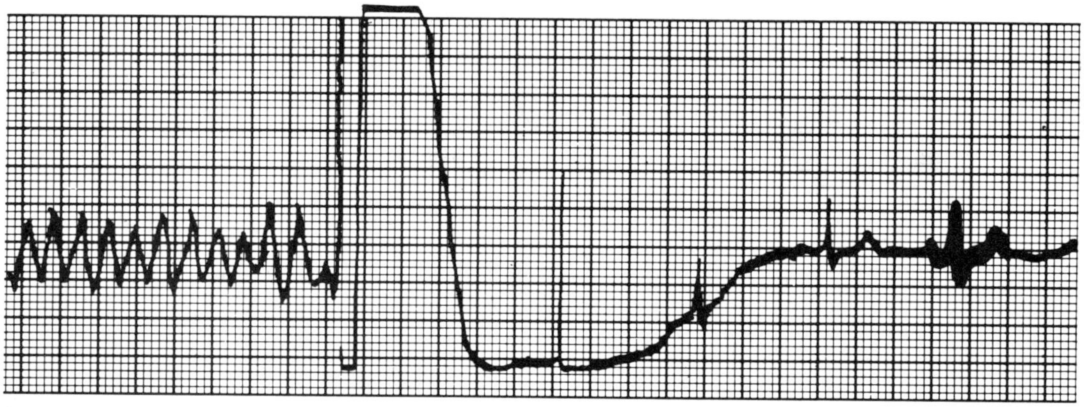

Practice strip A-63

RHYTHM:

RATE:

P WAVES:

PR INTERVAL:

QRS COMPLEX:

INTERPRETATION:

THERAPY:

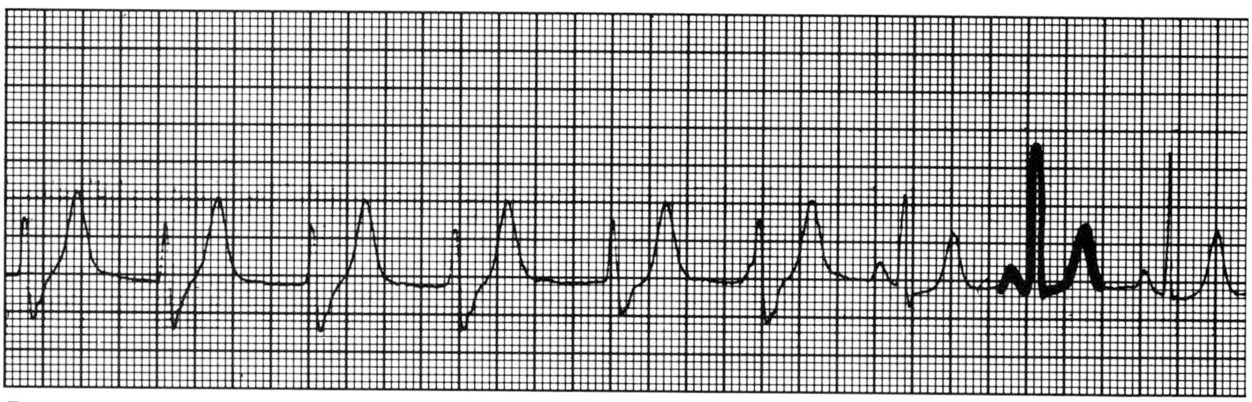

Practice strip A-64

RHYTHM:

RATE:

P WAVES:

PR INTERVAL:

QRS COMPLEX:

INTERPRETATION:

THERAPY:

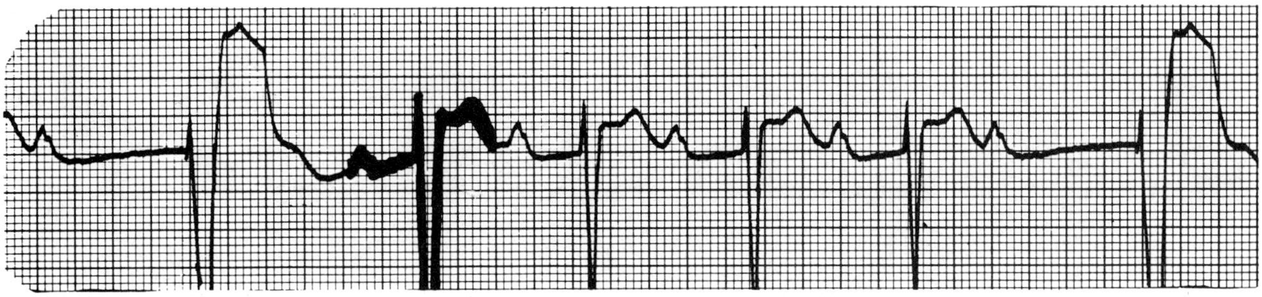

Practice strip A-65

RHYTHM:
RATE:
P WAVES:
PR INTERVAL:
QRS COMPLEX:
INTERPRETATION:
THERAPY:

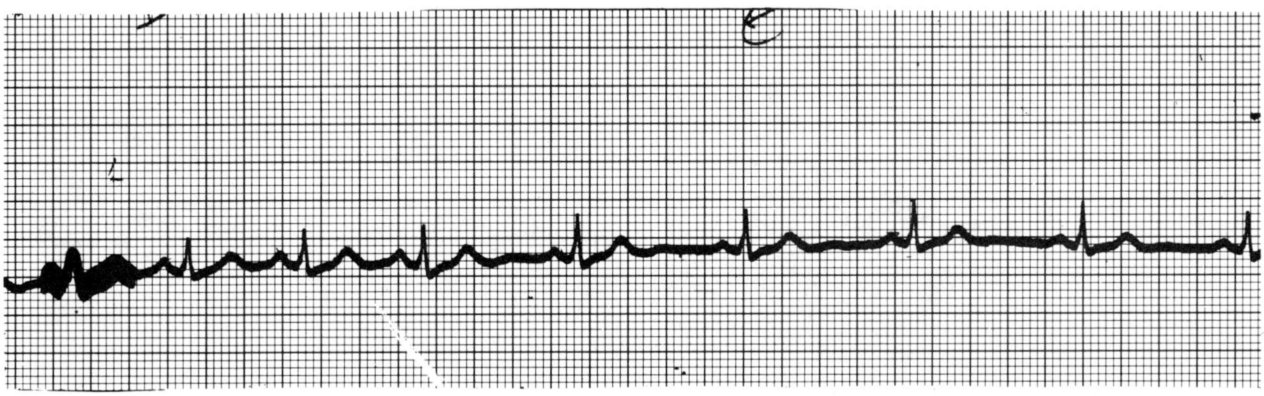

Practice strip A-66

RHYTHM:
RATE:
P WAVES:
PR INTERVAL:
QRS COMPLEX:
INTERPRETATION:
THERAPY:

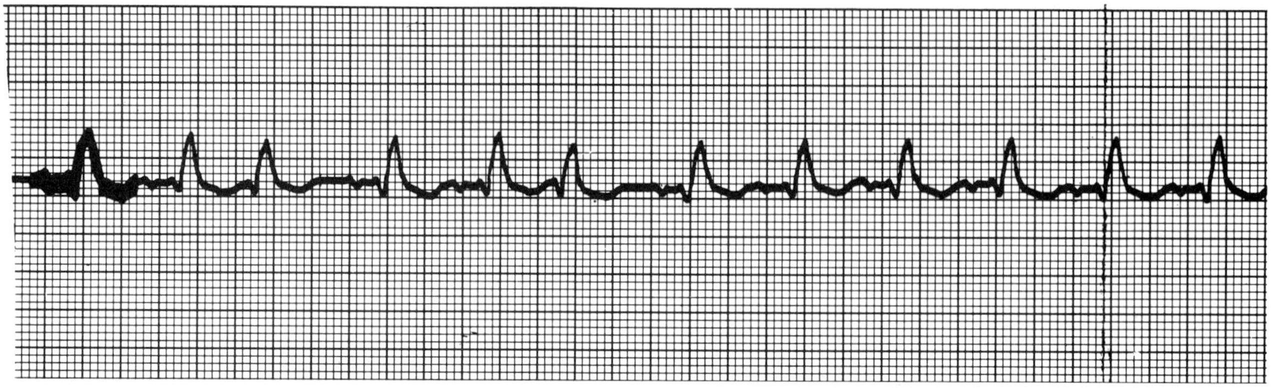

Practice strip A-67

RHYTHM:

RATE:

P WAVES:

PR INTERVAL:

QRS COMPLEX:

INTERPRETATION:

THERAPY:

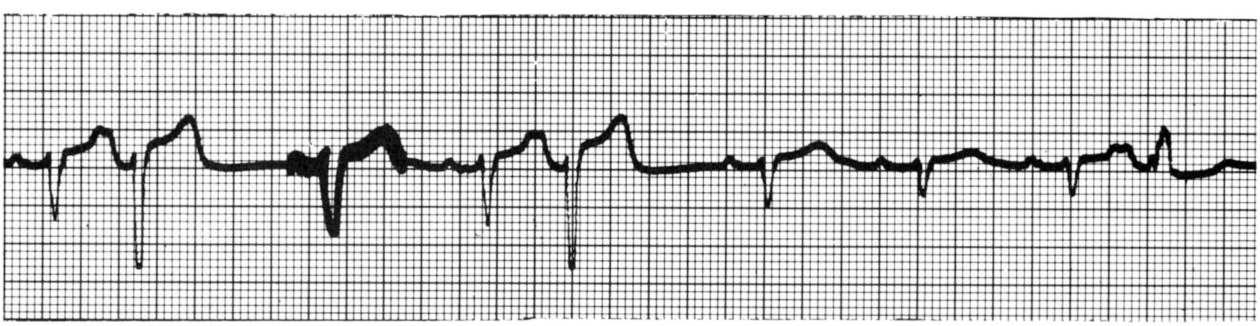

Practice strip A-68

RHYTHM:

RATE:

P WAVES:

PR INTERVAL:

QRS COMPLEX:

INTERPRETATION:

THERAPY:

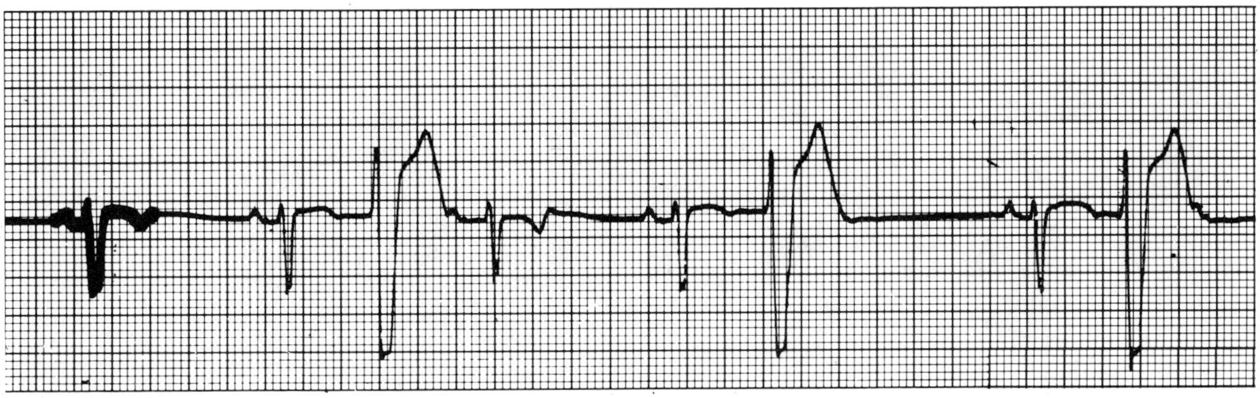

Practice strip A-69

RHYTHM:
RATE:
P WAVES:
PR INTERVAL:
QRS COMPLEX:
INTERPRETATION:
THERAPY:

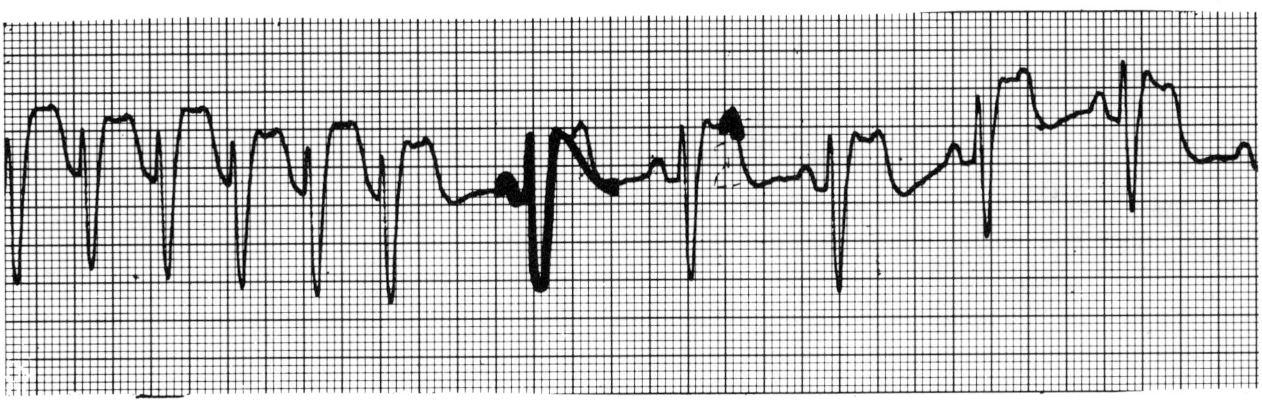

Practice strip A-70

RHYTHM:
RATE:
P WAVES:
PR INTERVAL:
QRS COMPLEX:
INTERPRETATION:
THERAPY:

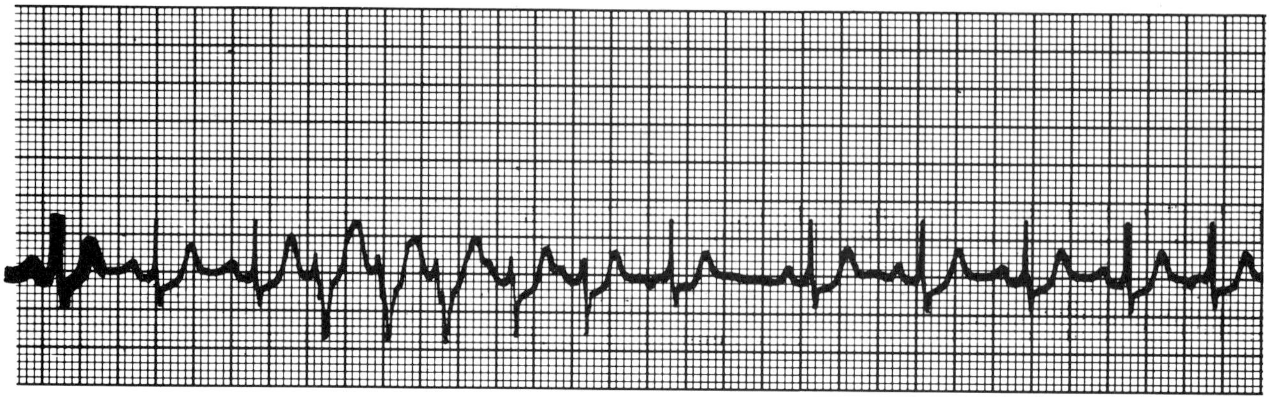

Practice strip A-71

RHYTHM:

RATE:

P WAVES:

PR INTERVAL:

QRS COMPLEX:

INTERPRETATION:

THERAPY:

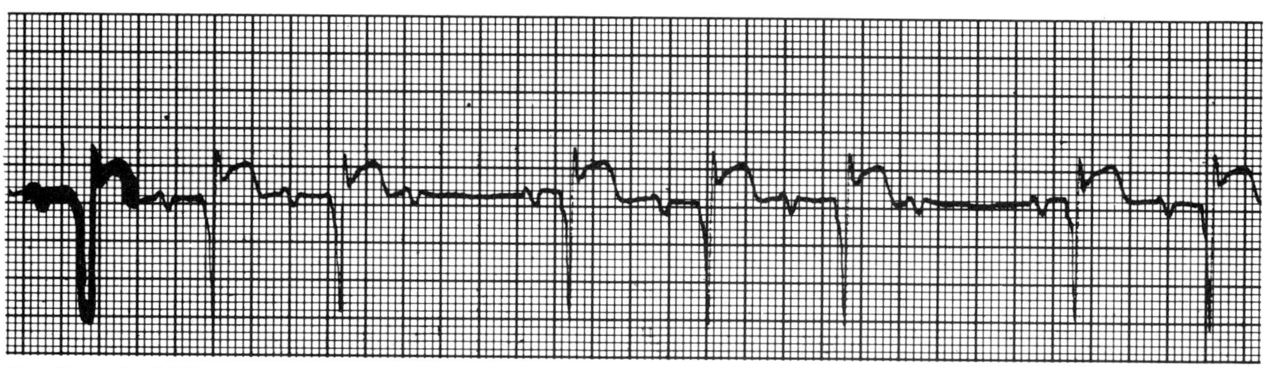

Practice strip A-72

RHYTHM:

RATE:

P WAVES:

PR INTERVAL:

QRS COMPLEX:

INTERPRETATION:

THERAPY:

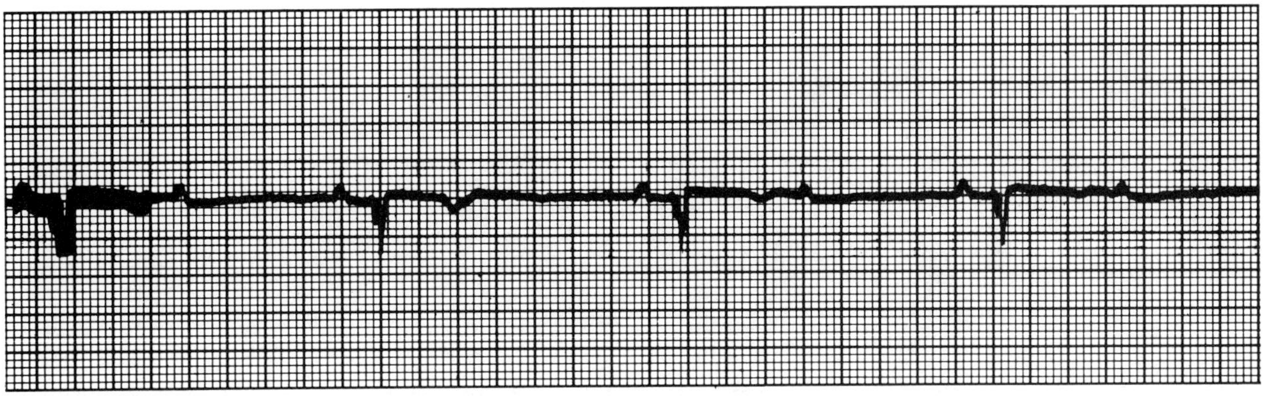

Practice strip A-73

RHYTHM:

RATE:

P WAVES:

PR INTERVAL:

QRS COMPLEX:

INTERPRETATION:

THERAPY:

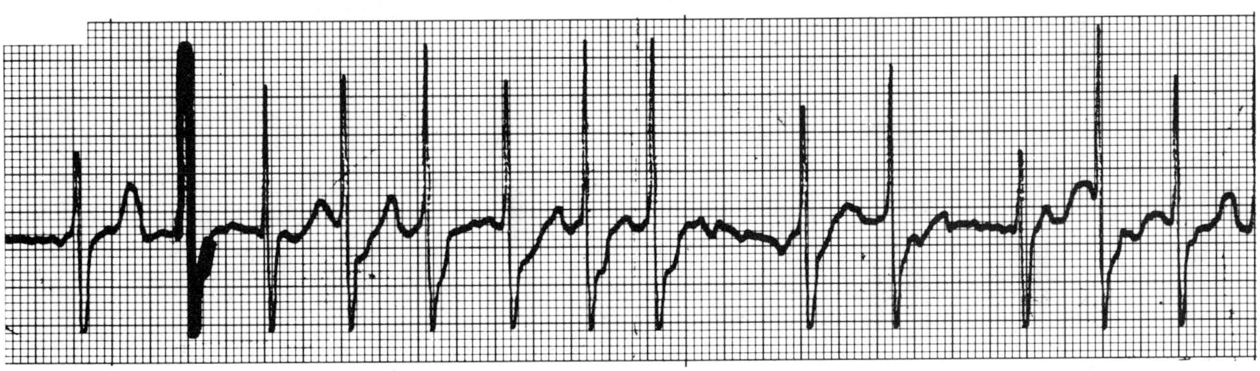

Practice strip A-74

RHYTHM:

RATE:

P WAVES:

PR INTERVAL:

QRS COMPLEX:

INTERPRETATION:

THERAPY:

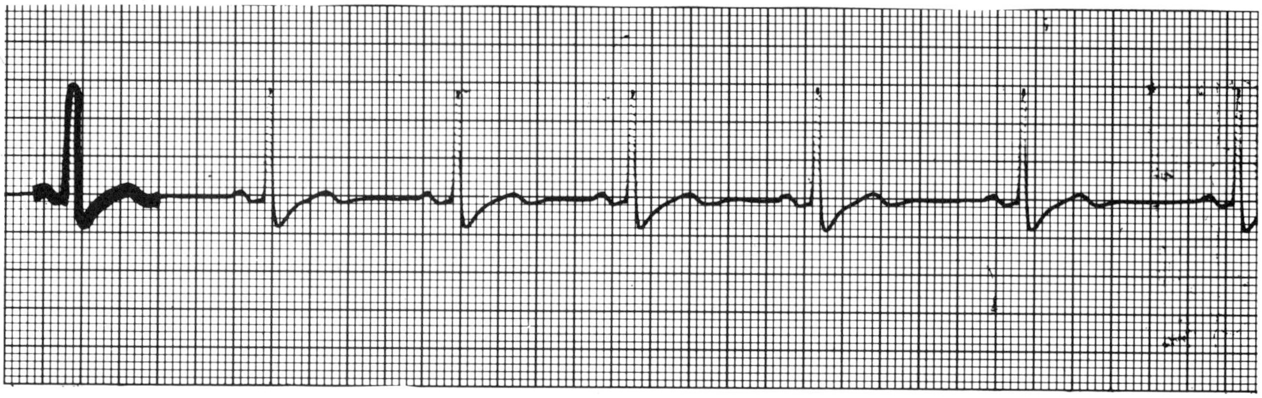

Practice strip A-75

RHYTHM:

RATE:

P WAVES:

PR INTERVAL:

QRS COMPLEX:

INTERPRETATION:

THERAPY:

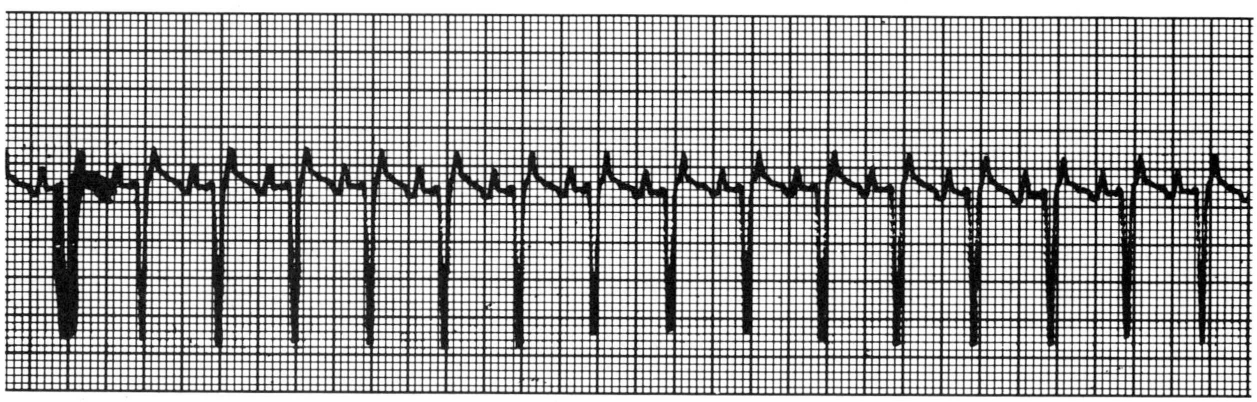

Practice strip A-76

RHYTHM:

RATE:

P WAVES:

PR INTERVAL:

QRS COMPLEX:

INTERPRETATION:

THERAPY:

ANSWER STRIPS

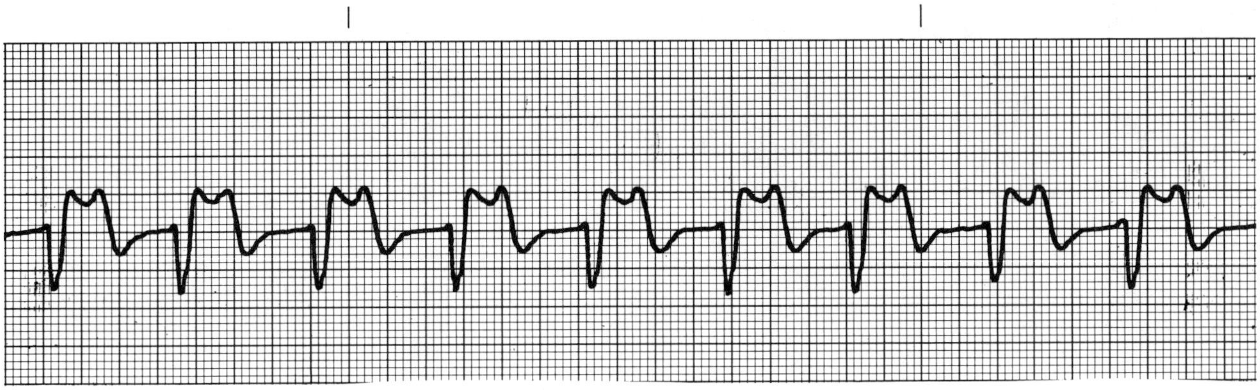

Answer strip A-1

RHYTHM: *Regular*

RATE: *85*

P WAVES: *None visible*

PR INTERVAL: —

QRS COMPLEX: *0.14 second*

INTERPRETATION: *Accelerated ventricular rhythm.*

THERAPY: *Check cause. Treat only if rate slows.*

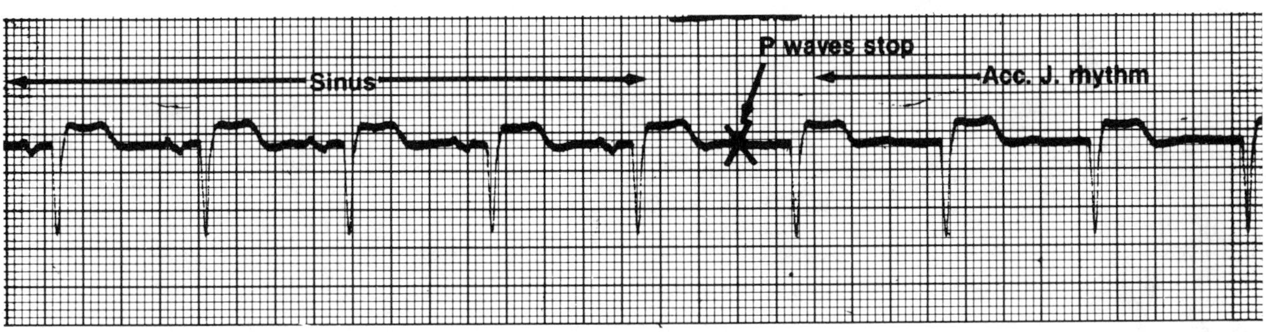

Answer strip A-2

RHYTHM: *Regular × 2*

RATE: *Sinus, 85; junctional, 75*

P WAVES: *Normal then absent*

PR INTERVAL: *0.18 second*

QRS COMPLEX: *0.10 second*

INTERPRETATION: *NSR → third-degree SA block (sinus arrest) → accelerated junctional rhythm*

THERAPY: *Check cause of suppression. Treat if rate slows.*

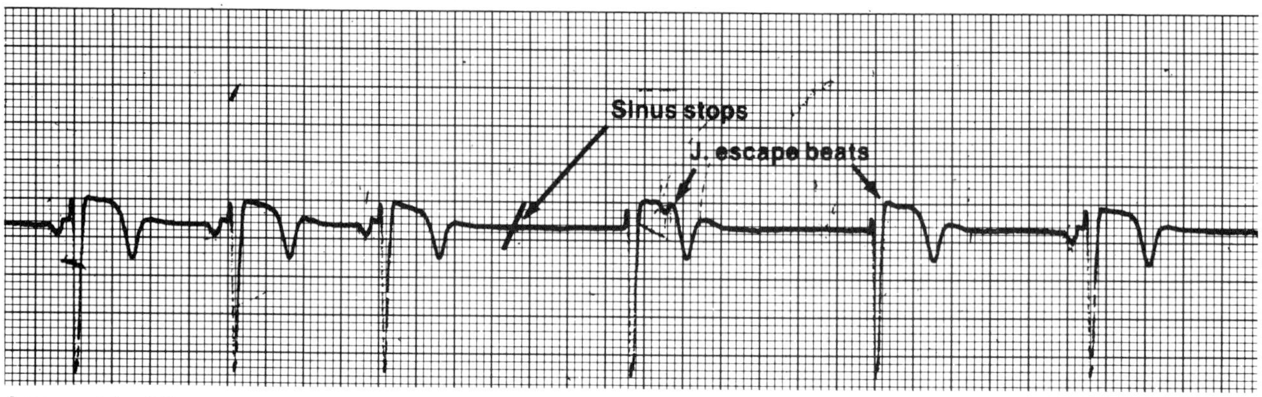

Answer strip A-3

RHYTHM: *Irregular due to pauses and late beats*

RATE: *Sinus, 75; Overall, 60*

P WAVES: *Present in sinus beats, missing in late beats*

PR INTERVAL: *0.14 second*

QRS COMPLEX: *0.10 second*

INTERPRETATION: *Sinus rhythm with third-degree SA block (sinus arrest) and junctional escape beats*

THERAPY: *Observe patient. Administer atropine if needed.*

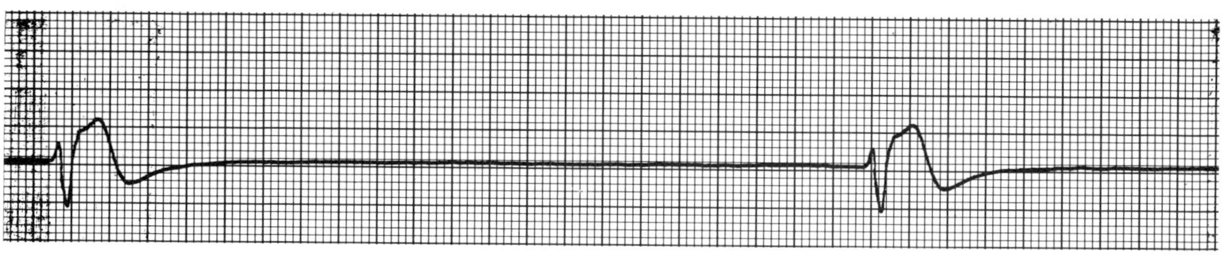

Answer strip A-4

RHYTHM: *Regular ?*

RATE: *Around 10*

P WAVES: *None*

PR INTERVAL: *None*

QRS COMPLEX: *0.16 second, wide and bizarre*

INTERPRETATION: *Secondary ventricular standstill (E.M.D.)*

THERAPY: *Code Blue; CPR; pacemaker; calcium chloride*

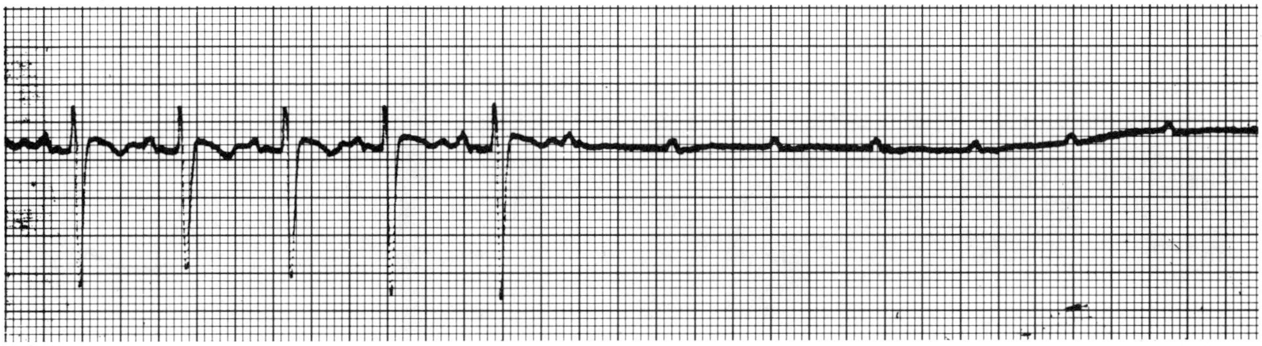

Answer strip A-5

RHYTHM: *Regular*

RATE: *Sinus, 110; ventricular, 110 → 0*

P WAVES: *Present—stop conducting*

PR INTERVAL: *0.18 second*

QRS COMPLEX: *0.10 second*

INTERPRETATION: *Sinus tachycardia → Primary ventricular standstill*

THERAPY: *CPR; Code Blue; pacemaker*

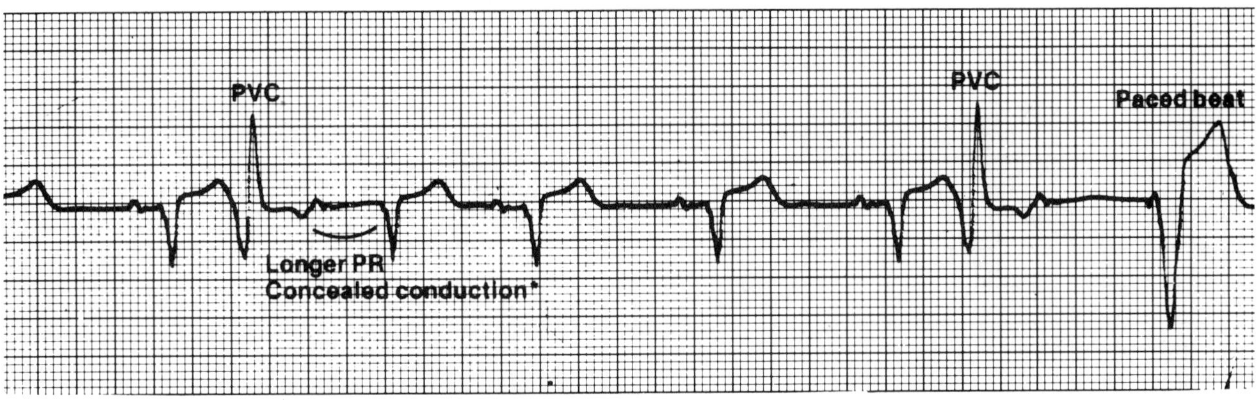

Answer strip A-6

RHYTHM: *Irregular due to premature beats, pauses, late beat*

RATE: *Sinus, 65*

P WAVES: *Present—none in premature beats or late beat*

PR INTERVAL: *0.16 second*

QRS COMPLEX: *0.12 second; premature and late beats, wide and bizarre*

INTERPRETATION: *NSR with unifocal PVCs. Pacer fires and captures in compensatory pause.*

THERAPY: *Lidocaine*

*Concealed conduction is shown when the PR of the sinus beat following an early beat is longer than normal. The early beat penetrates the AV node, causing it to have a longer refractory period.

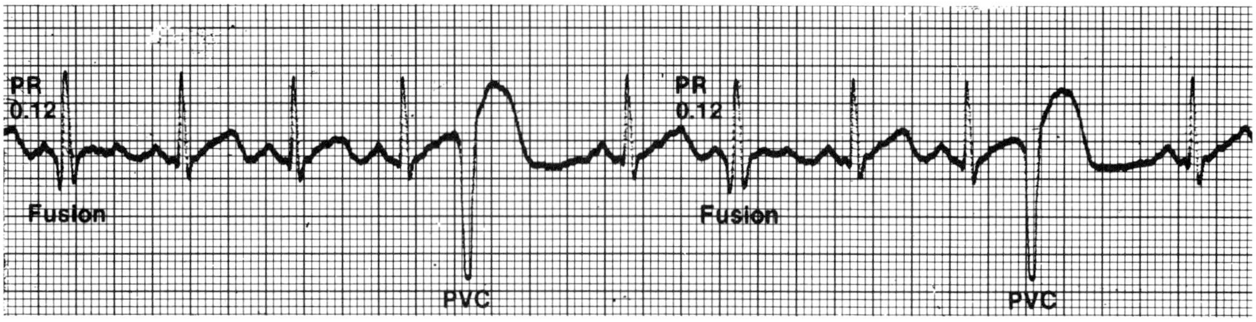

Answer strip A-7

RHYTHM: *Irregular due to premature beats*

RATE: *Sinus, 100*

P WAVES: *Present—none in premature beats*

PR INTERVAL: *0.16 second*

QRS COMPLEX: *0.08 second, wide and bizarre in premature beats*

INTERPRETATION: *NSR (or sinus tachycardia) with PVCs and fusion beats*

THERAPY: *Lidocaine*

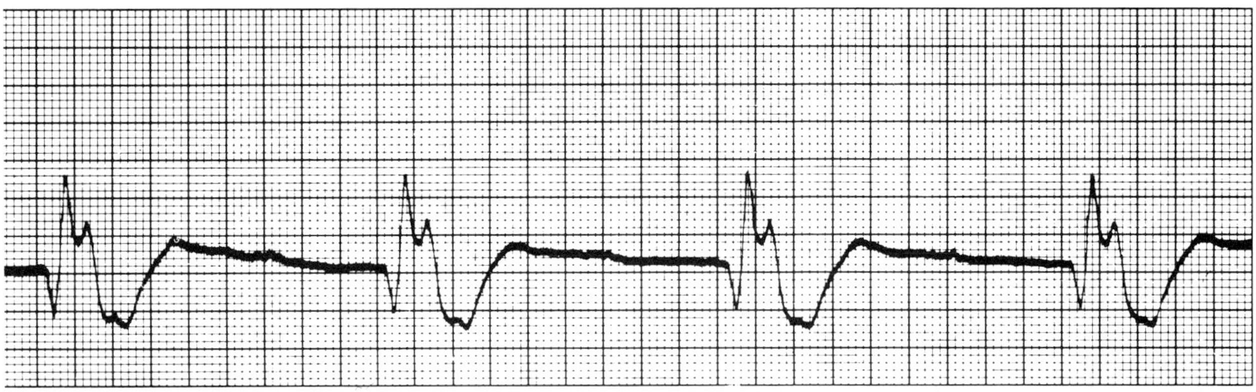

Answer strip A-8

RHYTHM: *Regular*

RATE: *33*

P WAVES: *None*

PR INTERVAL: *None*

QRS COMPLEX: *0.22 second*

INTERPRETATION: *Ventricular rhythm*

THERAPY: *Isoproterenol; pacemaker*

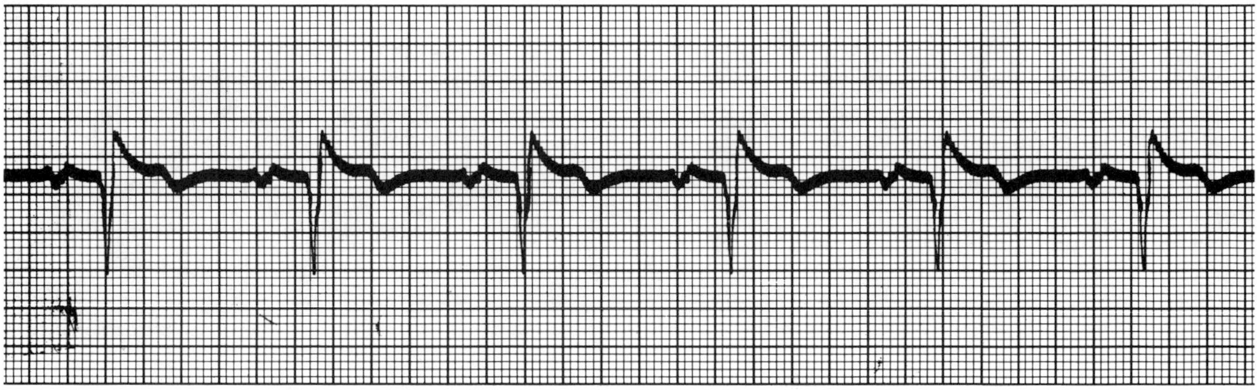

Answer strip A-9

RHYTHM: *Regular*

RATE: *56*

P WAVES: *Normal*

PR INTERVAL: *0.28 second*

QRS COMPLEX: *0.06 second*

INTERPRETATION: *Sinus bradycardia with first-degree AV block*

THERAPY: *Observe patient; administer atropine if rate slows.*

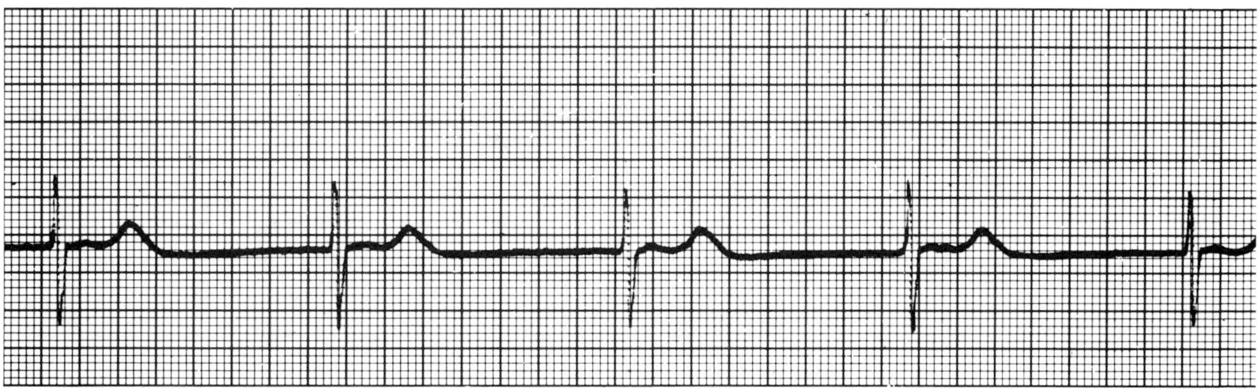

Answer strip A-10

RHYTHM: *Regular*

RATE: *40*

P WAVES: *None*

PR INTERVAL: *None*

QRS COMPLEX: *0.08 second*

INTERPRETATION: *Junctional rhythm*

THERAPY: *Atropine; pacemaker*

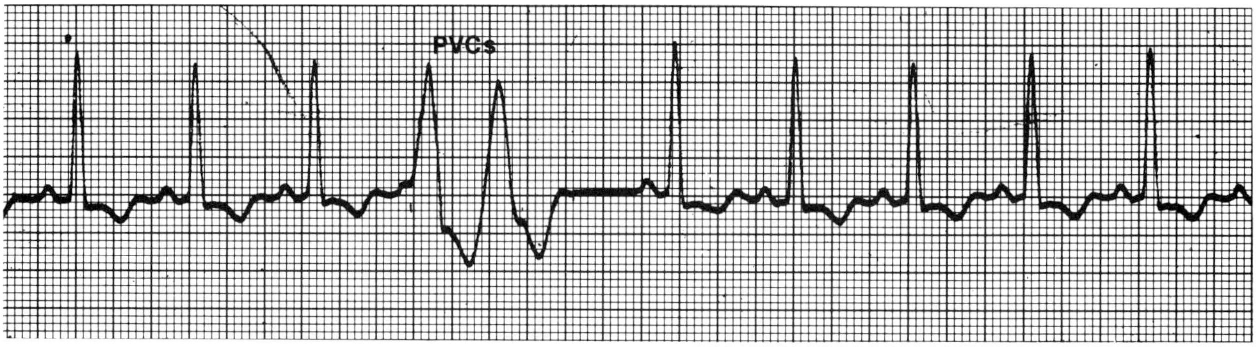

Answer strip A-11

RHYTHM: *Irregular due to premature beats*

RATE: *Sinus, 95*

P WAVES: *Present—none in premature beats*

PR INTERVAL: *0.18 second*

QRS COMPLEX: *0.08 second, wide and bizarre in early beats*

INTERPRETATION: *NSR with paired PVCs*

THERAPY: *Lidocaine*

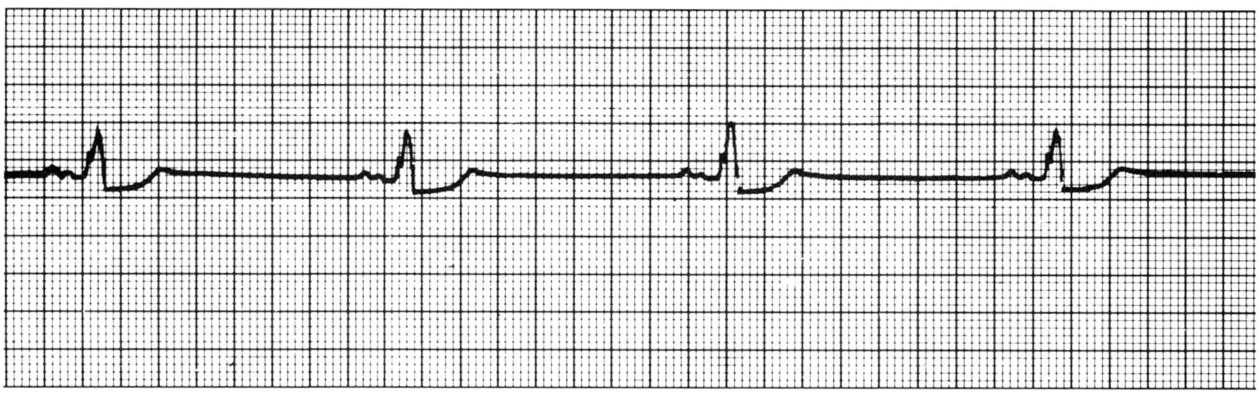

Answer strip A-12

RHYTHM: *Regular*

RATE: *40*

P WAVES: *Normal*

PR INTERVAL: *0.20 second*

QRS COMPLEX: *0.14 second*

INTERPRETATION: *Sinus bradycardia with bundle branch block (BBB)*

THERAPY: *Atropine; isoproterenol; pacemaker*

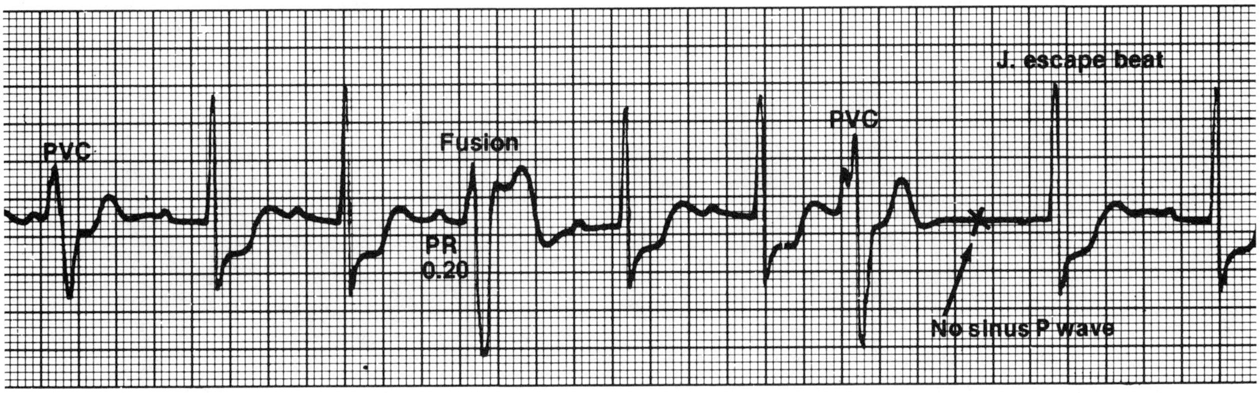

Answer strip A-13

RHYTHM: *Irregular due to premature beats, pauses, late beat.*

RATE: *Sinus, 85*

P WAVES: *Present—none with early or late beats*

PR INTERVAL: *0.24 second*

QRS COMPLEX: *0.10 second, wide and bizarre in early beats*

INTERPRETATION: *NSR with first-degree AV block, multifocal PVCs, fusion beats, third-degree SA block (sinus arrest), and junctional escape beat*

THERAPY: *Check digitalis and K^+ levels; Dilantin; lidocaine*

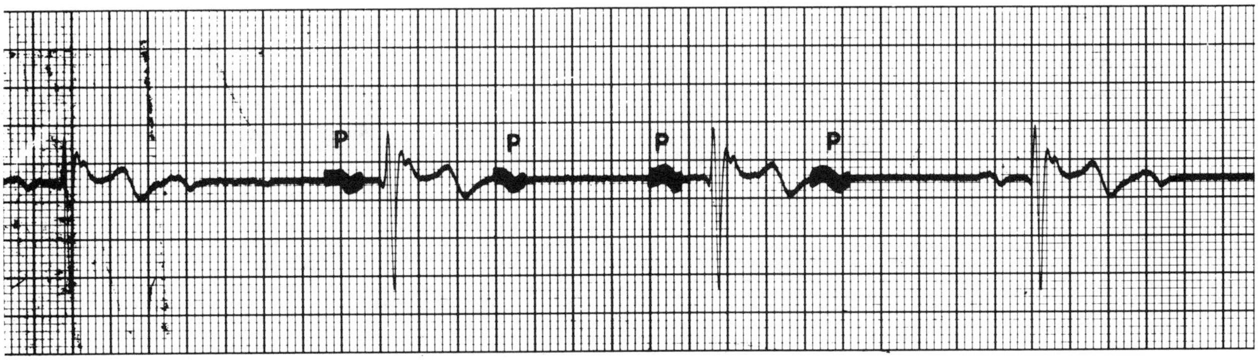

Answer strip A-14

RHYTHM: *Regular*

RATE: *Sinus, 70; ventricular, 35*

P WAVES: *Present—every other one not conducted*

PR INTERVAL: *0.26 second*

QRS COMPLEX: *0.14 second*

INTERPRETATION: *NSR with second-degree AV block, type II, 2:1 conduction and BBB*

THERAPY: *Atropine; isoproterenol; pacemaker*

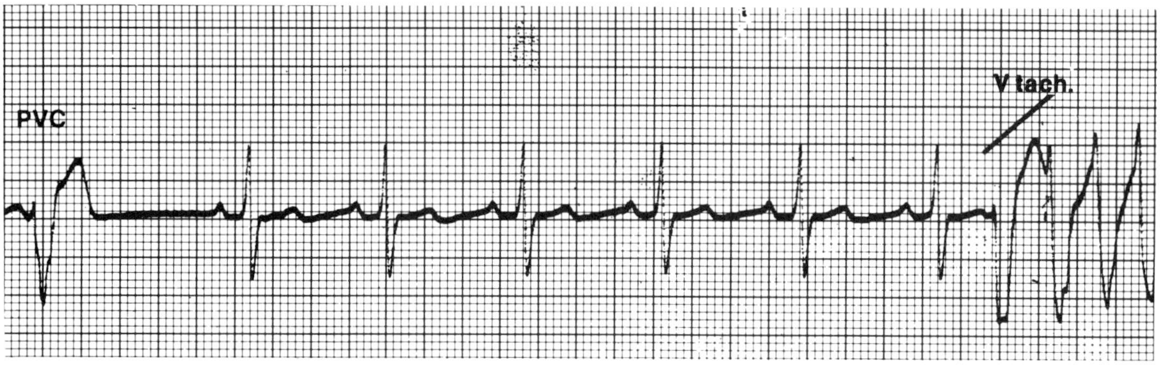

Answer strip A-15

RHYTHM: *Irregular due to premature beats and tachycardia*

RATE: *Sinus, 85*

P WAVES: *Present—none in premature beats*

PR INTERVAL: *0.16 second*

QRS COMPLEX: *0.12 second, wide and bizarre in early beats.*

INTERPRETATION: *NSR with PVC and short run of ventricular tachycardia*

THERAPY: *Lidocaine*

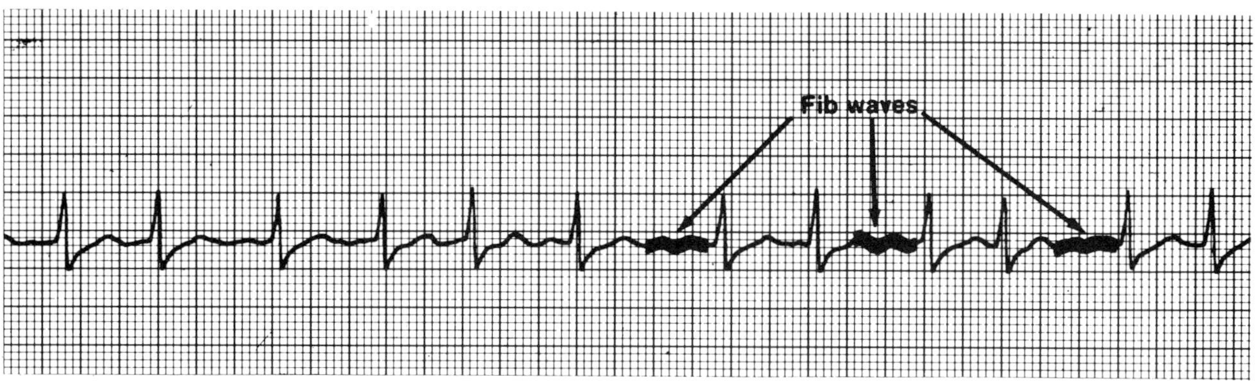

Answer strip A-16

RHYTHM: *Totally irregular*

RATE: *Ventricular, 110*

P WAVES: *None—fibrillation waves (fine)*

PR INTERVAL: *None*

QRS COMPLEX: *0.12 second*

INTERPRETATION: *Uncontrolled atrial fibrillation*

THERAPY: *Digitalis and a Class I agent or verapamil; cardioversion*

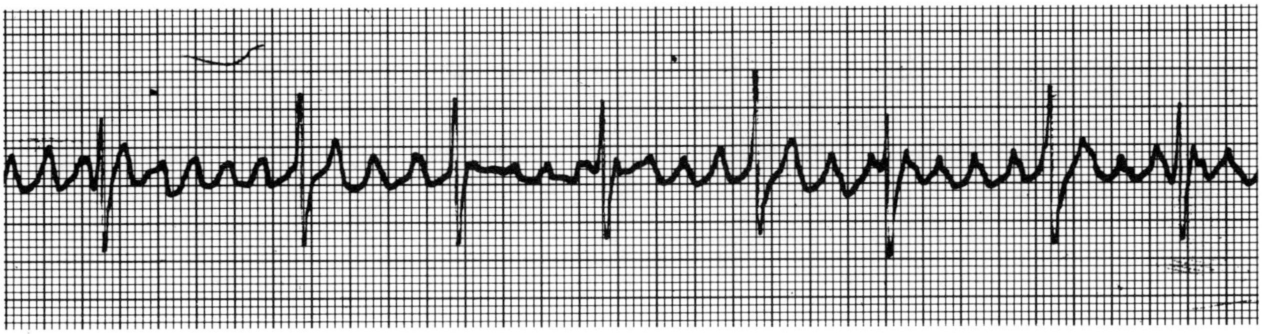

Answer strip A-17

RHYTHM: *Totally irregular*

RATE: *Ventricular, 80*

P WAVES: *None—fibrillation waves (coarse)*

PR INTERVAL: *None*

QRS COMPLEX: *0.08 second*

INTERPRETATION: *Controlled atrial fibrillation (fib–flutter)*

THERAPY: *Digitalis and a Class I agent; cardioversion*

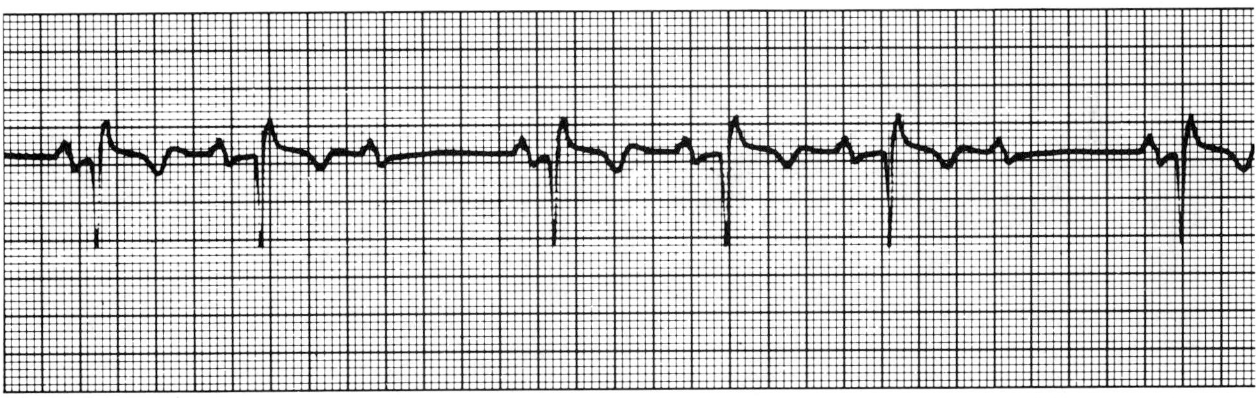

Answer strip A-18

RHYTHM: *Sinus, regular; ventricular, irregular*

RATE: *Sinus, 75; ventricular, 50*

P WAVES: *Present—some not conducted*

PR INTERVAL *Increases 0.20 → 0.24 second; QRS dropped.*

QRS COMPLEX: *0.12 second*

INTERPRETATION: *NSR with second-degree AV block, type I; Wenckebach with varying conduction*

THERAPY: *Observe for ↑ block.*

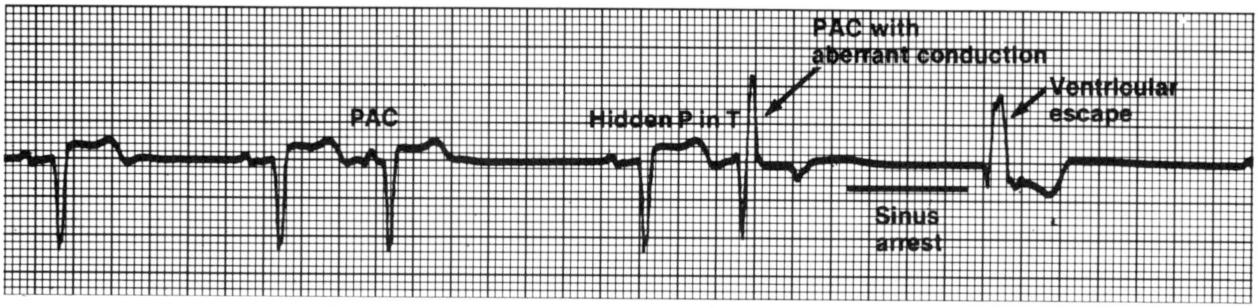

Answer strip A-19

RHYTHM: *Irregular due to premature beats, pauses, late beat*

RATE: *Sinus, 54*

P WAVES: *Present—change in shape in early beats, none in late beat*

PR INTERVAL: *0.16 second*

QRS COMPLEX: *0.08 second*

INTERPRETATION: *Sinus bradycardia with PACs (one with aberrant conduction and hidden P wave) and sinus arrest (third-degree SA block) and ventricular escape beat*

THERAPY: *Check digitalis and* K^+ *levels; atropine*

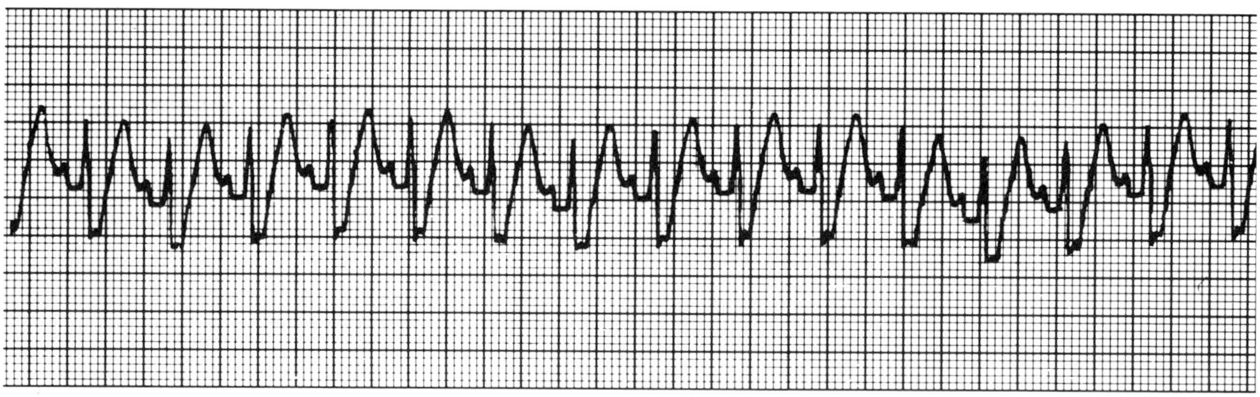

Answer strip A-20

RHYTHM: *Regular*

RATE: *145*

P WAVES: *Normal*

PR INTERVAL: *0.12 second*

QRS COMPLEX: *0.10 second*

INTERPRETATION: *Sinus tachycardia*

THERAPY: *Find cause and treat*

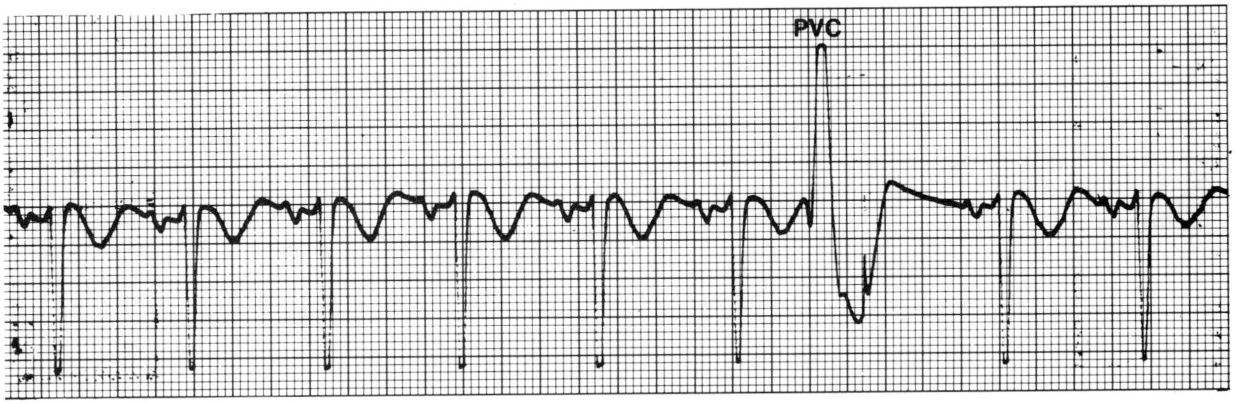

Answer strip A-21

RHYTHM: *Irregular due to one early beat*

RATE: *Sinus, 85*

P WAVES: *Present—none with early beat*

PR INTERVAL: *0.18 second*

QRS COMPLEX: *0.12 second, wide and bizarre in early beat*

INTERPRETATION: *NSR with one PVC*

THERAPY: *Lidocaine*

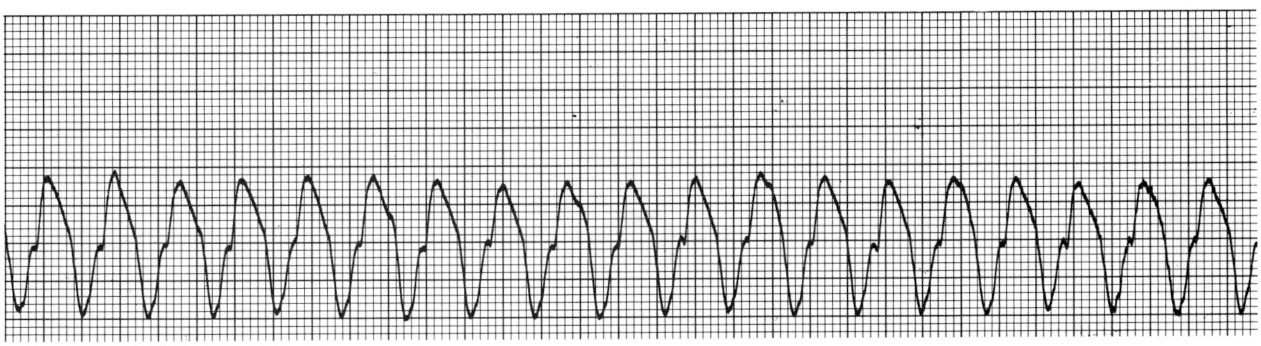

Answer strip A-22

RHYTHM: *Slightly irregular*

RATE: *210*

P WAVES: *None visible*

PR INTERVAL: —

QRS COMPLEX: *Wide and bizarre, change in configuration*

INTERPRETATION: *Ventricular tachycardia*

THERAPY: *Lidocaine; cardioversion*

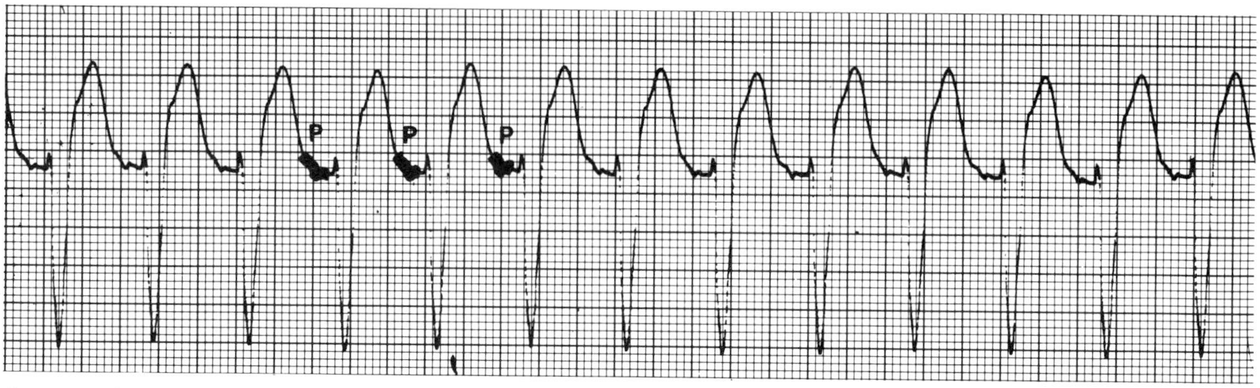

Answer strip A-23

RHYTHM: *Regular*

RATE: *125*

P WAVES: *Present at end of preceding T wave*

PR INTERVAL: *0.14 second*

QRS COMPLEX: *0.16 second*

INTERPRETATION: *Sinus tachycardia with BBB*

THERAPY: *Find cause and treat*

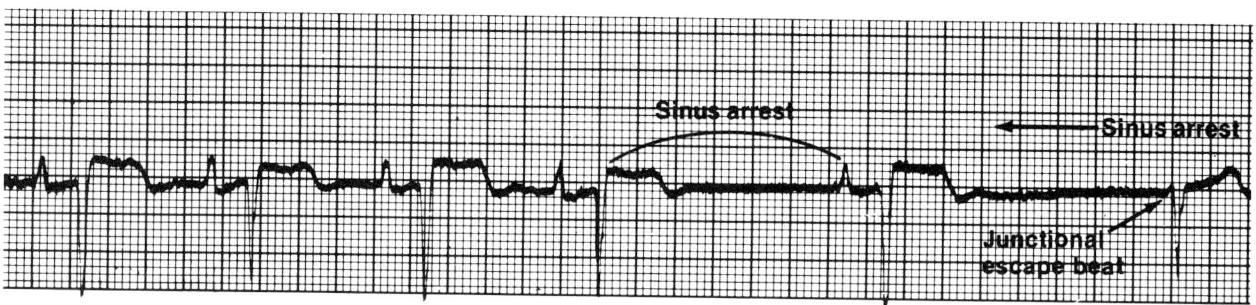

Answer strip A-24

RHYTHM: *Irregular due to pauses and late beats*

RATE: *Sinus, 66; Overall, 50*

P WAVES: *Present in first of strip, none with late beats*

PR INTERVAL: *0.20 second*

QRS COMPLEX: *0.10 second*

INTERPRETATION: *NSR with third-degree SA block (sinus arrests) and junctional escape beat*

THERAPY: *Atropine*

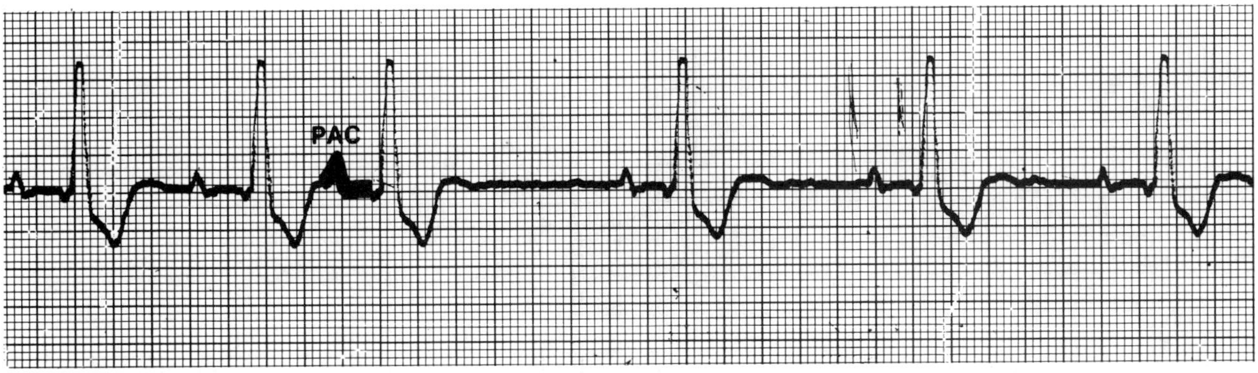

Answer strip A-25

RHYTHM: *Irregular due to early beats and slowing of SA*

RATE: *63 → 45*

P WAVES: *Present—changes before early beat*

PR INTERVAL: *0.26 second*

QRS COMPLEX: *0.16 second*

INTERPRETATION: *NSR with first-degree AV block and BBB with one PAC causing sinus bradycardia*

THERAPY: *Observe patient for ↑ suppression or block.*

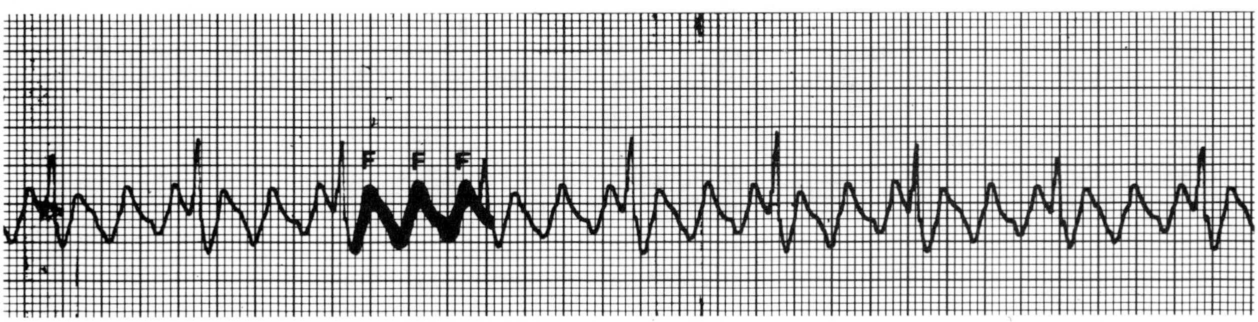

Answer strip A-26

RHYTHM: *Regular*

RATE: *Atrial, 270; ventricular, 80*

P WAVES: *None—flutter waves*

PR INTERVAL: *None*

QRS COMPLEX: *0.08 second*

INTERPRETATION: *Atrial flutter with 3:1 conduction*

THERAPY: *Digitalis and a Class I agent; cardioversion*

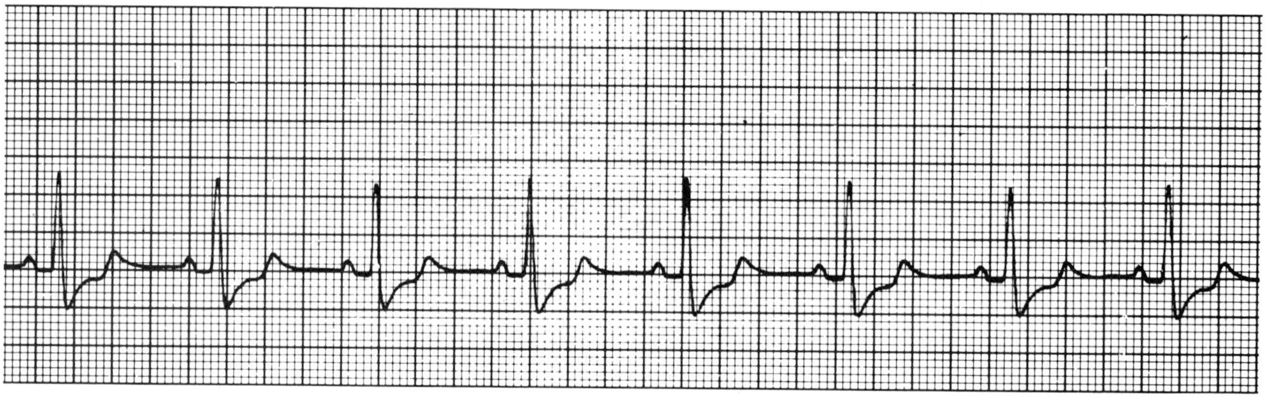

Answer strip A-27

RHYTHM: *Regular*

RATE: *72*

P WAVES: *Normal*

PR INTERVAL: *0.16 second*

QRS COMPLEX: *0.10 second*

INTERPRETATION: *NSR*

THERAPY: *None*

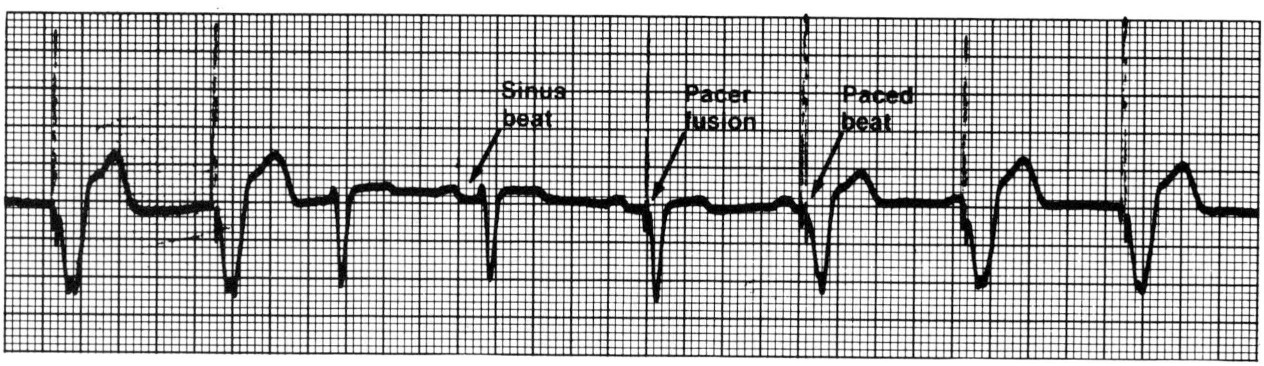

Answer strip A-28

RHYTHM: *Irregular due to change in rhythms*

RATE: *Pacer, 75*

P WAVES: *Present in sinus beats*

PR INTERVAL: *0.22 second*

QRS COMPLEX: *0.12 second, sinus; pacer, wide and bizarre*

INTERPRETATION: *Sinus rhythm with first-degree AV block and functioning demand ventricular pacemaker. (One beat is a fusion between pacer and sinus.)*

THERAPY: *None*

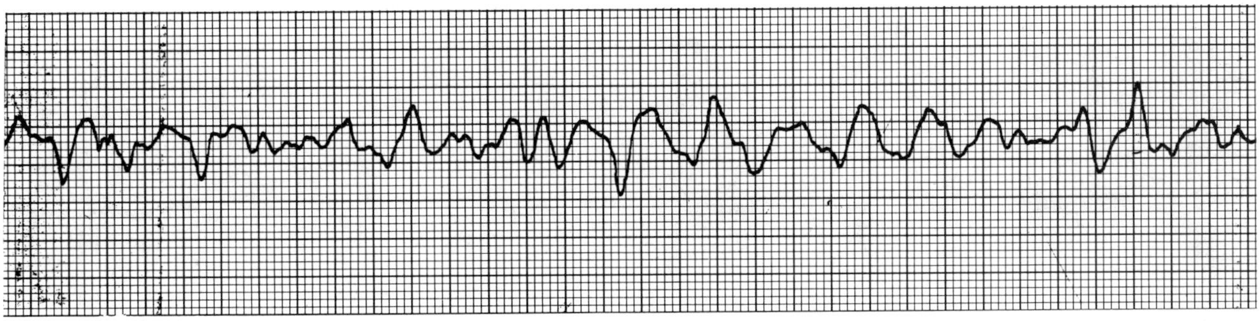

Answer strip A-29

RHYTHM: *Totally chaotic*

RATE: *?*

P WAVES: —

PR INTERVAL: —

QRS COMPLEX —

INTERPRETATION: *Ventricular fibrillation*

THERAPY: *Code Blue; CPR; defibrillation*

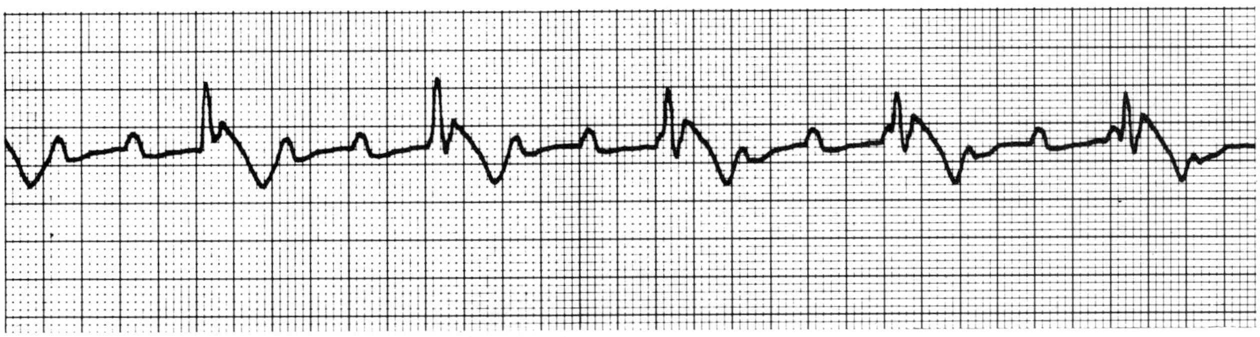

Answer strip A-30

RHYTHM: *Two regular rhythms*

RATE: *Sinus, 150; ventricular, 48*

P WAVES: *Present—none are conducted*

PR INTERVAL: *None—what appears to be a PR interval varies with each beat.*

QRS COMPLEX: *0.12 second*

INTERPRETATION: *Sinus tachycardia with third-degree AV block*

THERAPY: *Pacemaker*

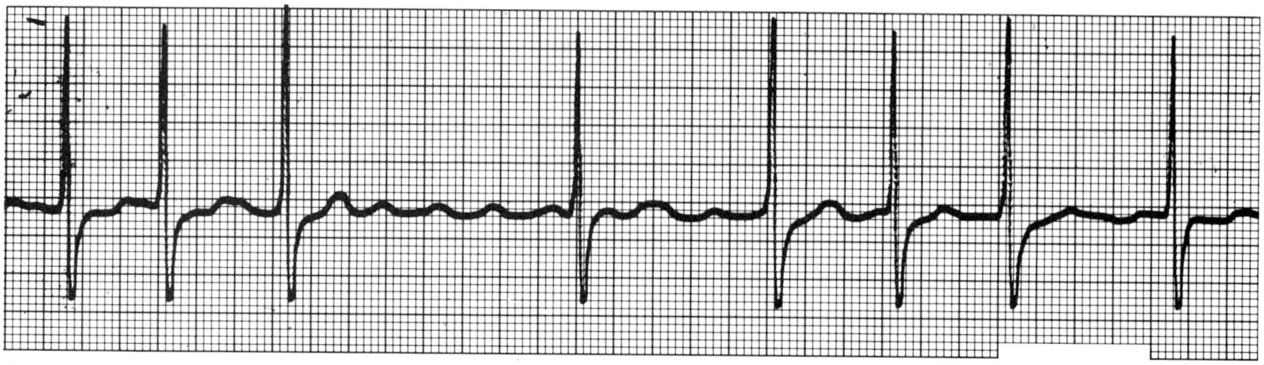

Answer strip A-31

RHYTHM: *Totally irregular*

RATE: *Ventricular, 70*

P WAVES: *None—fibrillation waves*

PR INTERVAL: *None*

QRS COMPLEX: *0.10 second*

INTERPRETATION: *Controlled atrial fibrillation*

THERAPY: *Digitalis and a Class I agent; cardioversion*

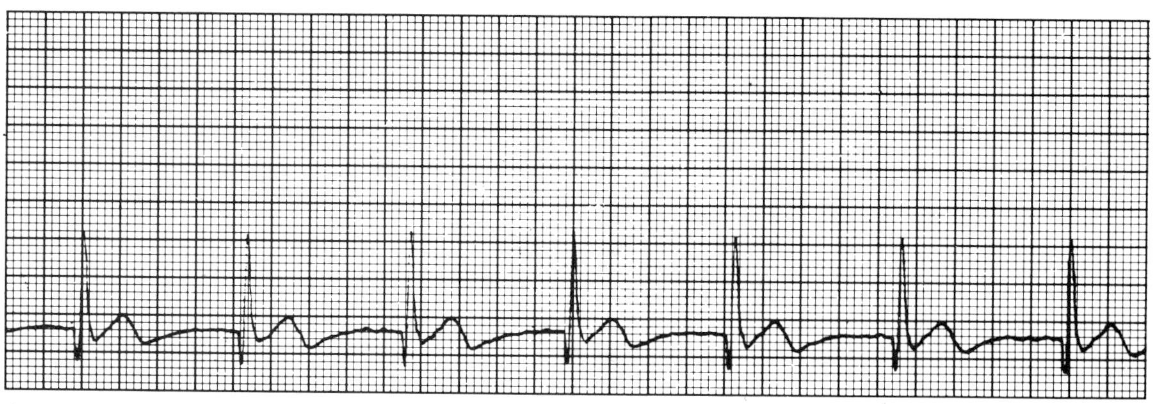

Answer strip A-32

RHYTHM: *Regular*

RATE: *69*

P WAVES: *None*

QRS COMPLEX: *0.10 second*

INTERPRETATION: *Accelerated junctional rhythm*

THERAPY: *Observe patient; atropine if rate slows*

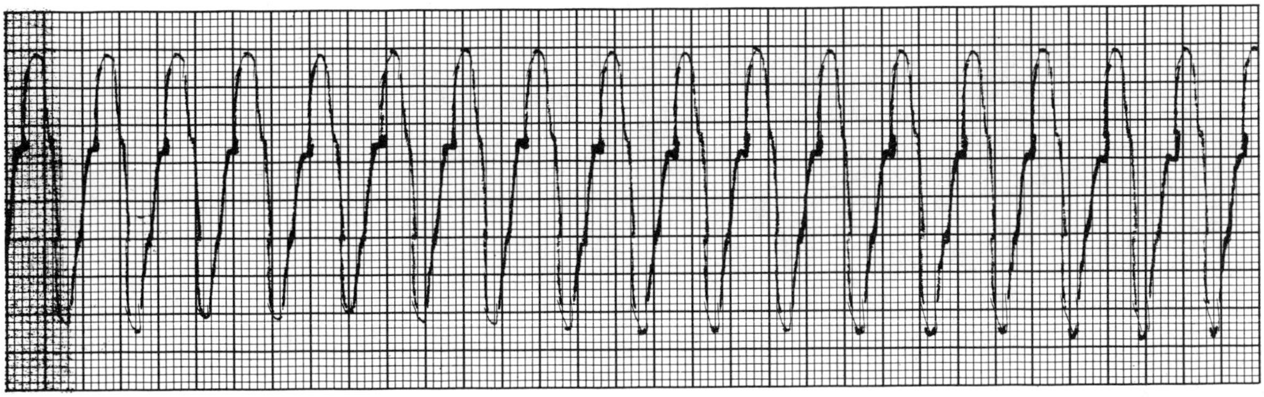

Answer strip A-33

RHYTHM: *Regular*

RATE: *150*

P WAVES: *Not visible*

PR INTERVAL: —

QRS COMPLEX: *Wide—each QRS is identical to all of the others*

INTERPRETATION: *Supraventricular tachycardia with aberration*

THERAPY: *Digitalis and a Class I agent, or verapamil; cardioversion*

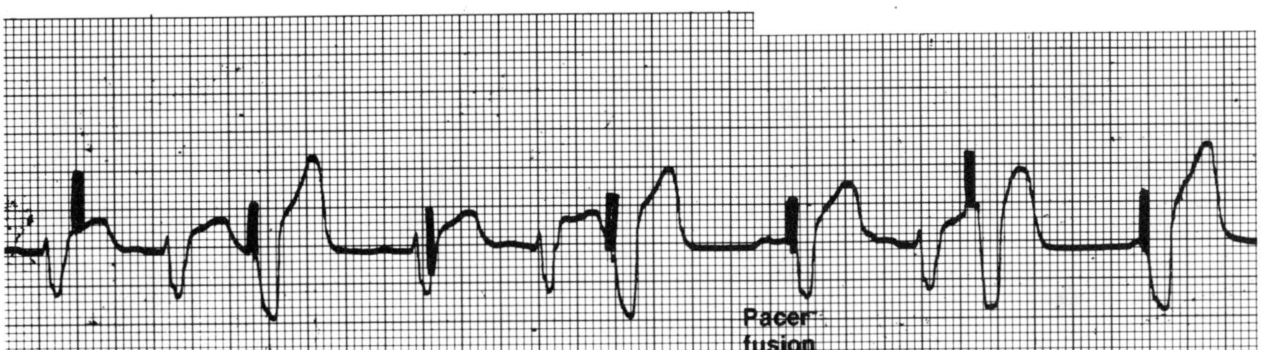

Answer strip A-34

RHYTHM: *Irregular with sinus and pacer competing*

RATE: *Sinus, 100; pacer, 68*

P WAVES: *Present in sinus beats*

PR INTERVAL: *0.20 second*

QRS COMPLEX: *0.16 second, paced beats, wide and bizarre*

INTERPRETATION: *NSR with BBB and ventricular demand pacemaker malfunction—not sensing*

THERAPY: *Turn off pacer.*

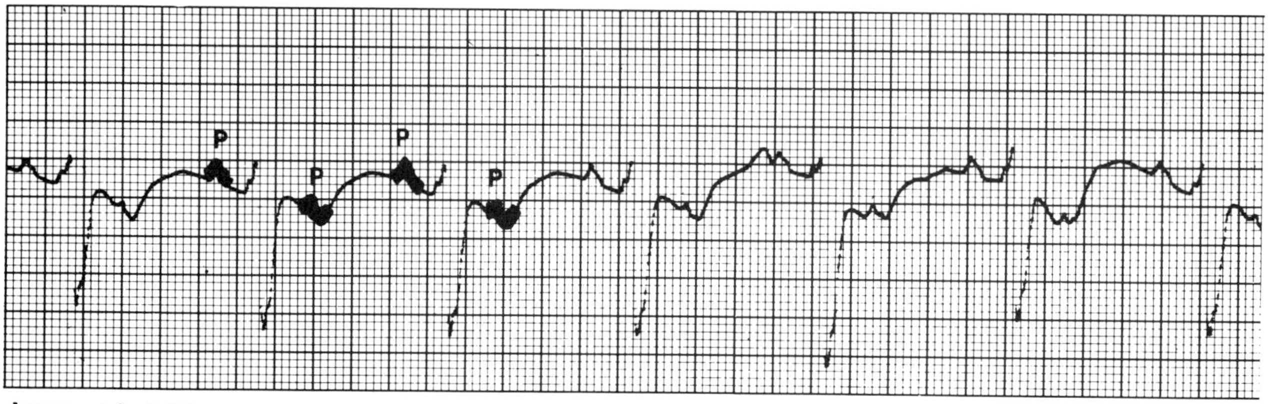

Answer strip A-35

RHYTHM: *Regular*

RATE: *Sinus, 120; ventricular, 60*

P WAVES: *Present—every other one not conducted*

PR INTERVAL: *0.20 second and constant*

QRS COMPLEX: *0.18 second*

INTERPRETATION: *Sinus tachycardia with second-degree AV block, type II 2:1 and BBB*

THERAPY: *Pacemaker*

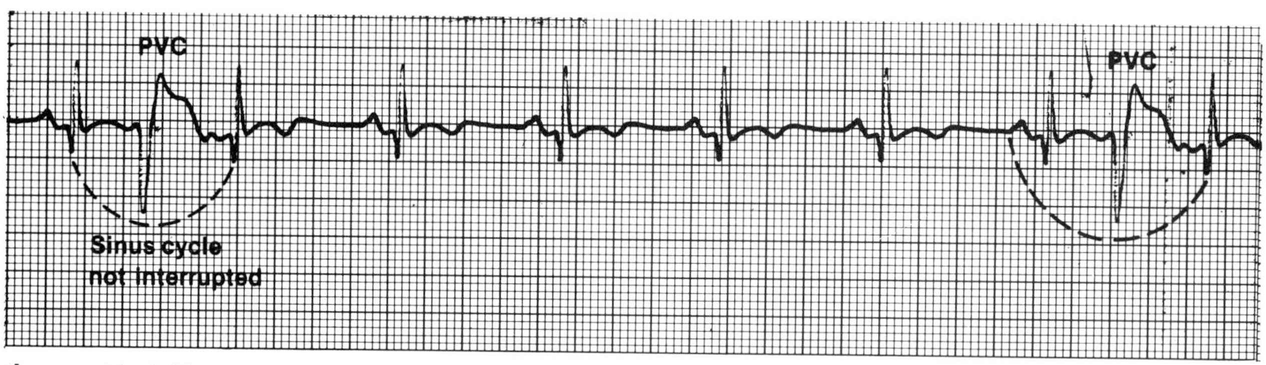

Answer strip A-36

RHYTHM: *Irregular due to premature beats*

RATE: *Sinus, 72*

P WAVES: *Present—none with early beats*

PR INTERVAL: *0.16 second*

QRS COMPLEX: *0.10 second, wide and bizarre in early beats*

INTERPRETATION: *NSR with interpolated unifocal PVCs*

THERAPY: *Lidocaine*

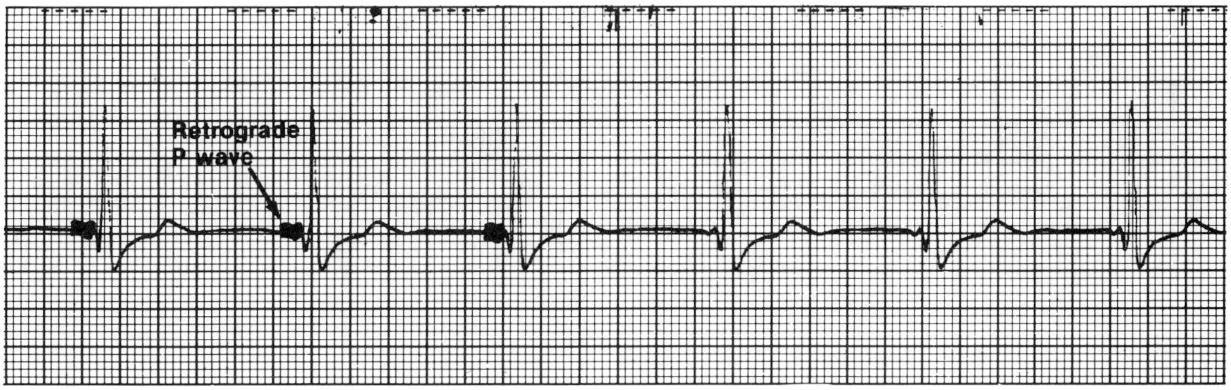

Answer strip A-37

RHYTHM: *Regular*

RATE: *56*

P WAVES: *Retrograde in front of QRS*

PR INTERVAL: *0.08 second*

QRS COMPLEX: *0.10 second*

INTERPRETATION: *Junctional rhythm*

THERAPY: *Observe patient; administer atropine if necessary.*

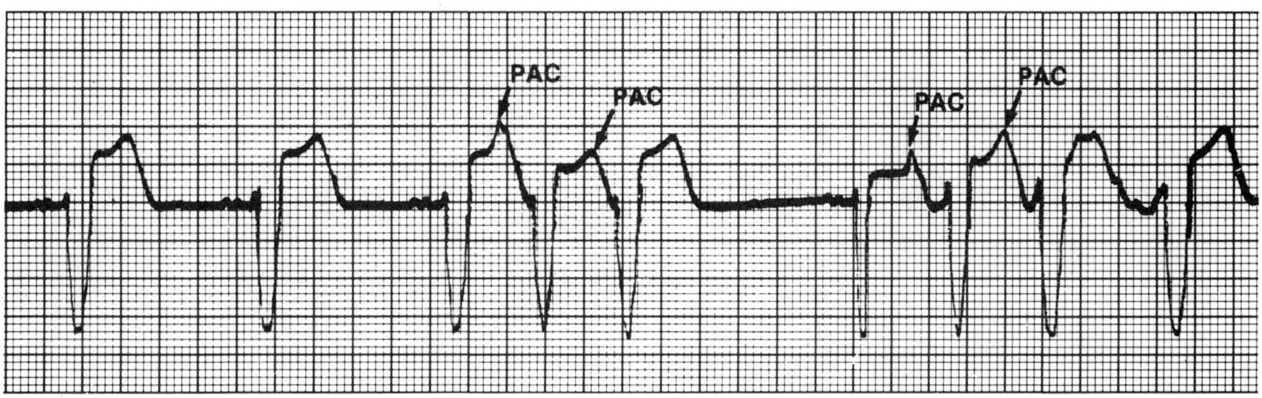

Answer strip A-38

RHYTHM: *Irregular due to premature beats*

RATE: *Sinus, 63*

P WAVES: *Present—change in shape in early beats*

PR INTERVAL: *0.18 second*

QRS COMPLEX: *0.16 second*

INTERPRETATION: *NSR with BBB with frequent PACs*

THERAPY: *Observe patient.*

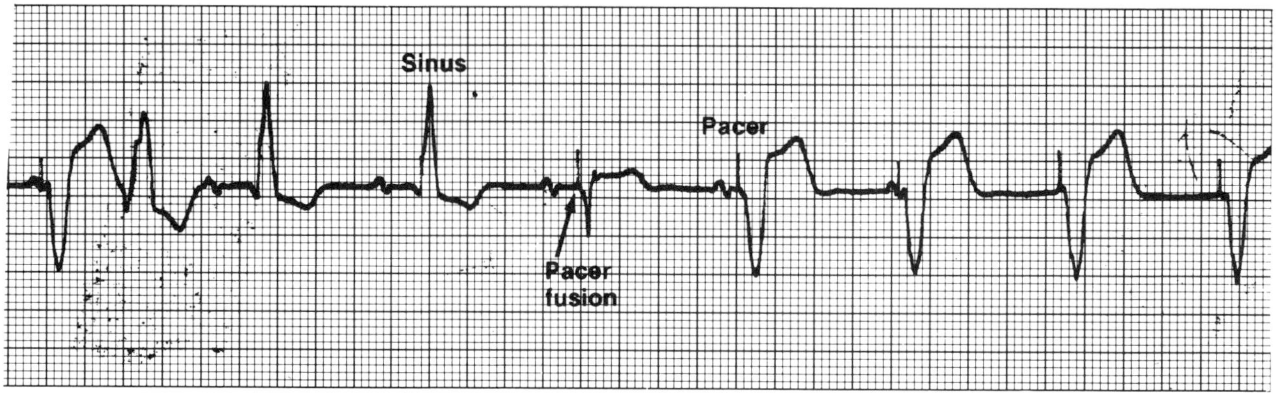

Answer strip A-39

RHYTHM: *Irregular due to pacemaker*

RATE: *Sinus, 69; pacer, 72*

P WAVES: *Present in sinus beats*

PR INTERVAL: *0.24 second*

QRS COMPLEX: *0.16 second*

INTERPRETATION: *NSR with first-degree AV block and BBB with functioning ventricular demand pacemaker*

THERAPY: *None needed*

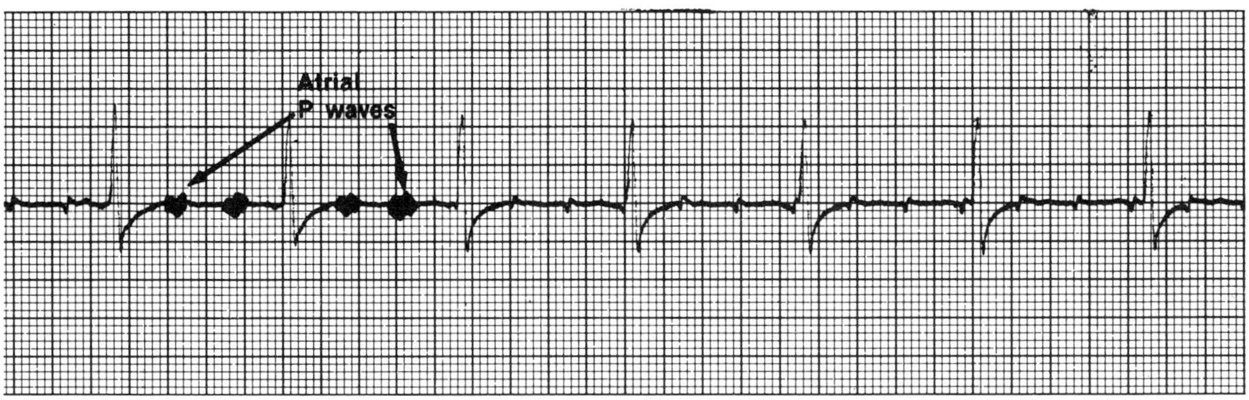

Answer strip A-40

RHYTHM: *Regular*

RATE: *Atrial, 210; ventricular, 70*

P WAVES: *Present—not all conducted*

PR INTERVAL: *0.28 second*

QRS COMPLEX: *0.06 second*

INTERPRETATION: *Atrial tachycardia with block (3:1)*

THERAPY: *Check digitalis and K^+ levels; Dilantin*

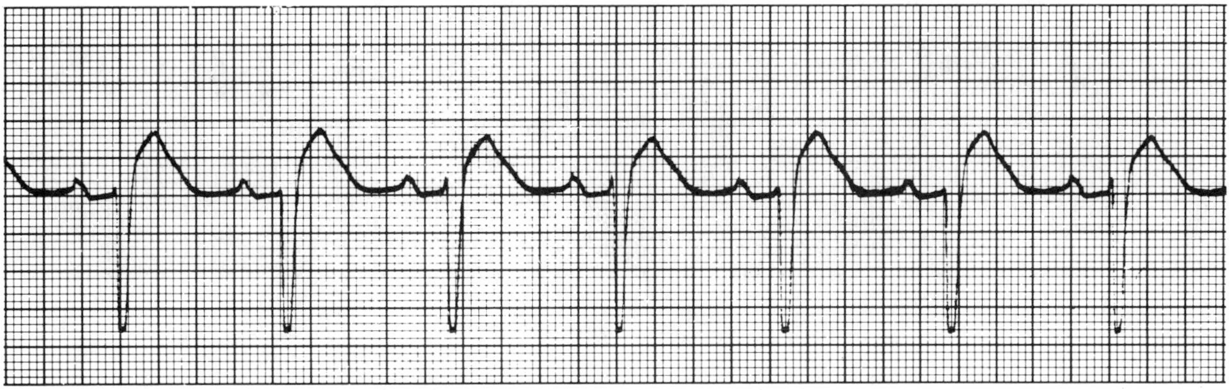

Answer strip A-41

RHYTHM: *Regular*

RATE: *69*

P WAVES: *Normal*

PR INTERVAL: *0.24 second*

QRS COMPLEX: *0.12 second*

INTERPRETATION: *NSR with first-degree AV block*

THERAPY: *Observe for ↑ block.*

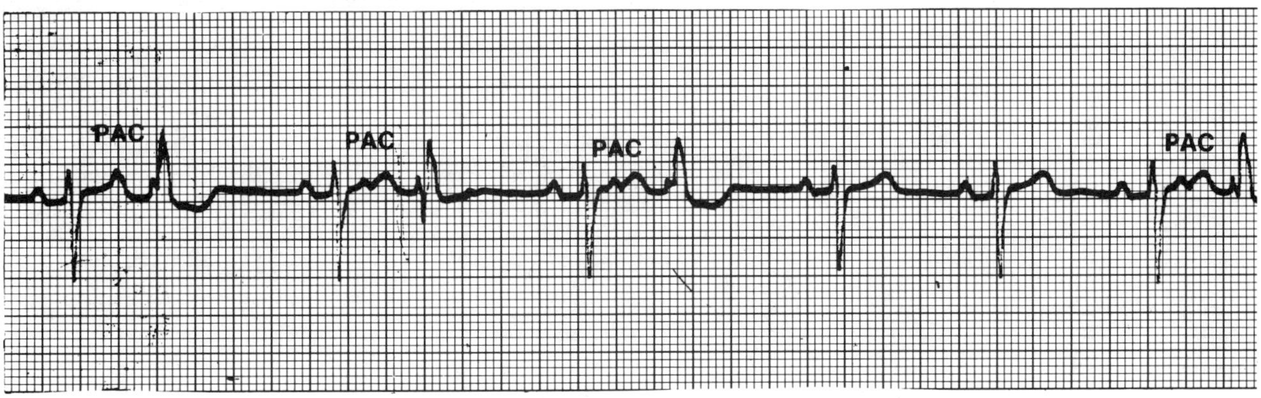

Answer strip A-42

RHYTHM: *Irregular due to early beats*

RATE: *Sinus, 72; overall, 90*

P WAVES: *Present—change in configuration in early beats*

PR INTERVAL: *0.16 second*

QRS COMPLEX: *0.10 second, early beats—wide and bizarre*

INTERPRETATION: *NSR with frequent PACs with aberrant ventricular conduction*

THERAPY: *Observe patient.*

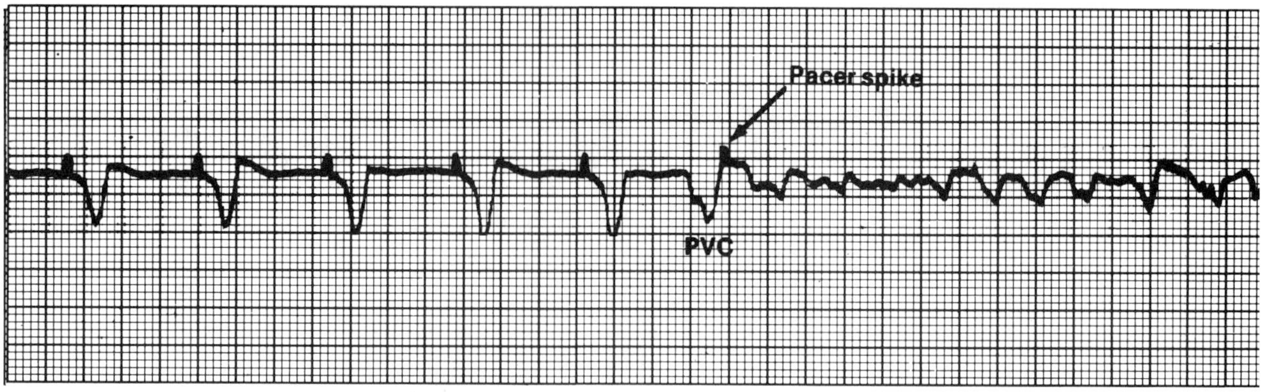

Answer strip A-43

RHYTHM: *Regular with an early beat then totally chaotic*

RATE: *Pacer, 90*

P WAVES: *None*

PR INTERVAL: *None*

QRS COMPLEX: *Wide, bizarre pacer complexes—early beat, wide and bizarre*

INTERPRETATION: *Ventricular demand pacer not sensing—fires on T wave of PVC → ventricular fibrillation*

THERAPY: *Code Blue; CPR; defibrillation; fix pacer malfunction*

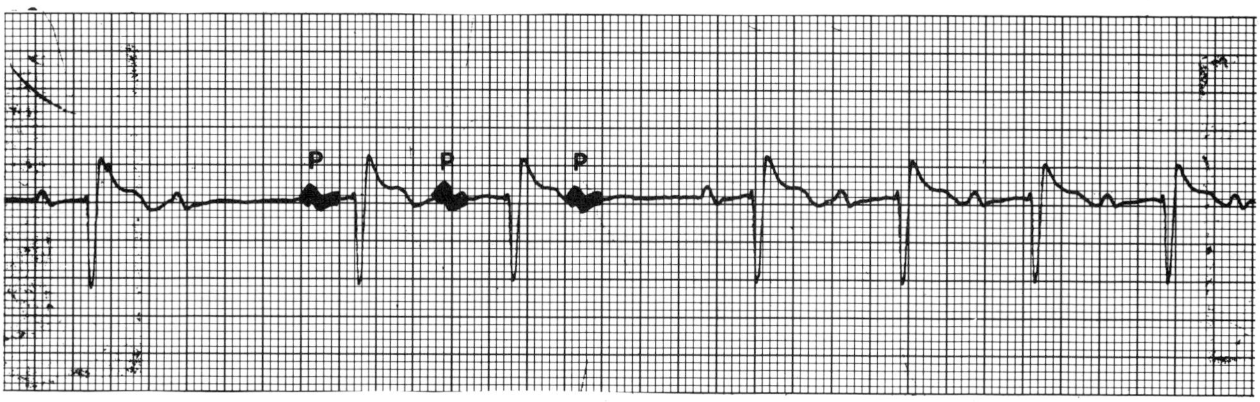

Answer strip A-44

RHYTHM: *Sinus, regular; ventricular, irregular due to pauses and changing P.R.*

RATE: *Sinus, 90; ventricular, 65*

P WAVES: *Present—not all are conducted*

PR INTERVAL: *Increases 0.26→0.36 second until beat is dropped*

QRS COMPLEX: *0.12 second*

INTERPRETATION: *NSR with second-degree AV block, type I (Wenkebach with varying conduction)*

THERAPY: *Observe for ↑ block*

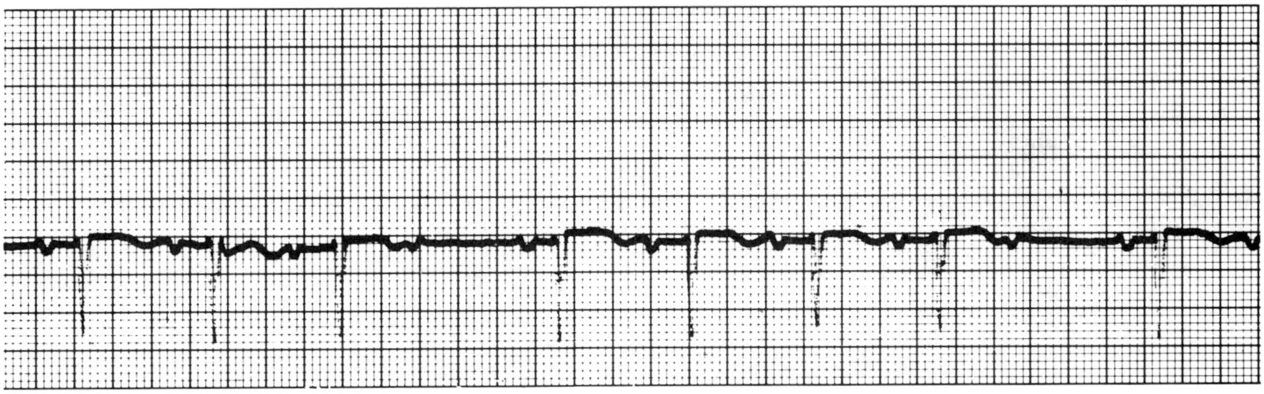

Answer strip A-45

RHYTHM: *Sinus, slightly irregular; ventricular, irregular*

RATE: *Sinus, 95*

P WAVES: *Present—not all conducted*

PR INTERVAL: *Increases 0.22 → 0.26 second until beat is dropped*

QRS COMPLEX: *0.08 second*

INTERPRETATION: *NSR with second-degree AV block, type I (Wenckebach) with varying conduction*

THERAPY: *Observe for ↑ block.*

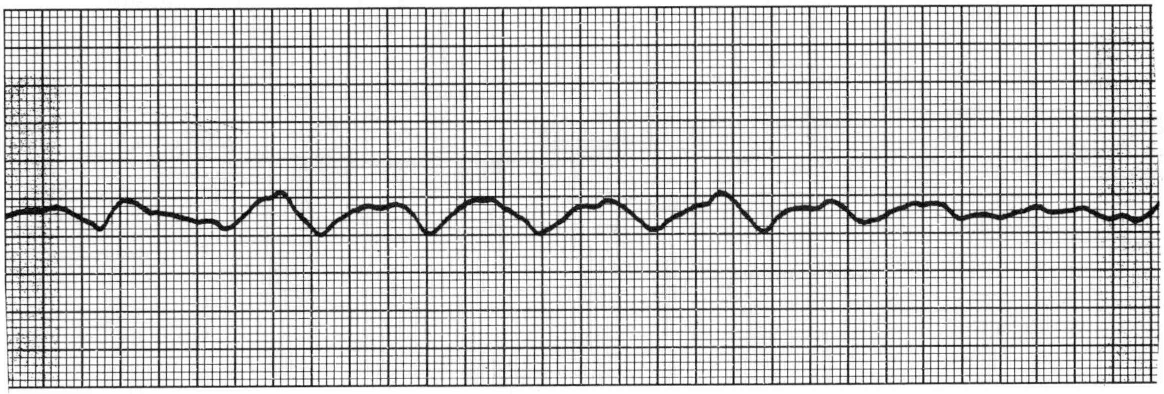

Answer strip A-46

RHYTHM: *Irregular*

RATE: *None*

P WAVES: *None*

PR INTERVAL: *None*

QRS COMPLEX: *Wide, irregular waveforms*

INTERPRETATION: *Agonal rhythm*

THERAPY: *Code Blue; CPR*

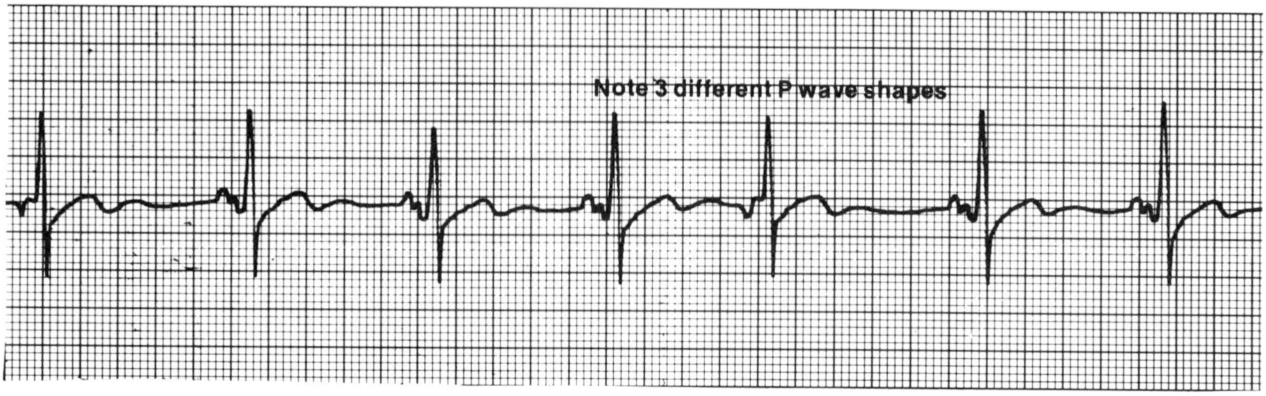

Answer strip A-47

RHYTHM: *Irregular due to changing rate of pacing cells*

RATE: *60*

P WAVES: *Present—changes configuration.*

PR INTERVAL: *0.16 second, changes as P wave changes*

QRS COMPLEX: *0.08 second*

INTERPRETATION: *Wandering atrial pacemaker*

THERAPY: *Observe patient*

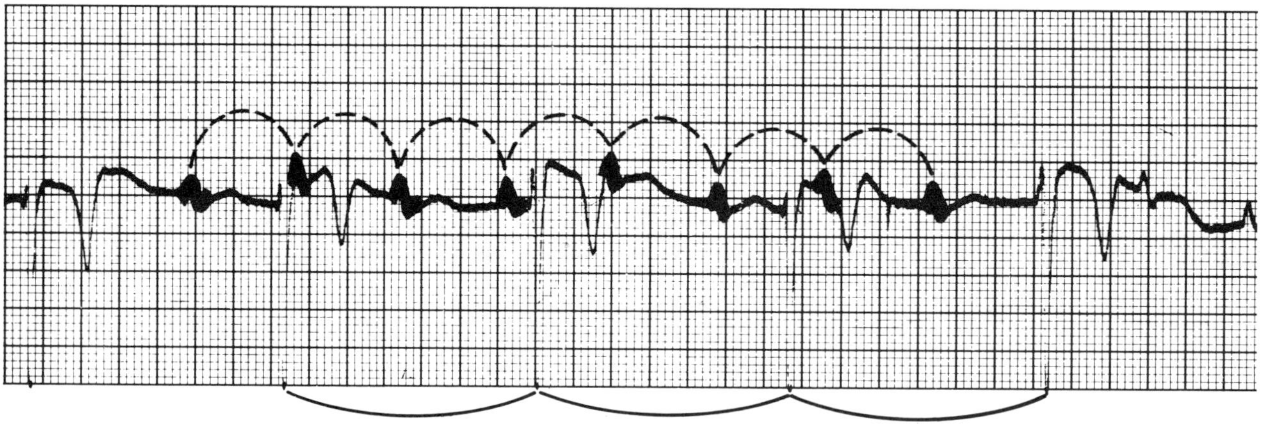

Answer strip A-48

RHYTHM: *Sinus, regular; ventricular, regular*

RATE: *Sinus, 110; ventricular, 45*

P WAVES: *Present—none are conducted*

PR INTERVAL: *Varies with each QRS*

QRS COMPLEX: *0.10 second*

INTERPRETATION: *Sinus tachycardia with third-degree AV block*

THERAPY: *Pacemaker*

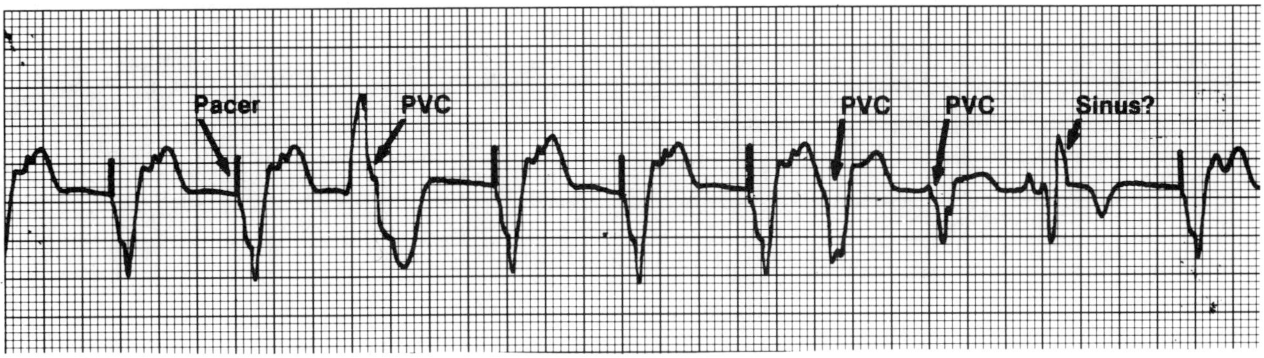

Answer strip A-49

RHYTHM: *Irregular due to pacer and early beats*

RATE: *Pacemaker, 95*

P WAVES: *None visible except one*

PR INTERVAL: —

QRS COMPLEX: *0.16 second pacer—early beats, wide and bizarre*

INTERPRETATION: *Functioning ventricular demand pacemaker with PVCs*

THERAPY: *Lidocaine*

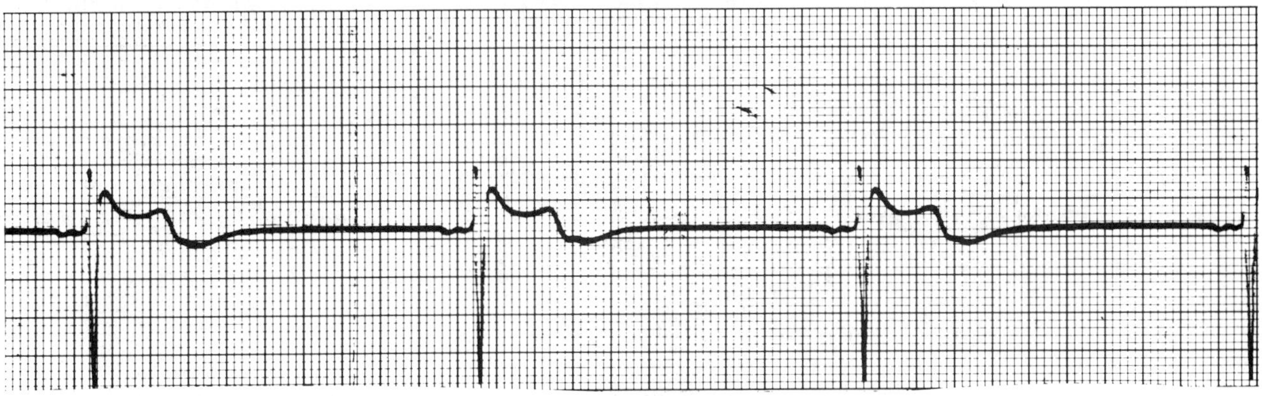

Answer strip A-50

RHYTHM: *Regular*

RATE: *30*

P WAVES: *Normal*

PR INTERVAL: *0.18 second*

QRS COMPLEX: *0.10 second*

INTERPRETATION: *Sinus bradycardia*

THERAPY: *Atropine; pacemaker*

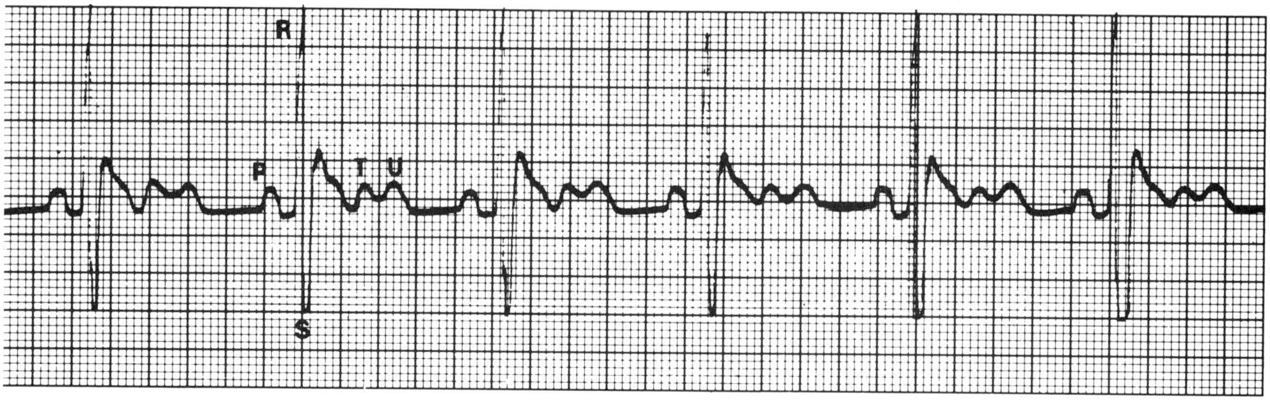

Answer strip A-51

RHYTHM: *Regular*

RATE: *56*

P WAVES: *Normal*

PR INTERVAL: *0.18 second*

QRS COMPLEX: *0.14 second*

INTERPRETATION: *Sinus bradycardia with BBB*

THERAPY: *Observe patient. Administer atropine if needed.*

Check K^+ level—presence of U waves can mean hypokalemia.

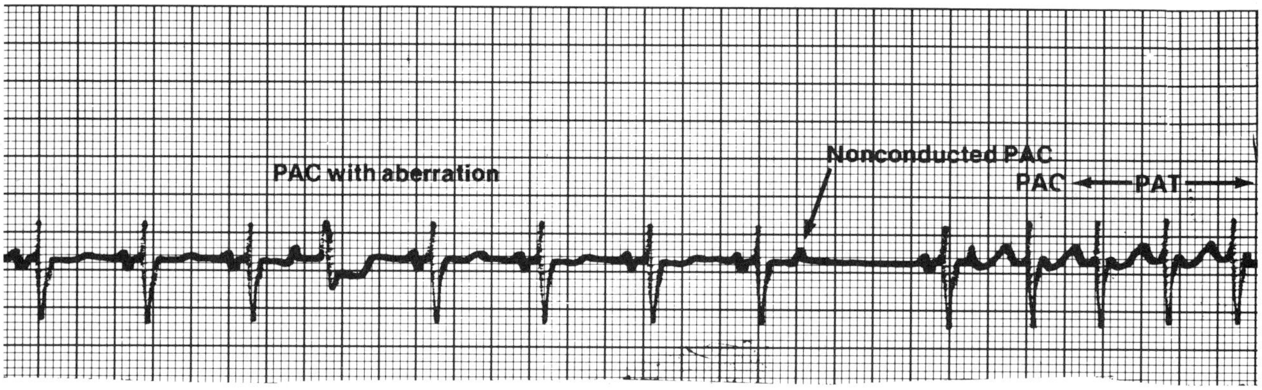

Answer strip A-52

RHYTHM: *Irregular due to early beats, pause, and tachycardia*

RATE: *Sinus, 110; tachycardia at end of strip, 180*

P WAVES: *Present—change in shape, early beats and tachycardia*

PR INTERVAL: *0.16 second*

QRS COMPLEX: *0.10 second*

INTERPRETATION: *Sinus tachycardia with PACs (one aberrant, one nonconducted) and paroxysmal atrial tachycardia (PAT)*

THERAPY: *Digitalis, and a Class I agent, or Verapamil; cardioversion*

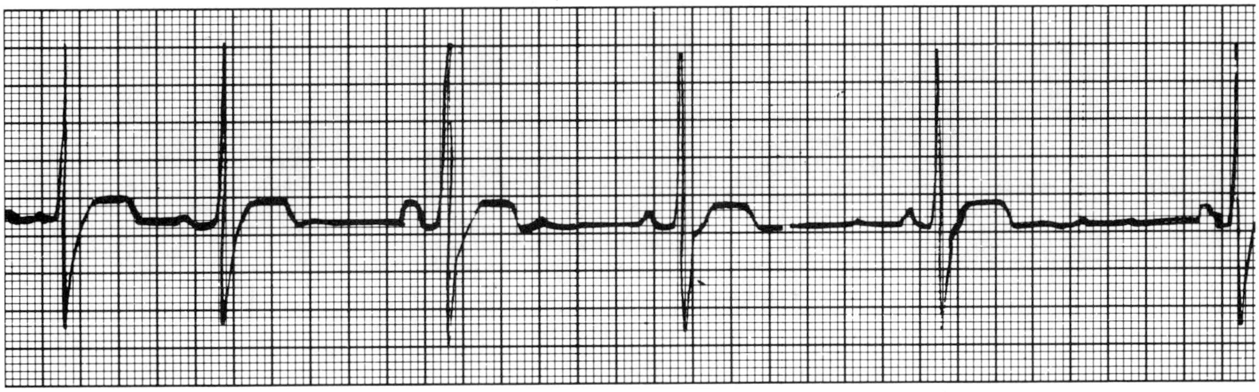

Answer strip A-53

RHYTHM: *Irregular due to changing cycle lengths*

RATE: *50*

P WAVES: *Present change in configuration*

PR INTERVAL: *Varies with each shape of P wave*

QRS COMPLEX: *0.10 second*

INTERPRETATION: *Wandering atrial pacemaker*

THERAPY: *Observe patient; administer atropine if needed*

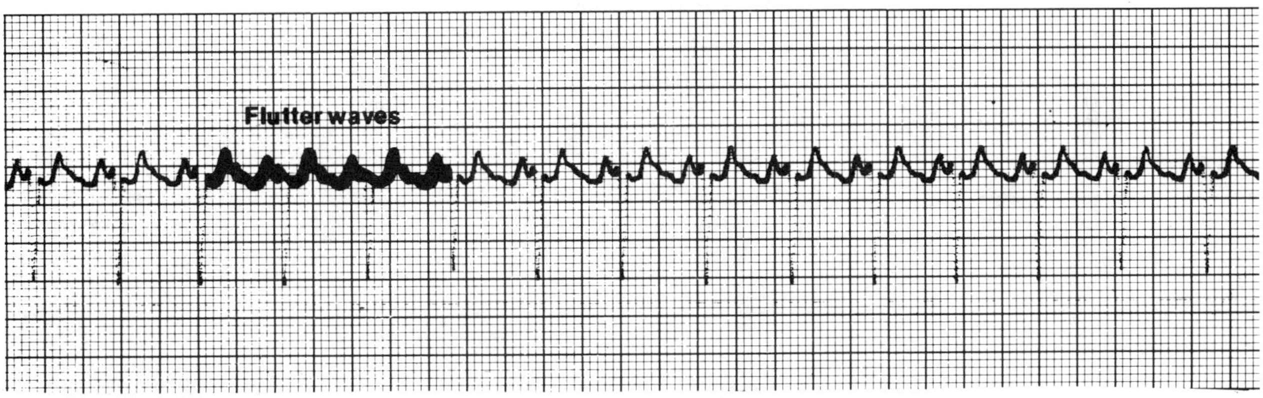

Answer strip A-54

RHYTHM: *Regular*

RATE: *Atrial, 280; ventricular, 140*

P WAVES: *None—flutter waves*

PR INTERVAL: —

QRS COMPLEX: *0.08 second*

INTERPRETATION: *Atrial flutter with 2:1 conduction*

THERAPY: *Administer digitalis and a Class I agent, or verapamil; cardioversion.*

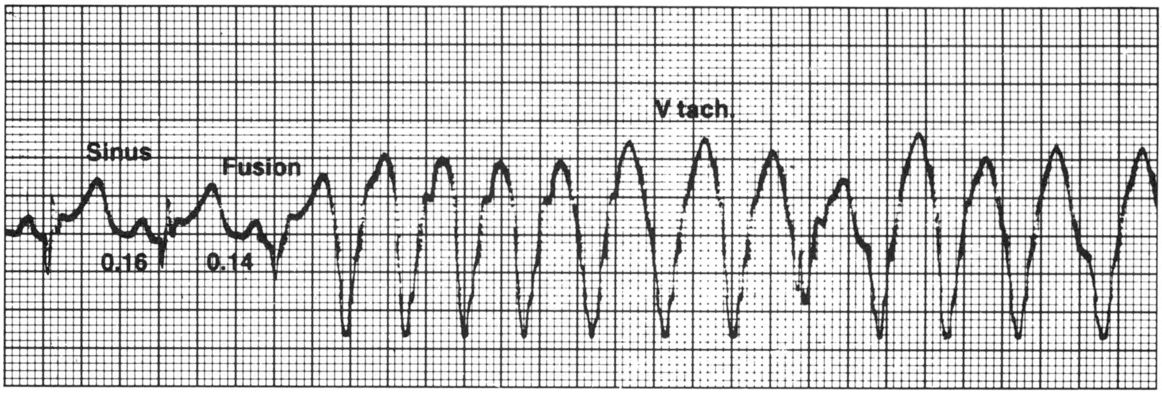

Answer strip A-55

RHYTHM: *Regular then irregular*

RATE: *Sinus, 100; tachycardia, 150*

P WAVES: *Present initially then none visible*

PR INTERVAL: *0.16 second; 0.14 second on fusion beat*

QRS COMPLEX: *0.10 second, wide and bizarre*

INTERPRETATION: *NSR → Ventricular tachycardia (starts with a fusion beat)*

THERAPY: *Lidocaine; cardioversion*

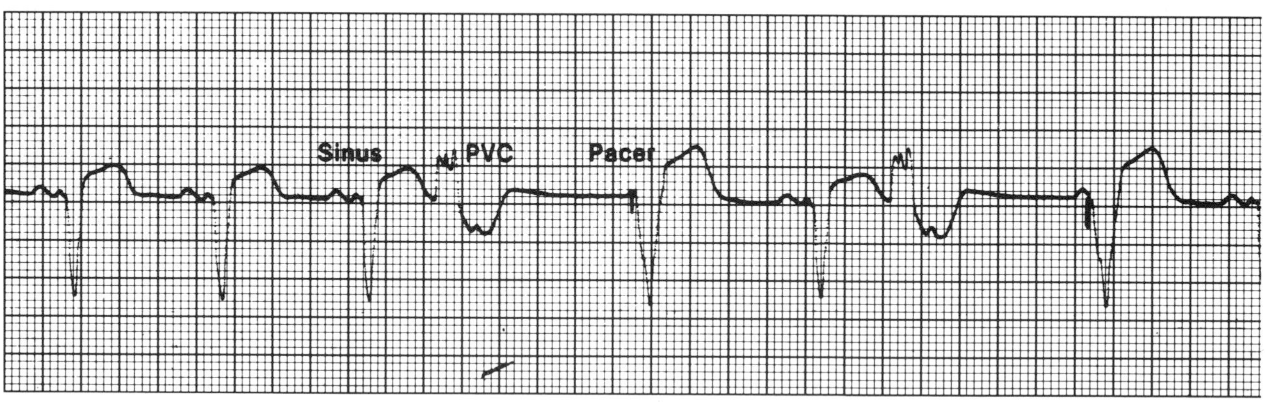

Answer strip A-56

RHYTHM: *Irregular due to early beats and paced rhythms*

RATE: *Sinus, 75; pacer, 60 (escape interval)*

P WAVES: *Present—none with early beats or pacer*

PR INTERVAL: *0.16 second*

QRS COMPLEX: *0.12 second*

INTERPRETATION: *NSR with PVCs and ventricular demand pacer firing during compensatory pause following PVCs*

THERAPY: *Lidocaine*

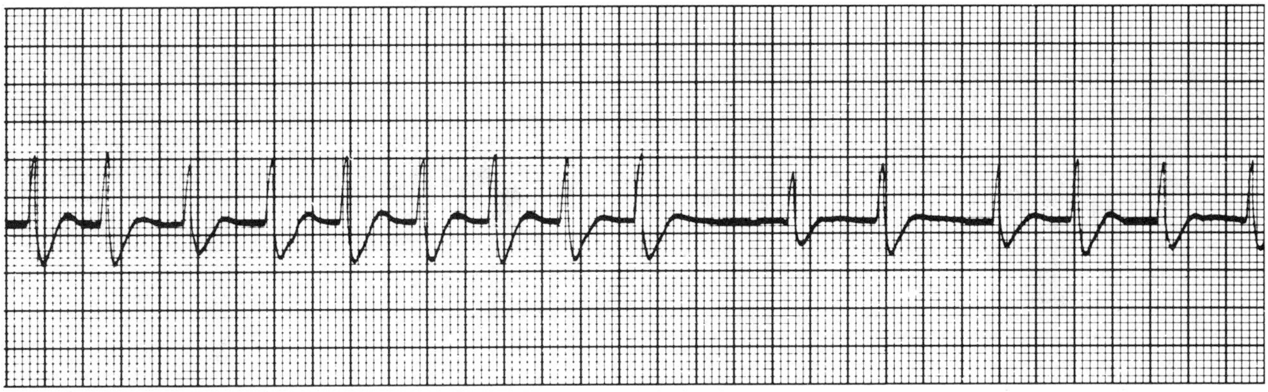

Answer strip A-57

RHYTHM: *Totally irregular*

RATE: *150*

P WAVES: *None—fibrillation waves present but too fine to be seen.*

PR INTERVAL: *None*

QRS COMPLEX: *0.12 second*

INTERPRETATION: *Uncontrolled atrial fibrillation (straight-line atrial fibrillation)*

THERAPY: *Administer digitalis and a Class I agent, or verapamil, cardioversion.*

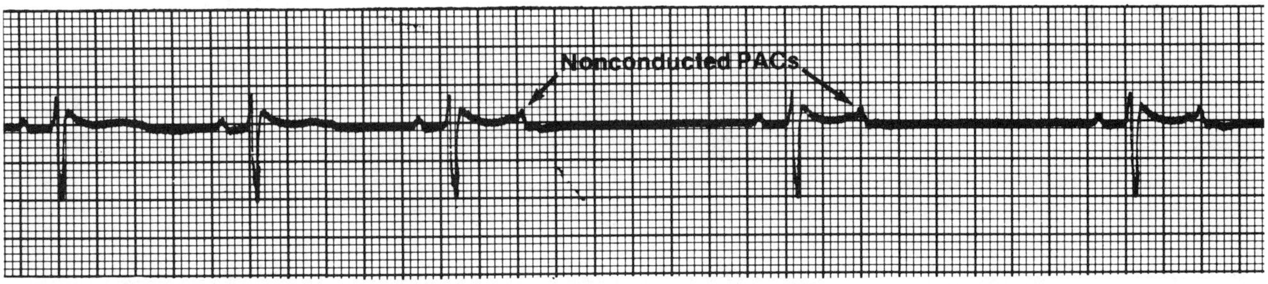

Answer strip A-58

RHYTHM: *Regular then regularly irregular due to pauses*

RATE: *Sinus, 58; overall, 40*

P WAVES: *Present—change in shape before each pause*

PR INTERVAL: *0.20 second*

QRS COMPLEX: *0.08 second*

INTERPRETATION: *Sinus bradycardia with bigeminal nonconducted PACs*

THERAPY: *Observe patient; administer atropine if needed.*

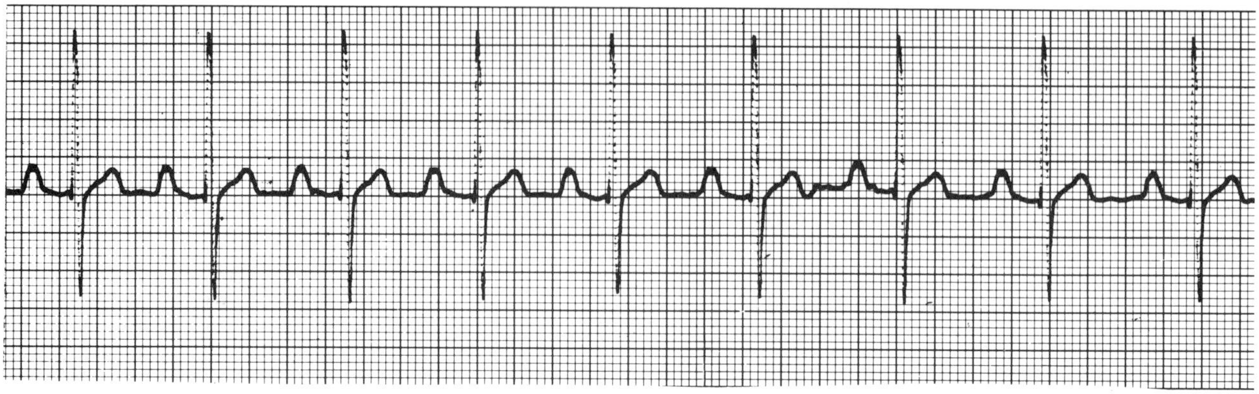

Answer strip A-59

RHYTHM: *Regular but slowing down*

RATE: *85 → 75*

P WAVES: *Normal*

PR INTERVAL: *0.26 second*

QRS COMPLEX: *0.08 second*

INTERPRETATION: *NSR with first-degree AV block*

THERAPY: *Observe for ↑ block.*

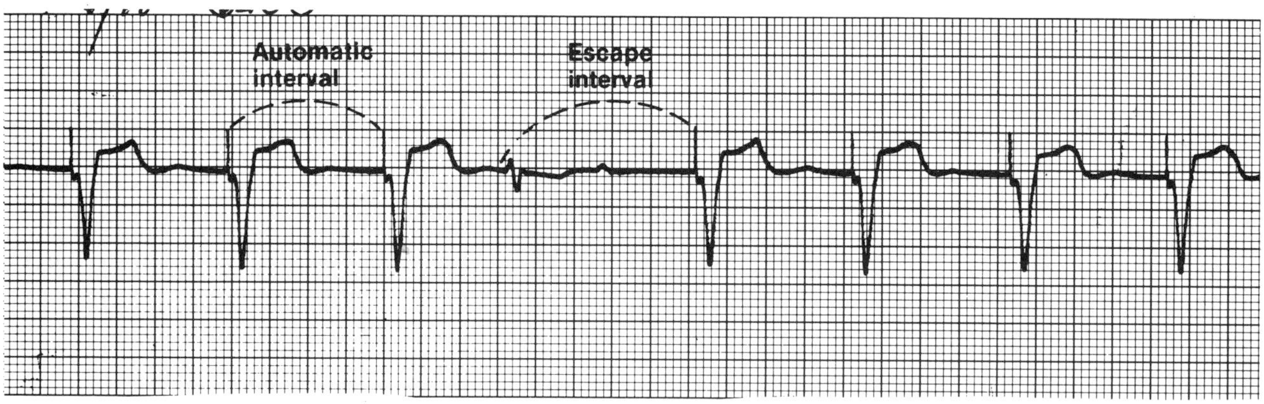

Answer strip A-60

RHYTHM: *Irregular due to paced rhythm*

RATE: *Pacer, 75*

P WAVES: *None visible*

PR INTERVAL: —

QRS COMPLEX: *Wide paced complexes*

INTERPRETATION: *Demand ventricular pacemaker that is functioning properly—has hysteresis*

THERAPY: *None*

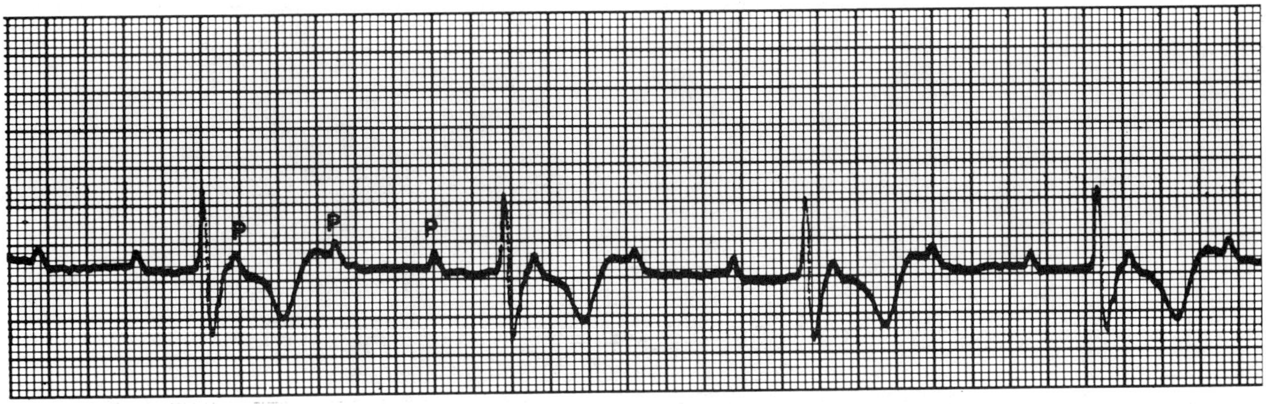

Answer strip A-61

RHYTHM: *Regular*

RATE: *Atrial, 120; ventricular, 40*

P WAVES: *Present—not all are conducted*

PR INTERVAL: *0.36 second, constant*

QRS COMPLEX: *0.12 second*

INTERPRETATION: *Sinus tachycardia with second-degree AV block, type II 3:1 Block*

THERAPY: *Pacemaker*

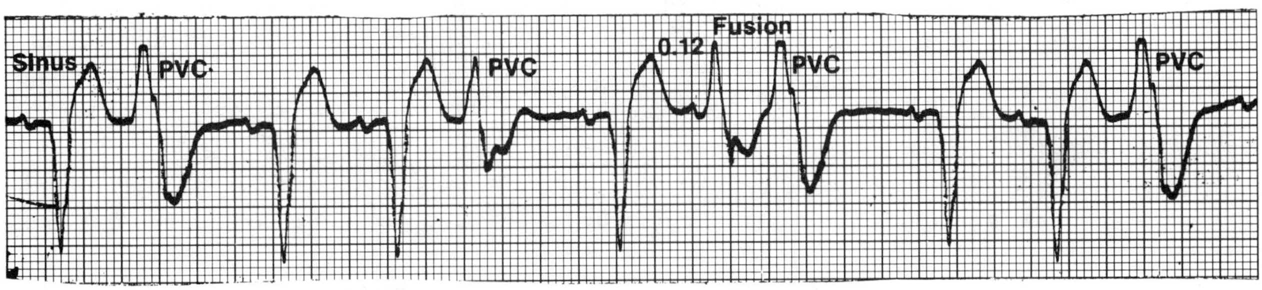

Answer strip A-62

RHYTHM: *Irregular due to early beats*

RATE: *Sinus, 100*

P WAVES: *Present—none in some of the early beats*

PR INTERVAL: *0.16–0.12 second in fusion*

QRS COMPLEX: *0.12 second, wide and bizarre in early beats*

INTERPRETATION: *NSR with multifocal PVCs and fusion beats.*

THERAPY: *Lidocaine*

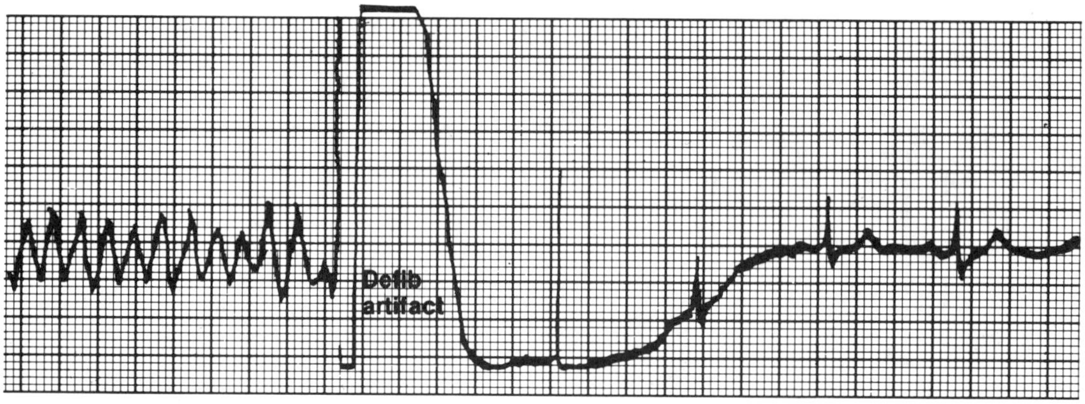

Answer strip A-63

RHYTHM: *Totally chaotic → regular*

RATE: *Sinus, 85*

P WAVES: *Present at end; none at beginning*

PR INTERVAL: *0.18 second, at end of strip*

QRS COMPLEX: *0.10 second at end of strip*

INTERPRETATION: *Ventricular fibrillation → defibrillation → NSR*

THERAPY: *Lidocaine; sodium bicarbonate*

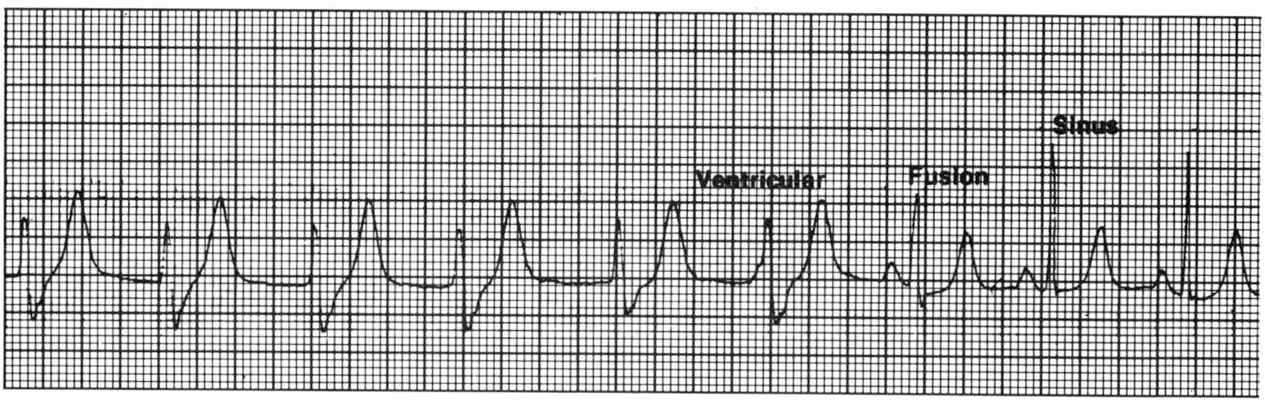

Answer strip A-64

RHYTHM: *Slightly irregular due to changing pacemaker*

RATE: *Ventricular, 80; sinus, 85*

P WAVES: *Present—some are hidden, conduct at end of strip*

PR INTERVAL: *0.16–0.14 second on fusion beat*

QRS COMPLEX: *0.14 second at first; 0.08 second at end*

INTERPRETATION: *Accelerated ventricular rhythm competing with NSR; fusion beat*

THERAPY: *None needed; observe patient.*

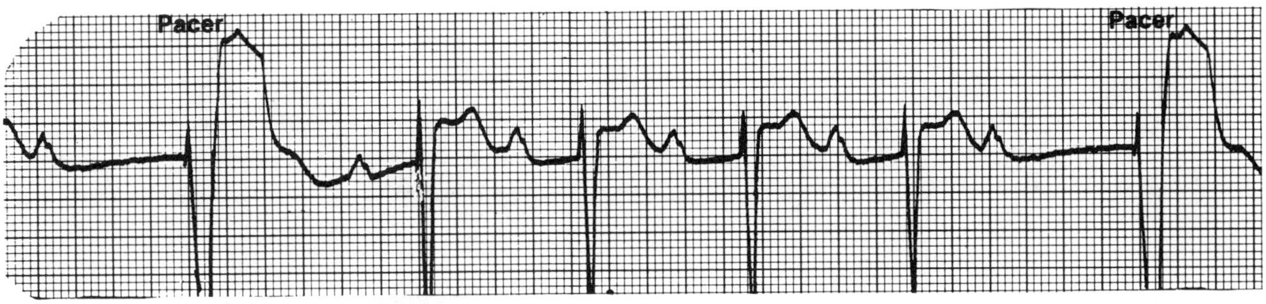

Answer strip A-65

RHYTHM: *Sinus, regular; ventricular, irregular due to missing QRSs and late beats*

RATE: *Sinus, 72; ventricular, 50*

P WAVES: *Present—not all conducted*

PR INTERVAL: *Increases 0.32 → 0.40 second until beat is dropped*

QRS COMPLEX: *0.08 second, late beats, wide and bizarre*

INTERPRETATION: *NSR with second-degree AV block, type I (5:4 Wenckebach) with a functioning ventricular demand pacemaker that fires in Wenckebach pause*

THERAPY: *Observe patient.*

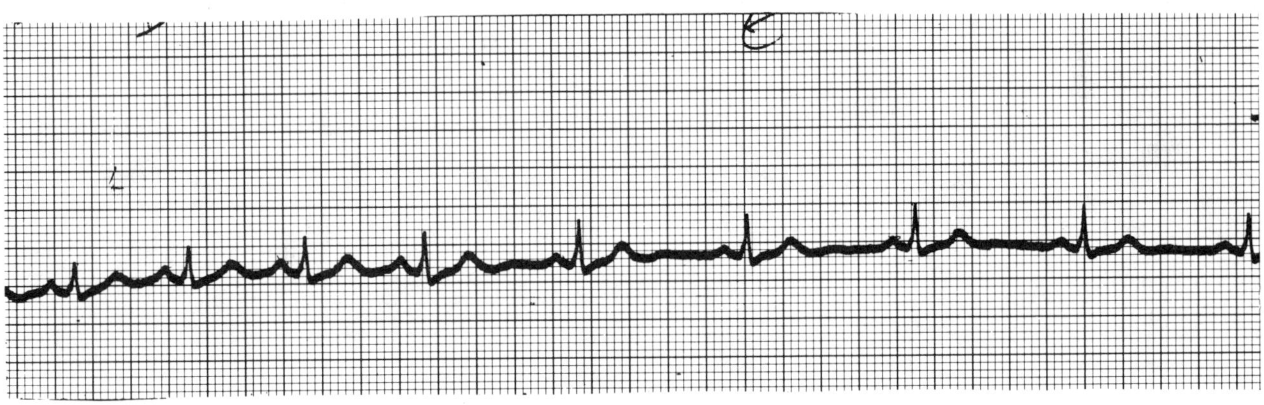

Answer strip A-66

RHYTHM: *Irregular due to slowing and speeding in cycles*

RATE: *80*

P WAVES: *Normal*

PR INTERVAL: *0.16 second*

QRS COMPLEX: *0.08 second*

INTERPRETATION: *Sinus arrhythmia*

THERAPY: *None*

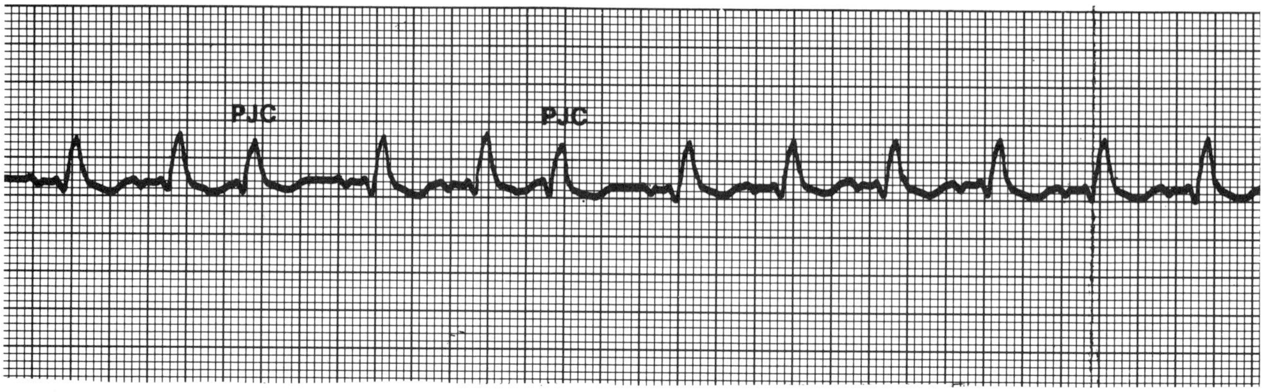

Answer strip A-67

RHYTHM: *Irregular due to premature beats*

RATE: *Sinus—110*

P WAVES: *Present—none in early beats*

PR INTERVAL: *0.18 second*

QRS COMPLEX: *0.14 second*

INTERPRETATION: *Sinus tachycardia with BBB and PJCs*

THERAPY: *Observe patient; may need to find cause of tachycardia and treat.*

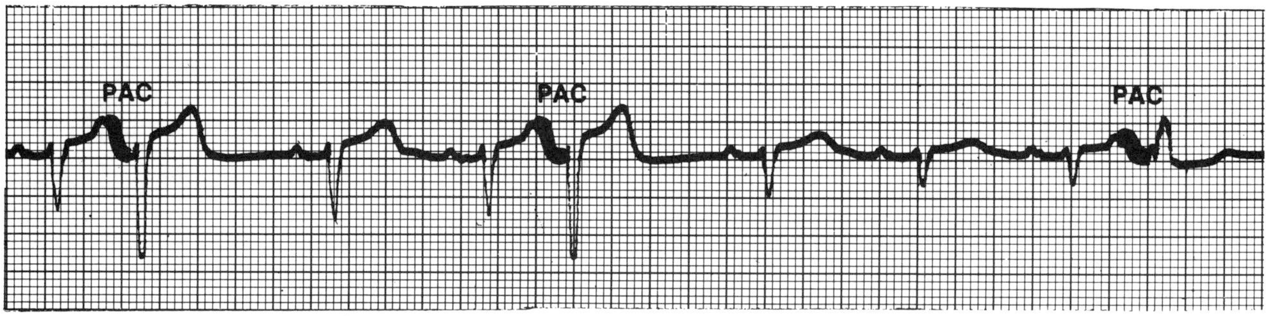

Answer strip A-68

RHYTHM: *Irregular due to early beats*

RATE: *Sinus, 75*

P WAVES: *Present—change in shape in early beats*

PR INTERVAL: *0.20 second*

QRS COMPLEX: *0.10 second, differs in early beats*

INTERPRETATION: *NSR with PACs with aberrant ventricular conduction*

THERAPY: *Observe patient.*

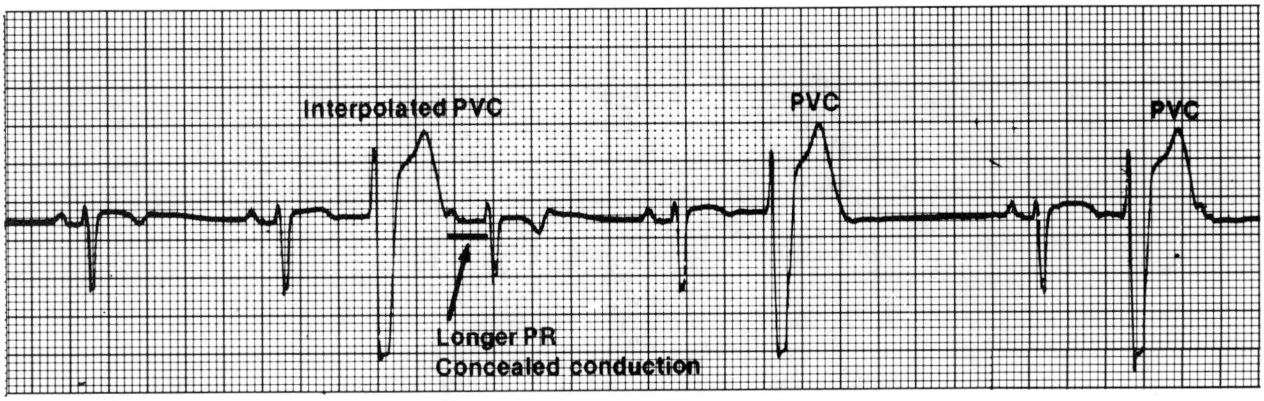

Answer strip A-69

RHYTHM: *Irregular due to premature beats*

RATE: *Sinus, 58*

P WAVES: *Present—none in premature beat*

PR INTERVAL: *0.16 second*

QRS COMPLEX: *0.10 second, wide and bizarre in premature beats*

INTERPRETATION: *Sinus bradycardia with unifocal PVCs*

THERAPY: *Atropine(?); lidocaine*

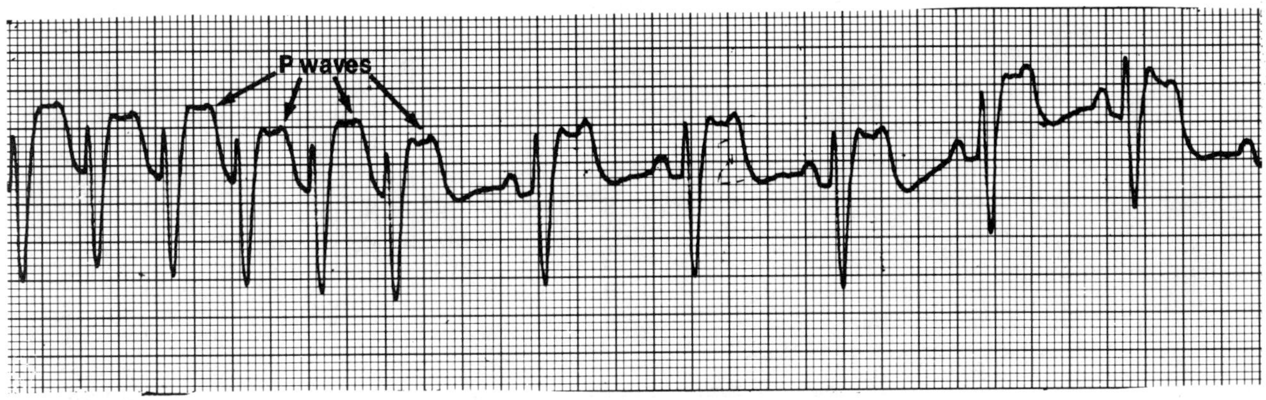

Answer strip A-70

RHYTHM: *Regular*

RATE: *Atrial, 150; ventricular, 150 → 75*

P WAVES: *Present—not all conducted*

PR INTERVAL: *0.16 second*

QRS COMPLEX: *0.16 second*

INTERPRETATION: *Atrial tachycardia with 1:1 → 2:1 conduction and BBB*

THERAPY: *Check digitalis and K^+ levels; Dilantin*

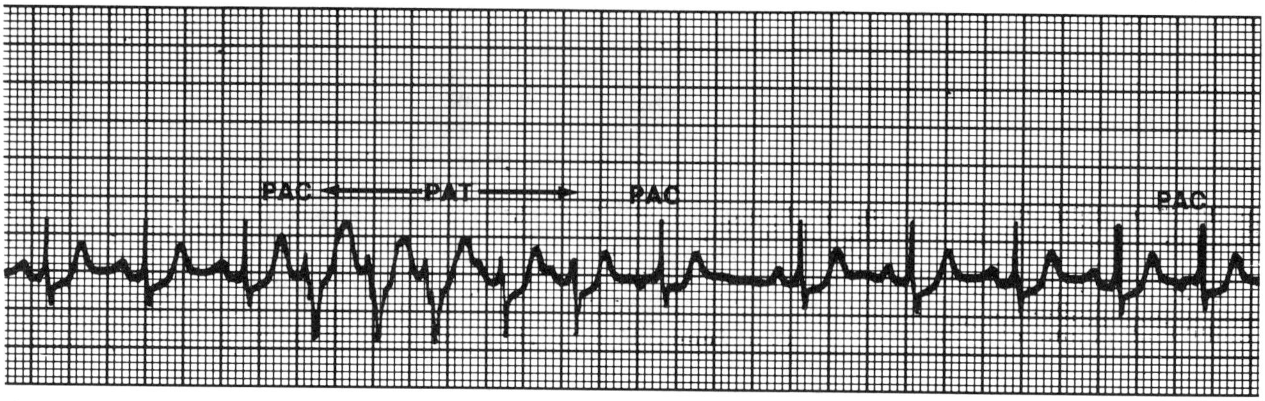

Answer strip A-71

RHYTHM: *Irregular due to tachycardias and premature beats*

RATE: *Sinus, 110; Tachycardia, 180*

P WAVES: *Present—change in shape in tachycardia and early beats*

PR INTERVAL: *0.14 second*

QRS COMPLEX: *0.08 second, wider in tachycardia*

INTERPRETATION: *Sinus tachycardia with PACs and short run of PAT with aberration*

THERAPY: *Digitalis and a Class I agent*

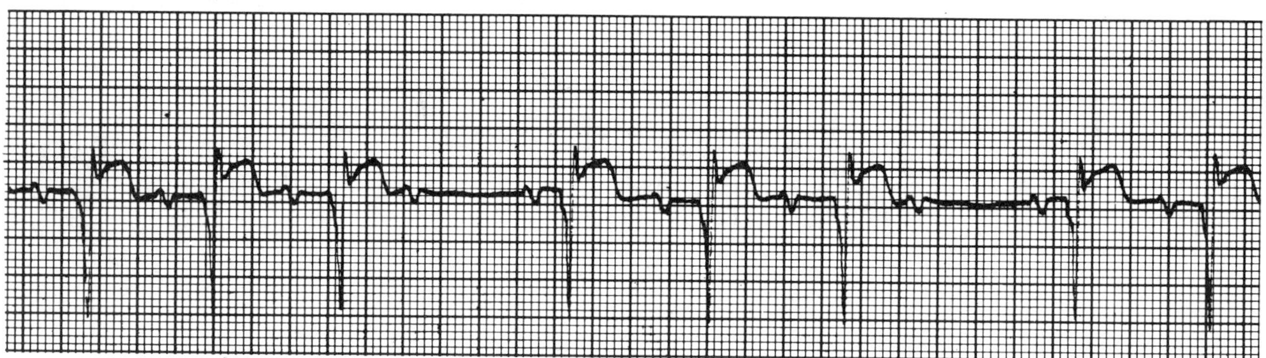

Answer strip A-72

RHYTHM: *Sinus, regular; ventricular, irregular*

RATE: *Sinus, 90; ventricular, 70*

P WAVES: *Present—not all are conducted*

PR INTERVAL: *Increases 0.20 → 0.28 second until beat is dropped*

QRS COMPLEX: *0.10 second*

INTERPRETATION: *NSR with second-degree AV block, type I (Wenckebach with varying conduction)*

THERAPY: *Observe for ↑ block.*

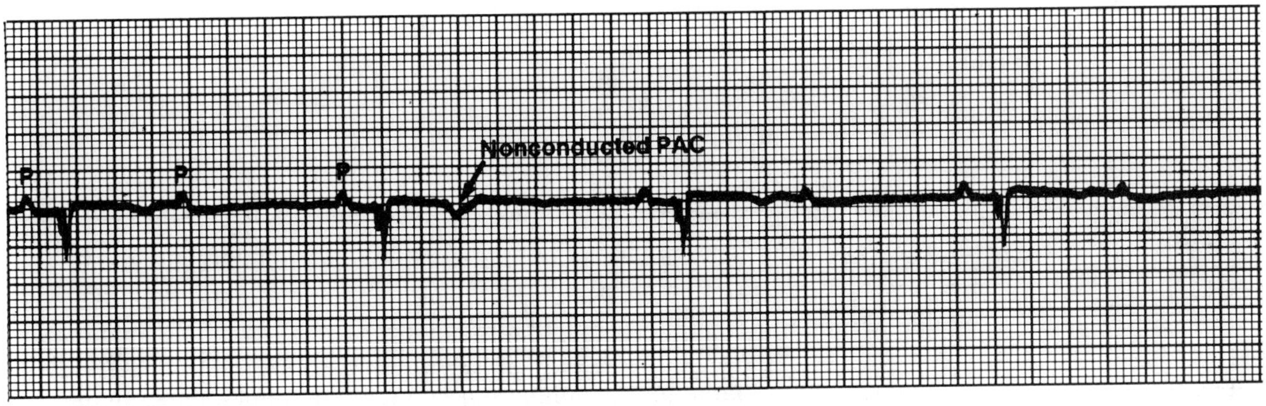

Answer strip A-73

RHYTHM: *Irregular due to early beat*

RATE: *Sinus, 72; ventricular, 36*

P WAVES: *Present—not all conducted; early P wave differs in shape*

PR INTERVAL: *0.20 second*

QRS COMPLEX: *0.08 second*

INTERPRETATION: *NSR with second-degree AV block, Type II; 2:1 with one nonconducted PAC*

THERAPY: *Atropine, isoproterenol; pacemaker*

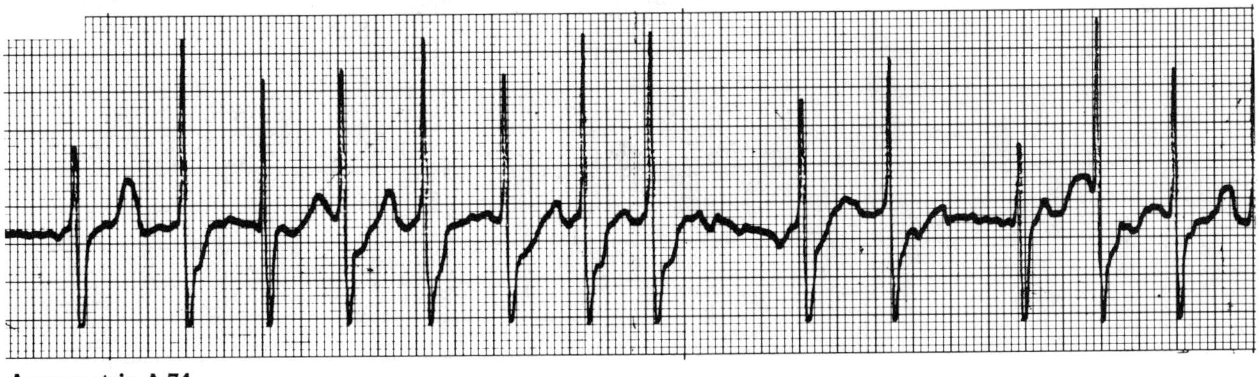

Answer strip A-74

RHYTHM: *Totally irregular*

RATE: *Ventricular, 120*

P WAVES: *None—fibrillation waves*

PR INTERVAL: *None*

QRS COMPLEX: *0.08 second*

INTERPRETATION: *Uncontrolled atrial fibrillation*

THERAPY: *Digitalis and a Class I agent, or verapamil; cardioversion*

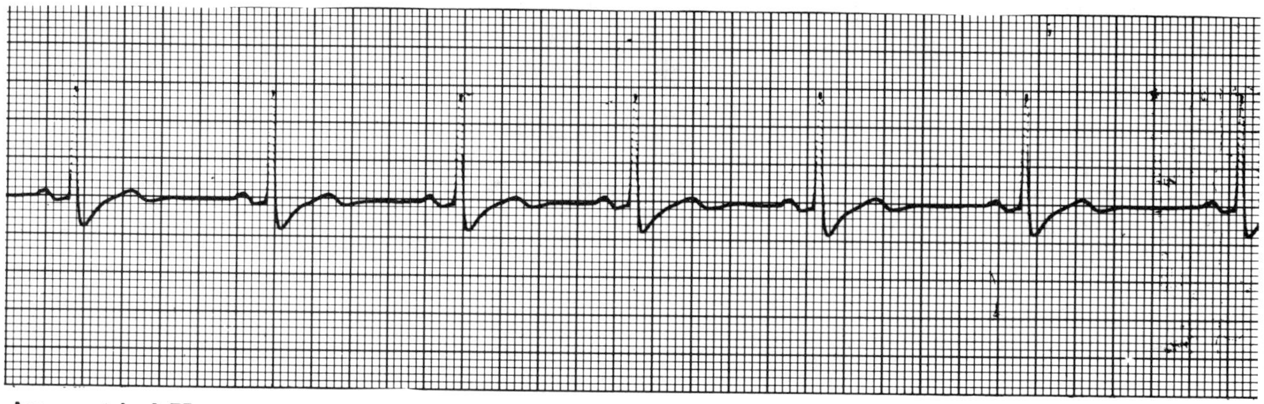

Answer strip A-75

RHYTHM: *Irregular—speeds and slows*

RATE: *60*

P WAVES: *Normal*

PR INTERVAL: *0.18 second*

QRS COMPLEX: *0.12 second*

INTERPRETATION: *Sinus arrhythmia*

THERAPY: *None*

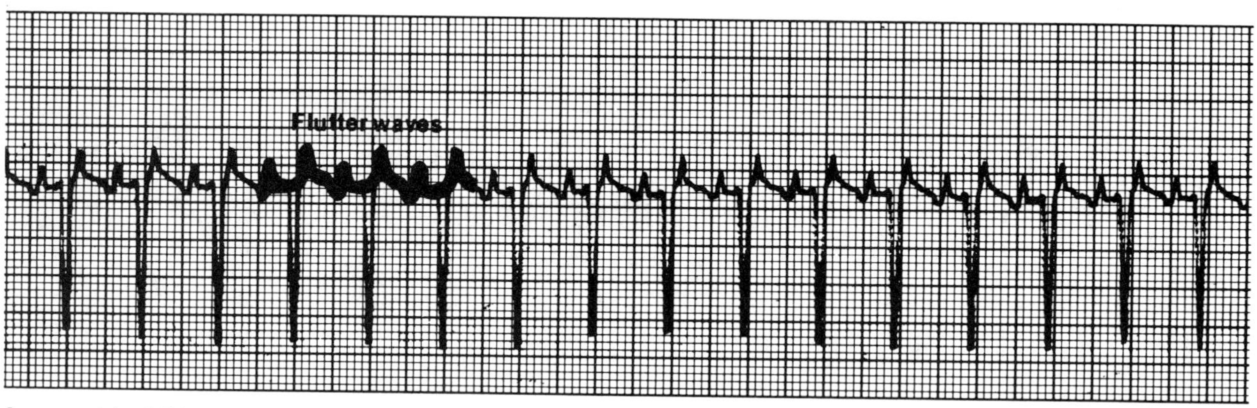

Answer strip A-76

RHYTHM: *Regular*

RATE: *Atrial, 300; ventricular, 150*

P WAVES: *None—flutter waves*

PR INTERVAL: —

QRS COMPLEX: *0.08 second*

INTERPRETATION: *Atrial flutter with 2:1 conduction*

THERAPY: *Digitalis and a Class I agent or Verapamil; cardioversion*

INDEX

Page numbers followed by *f* indicate illustrations; *t* following a page number indicates tabular material.